O╳FORD MEDICAL PUBLICATIONS

Prison Medicine and Health

T0073775

Oxford Specialist Handbooks

Oxford Specialist Handbooks published and forthcoming

Prison Medicine and Health

EDITED BY

Emily Phipps

MBChB (Hons), MSc, PGDip, MFPH
Consultant in Communicable Disease Control, UK Health
Security Agency, Oxford, UK

Éamonn O'Moore FFPH

Director of National Health Protection, HSE National Health
Protection Service of Ireland, Dublin, Ireland.
Former National Lead for Health & Justice & Deputy Director for
Vulnerable People & Inclusion Health, UK Health Security Agency,
London, UK.
Former Director UK Collaborating Centre, WHO Health in
Prisons Programme, WHO EURO, Copenhagen, Denmark.

Emma Plugge

Senior Research Fellow, the Health and Justice Team, UK Health
Security Agency, London, and Associate Professor of Public
Health, University of Southampton, Southampton, UK
and

Jake Hard

Clinical Director HMP Cardiff, Former Chair of the RCGP
Secure Environments Group, Clinical Lead for Health and Justice
Information Service, NHS England

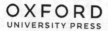

OXFORD
UNIVERSITY PRESS

OXFORD
UNIVERSITY PRESS

Great Clarendon Street, Oxford, OX2 6DP,
United Kingdom

Oxford University Press is a department of the University of Oxford.
It furthers the University's objective of excellence in research, scholarship,
and education by publishing worldwide. Oxford is a registered trade mark of
Oxford University Press in the UK and in certain other countries

© Oxford University Press 2024

The moral rights of the authors have been asserted

First Edition published in 2024

Published in the United States of America by Oxford University Press
198 Madison Avenue, New York, NY 10016, United States of America

British Library Cataloguing in Publication Data
Data available

Library of Congress Control Number:2023931687

ISBN 978-0-19-883453-3

DOI: 10.1093/med/9780198834533.001.0001

Printed in the UK by
Ashford Colour Press Ltd, Gosport, Hampshire

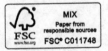

Foreword

Language matters

Individuals who experience the criminal justice system often face multiple areas of stigma. Reasons for arrest and incarceration can include factors that have negative connotations in the views of the general public, such as mental health conditions, the use of drugs, or contested immigration status. Internationally, these reasons can also include sexual orientation or behaviour and HIV status. Stereotypes that become ingrained in institutional structures and systems can mask the negative effects on the marginalized group.

Such stigma and discrimination can affect the identities of incarcerated individuals, both in how they see themselves (from perceived to internalized stigma), and in how society perceives *them*. Words matter when describing incarcerated people.

The words used can shape their life experiences, behaviours, health risk factors, and medical conditions, because language can have a significant impact on health and well-being. The words used can affect the ability of a person to access health information and services. However, terminology used in policies, programmes, and research publications is often derogatory, stigmatizing, and dehumanizing (e.g. criminal, felon, offender, and drug addict). Therefore, respectful language is a cornerstone of reducing harm and suffering. Four principles that foster constructive and humanizing language can guide healthcare professionals, researchers, and policymakers working with people involved in the criminal justice system. These principles are:

- engaging people and respect their preferences by asking them about the language they prefer using to identify themselves
- using stigma-free and accurate language
- prioritizing individuals over their characteristics by using a person-oriented language
- cultivating self-awareness by developing cultural humility and self-reflection, being mindful, and refraining from repeating negative terms that discriminate, devalue, and perpetuate harmful stereotypes and power imbalances.

The following table offers examples of problematic terms to avoid because they do not convey respect for incarcerated people and proposes preferred wording that requires contextualization to local language, culture, and environment.

Examples of terminology to avoid (in alphabetical order), problems related to its use, and preferred wording to describe people who are incarcerated

Terminology to avoid	Problems	Preferred wording
Abuse; misuse	Judgemental; negates the fact that substance use disorders are a medical condition; not conducive to fostering the trust and respect required when engaging with people who use psychoactive substances	(Heavy) substance use; substance use disorder (*Diagnostic and Statistical Manual of Mental Disorders*, fifth edition); dependence syndrome (International Classification of Diseases, tenth revision)
Body-packer, drug mule, drug smuggler	Not person-centred language, judgemental	Person with body-packing, or with internal concealment of psychoactive substance
Body-stuffer	Not person-centred language, judgemental	Person diagnosed with acute ingestion of psychoactive substance
Correctional, offender, penitentiary, prison health services	Reinforces stereotypes, moralistic, ambiguous	Health services in detention settings; healthcare in prison
Crazy; mental; insane; psycho; mentally ill; emotionally disturbed; demented	Not person-centred language, judgemental	Person living with a mental health condition; person living with dementia
Dungeon, hole	Derogatory, inaccurate, reinforces self-stigma	Solitary confinement
Drug user; abuser; addict; junkie; dependent	Not person-centred language, judgemental	Person with a substance use disorder; person with dependence syndrome; person who uses psychoactive substances
Ex-prisoner; ex-offender; ex-inmate; ex-felon; ex-con; criminal; thug; post-carceral	Not person-centred language, judgemental	Person who was in contact with, involved in, interacted with, or experienced the criminal justice system; person with convictions; person who was formerly incarcerated

High(er)-risk group	Implies that the risk is contained within the group; can increase stigma and discrimination against the designated groups; membership of groups does not place individuals at risk, behaviours may	Key populations; priority population; high-risk behaviour (e.g. sharing needles, condomless sex)
Hunger striker	Not person-centred language, judgemental	Person on hunger strike
Illegal immigrant; illegal; unlawful non-citizen; visa overstayer; undocumented alien	Not person-centred language, judgemental	Person who lacks resident documentation
Prisoner; inmate; felon; offender	Not person-centred language, judgemental	Person who is incarcerated; person who experience incarceration; person in detention/ jail/prison; person living in detention/jail/prison; person involved in, or experiencing the criminal justice system
Prisoner-patient	Health staff care for patients, irrespective of their status	Patient; person in treatment
Prostitute or prostitution	Not person-centred language, judgemental	Person involved in sex work, or in sale or trade of sexual services; sex worker
Probationer; parolee	Not person-centred language, judgemental	Person on parole; person on probation
Substitution therapy or opioid substitution therapy (OST)	Misleading: gives the impression to politicians, civil servants, and other laypeople that this therapy is replacing 'street drugs' with 'state drugs'; and therefore, this language counteracts availability of therapy	Opioid agonist therapy (OAT); opioid agonist therapy for the treatment of substance use disorder; treatment

Nguyen Toan Tran
Australian Centre for Public and Population Health Research,
Faculty of Health, University of Technology, Sydney, Australia

Words matter when describing people involved in the criminal justice system. Language can have a significant impact upon health, well-being, and access to health information and services.[1] As healthcare professionals, as well as a duty of care for our patients, we also have a responsibility to treat people with respect which includes using appropriate person-first language which reflects their humanity rather than their circumstances. So, we encourage all clinicians working with people in prison to adopt this approach and remember that you are not 'the prison doctor/nurse' but a healthcare professional who provides care for people in prison settings.

1. Tran NT, Baggio S, Dawson A, et al. Words matter: a call for humanizing and respectful language to describe people who experience incarceration. BMC Int Health Hum Rights, 2018;18(1):41.

Preface

It is estimated that around 10 million people across the globe are imprisoned in places of detention. Rates of incarceration vary significantly between countries; the US has the highest rate of detained individuals worldwide (419/100,000 in 2019), and the UK nations have the highest rate of incarcerated people in Western Europe—much higher than other European countries of a similar size (England and Wales 132/100,000 versus Germany 71/100,00 and France 102/100,000 in 2021/2022). People in prison have some of the most challenging health and social care needs out of the whole of society. They have higher rates of complex comorbid physical and mental health disorders, cardiovascular disease, substance misuse problems, and infectious diseases, and die on average around 15 years earlier than their counterparts in the community. Healthcare staff working within detention settings not only need a specific set of skills to manage the broad and complex range of health issues experienced by their patients, but also a knowledge of how to navigate the policies and constraints of the complex justice regimes they are working in.

Because of these factors, it is becoming well recognized that prison medicine is a clinical speciality in itself. Health research and expertise in places of detention is on the rise, and is being translated into significant improvements in the health and well-being of people in detention. The International Committee of the Red Cross, World Health Organization, and the United Nations Office on Drugs and Crime are publishing and training widely on the issues of prison health, demonstrating the commitment of the international community to improving the quality of care provided in detention settings across the world.

Swept on by this wave of change, we are therefore delighted to present to you the first ever Oxford Specialist Handbook of *Prison Medicine and Health*, which we hope will become an essential resource for your day-to-day clinical practice in prisons and other places of detention. Not only that, we also see this publication as a crucial cultural and academic statement, helping to cement the definition of prison medicine and health as a clinical and public health subspecialism, which we hope will contribute towards shaping further improvements in care.

An important factor for us as editors was promoting equivalence of care and evidence-based practice in detention settings, which is something we and our contributors have strived to embed throughout the book. We would strongly encourage all readers to reflect on these principles themselves when implementing the guidance in these pages. Furthermore, as discussed in the Foreword, language matters. Everything we have written and edited has been carefully considered in terms of the impact words may have on healthcare professionals and their patients.

This book will follow the general approach of Oxford Specialist Handbooks, with an introduction to the field, explanation of key terms, and chapters dedicated to common clinical scenarios seen in prisons and immigration removal centres. We hope that it will become a much-loved and well-read resource for anyone working in a health capacity within detention settings.

Contents

Contents

Contributors

Gareth Alderson

Abi Barlet

Ruth Bastable

Marcus Bicknell

Iain Brew

Alex Bunn

Richard Byng

Rob Callingham

Sophie Candfield

Ellie Carslake

Saeed Chaudhary

Yimmy Chow

Lindsey Cockerill

Nic Coetzee

Erin Dexter

Lisa Duff

Chantal Edge

Stefan Enggist

Denise Farmer

Seena Fazel

Sir Robert Francis QC

Elish Gilvarry

Catherine Glover

Lauren Grant

Don Grubin

Jake Hard

Tierney Harris

Ellie Henderson

Anna Hiley

Stacey Hilton

Laura Hinchliffe

Nick Hindley

Anna Hinley

Susanne Howes

Jane Hunt

Sarah Jarvis

Sheila Jenkins

Dave Jones

Kate Jones

Cornelius Katona

Mike Kelleher

Jane Leamann

Alexandra Lewis

Craig Lintern

Ruth Lloyd

Emma Mastracoola

Alan Mitchell

Pippa Morris

Éamonn O'Moore

Husein Oozeerally

Emily Phipps

Emma Plugge

Chris Pocock

Jörg Pont

Lucy Potter

Jan Rix

Anjana Roy

Howard Ryland

Lynne Saunders

Wayne Sturley

Sunita Sturup-Toft

Mary Tuner

Caroline Watson

Sandra White

Abbreviations

A&E	accident and emergency	FBC	full blood count
ACCT	Assessment, Care in Custody and Teamwork	FNP	foreign national person in prison
ADHD	attention deficit hyperactivity disorder	GC	Neisseria gonorrhoeae
		GIC	gender identity clinic
ADL	activity of daily living	GP	general practitioner
ANP	advanced nurse practitioner	HbA1c	glycated haemoglobin
ASC	autism spectrum condition	HBV	hepatitis B virus
AUDIT	Alcohol Use Disorders Identification Test	HCV	hepatitis C virus
		HIV	human immunodeficiency virus
BAME	black and minority ethnic	HMIP	His Majesty's Inspectorate of Prisons
BBV	blood-borne virus		
BMA	British Medical Association	HMPPS	His Majesty's Prison and Probation Service
BMI	body mass index		
BP	blood pressure	HPV	human papillomavirus
BV	bacterial vaginosis	ICD-11	International Classification of Diseases, 11th revision
CAMHS	child and adolescent mental health services		
		IDTS	Integrated Drug Treatment System
CBT	cognitive behavioural therapy		
CHAT	Comprehensive Health Assessment Tool	IRC	immigration removal centre
		IT	information technology
CIWA-Ar	Clinical Institute Withdrawal Assessment—Alcohol, revised	IV	intravenous
		LARC	long-acting reversible contraception
CMHS-M	Correctional Mental Health Screen for Men		
		LFT	liver function test
CMHS-W	Correctional Mental Health Screen for Women	LGBT	lesbian, gay, bisexual, and transgender
CNS	central nervous system		
COPD	chronic obstructive pulmonary disease	LTBI	latent tuberculosis infection
		MAP	medicines administration point
COVID-19	coronavirus disease 2019	MASH	Multi-Agency Safeguarding Hub
CPR	cardiopulmonary resuscitation		
CQC	Care Quality Commission	MBU	mother and baby unit
CT	Chlamydia trachomatis	MCS	microscopy, culture, and sensitivity
CYPSE	children and young people's secure estate		
		MDR	multiple drug-resistant
DNACPR	do not attempt cardiopulmonary resuscitation	MDT	multidisciplinary team
		MMSA	Medication to Manage Sexual Arousal
DSH	deliberate self-harm		
DSM-5	Diagnostic and Statistical Manual of Mental Disorders, fifth edition	MRC	Medical Research Council
		MSM	men who have sex with men
		MSU	medium secure unit
DXA	dual-energy X-ray absorptiometry	NAAT	nucleic acid amplification test
		NHS	National Health Service
ECG	electrocardiogram	NICE	National Institute for Health and Care Excellence

NMR	Nelson Mandela Rules	RCGP	Royal College of General Practitioners
NPM	National Preventive Mechanism	SARC	sexual assault referral centre
NSAID	non-steroidal anti-inflammatory drug	SCH	secure children's home
		SMART	specific, measurable, agreed-upon, realistic, time-limited
NSI	needlestick injury		
OCT	outbreak control team	SMR	United Nations Standard Minimum Rules for the Treatment of Prisoners
OHCA	out-of-hospital cardiac arrest		
OPCAT	Optional Protocol to the Convention against Torture and Other Cruel, Inhuman or Degrading Treatment or Punishment		
		SOE	significant occupational exposure
		SSRI	selective serotonin reuptake inhibitor
		STC	secure training centre
OST	opioid substitution therapy	STI	sexually transmitted infection
PCR	polymerase chain reaction	t½	half-life
PD	personality disorder	TB	tuberculosis
PGD	Patient Group Direction	TBI	traumatic brain injury
PHE	Public Health England (now UK Health Security Agency)	TFT	thyroid function test
		TV	Trichomonas vaginalis
PPE	personal protective equipment	U&E	urea and electrolytes
		UDS	urine drug screen
PReP	pharmacological relapse prevention	UKVI	UK Visas and Immigration
		UN	United Nations
PS	psychoactive substance	UNODC	United Nations Office on Drugs and Crime
PSD	Patient Specific Direction		
PSI	Prison Service Instruction	VZV	varicella zoster virus
PSO	Prison Service Order	WHO	World Health Organization
PTSD	post-traumatic stress disorder	YCS	youth custody service
		YOI	young offender institution
QTc	QT interval corrected for heart rate		

Chapter 1

Introduction to prison medicine

Introduction to healthcare in prisons: a person-centred approach

The challenge of healthcare in prisons

People in prison often have multiple and complex health needs, compounded by experience of significant social disadvantages such as persistent unemployment and housing problems, and may have experienced barriers to accessing preventive, diagnostic, and therapeutic services prior to imprisonment.[1] Prison can be an opportunity to address health and social care needs but it can also be an environment where pre-existing health needs are exacerbated and new health needs emerge. The operational prison environment can have both facilitating and impeding impacts on the ability of individuals in prison, and their healthcare team, to promote, enable, and maintain good health.

Fig. 1.1 illustrates the complex interplay of health and social care needs and the prison environment.

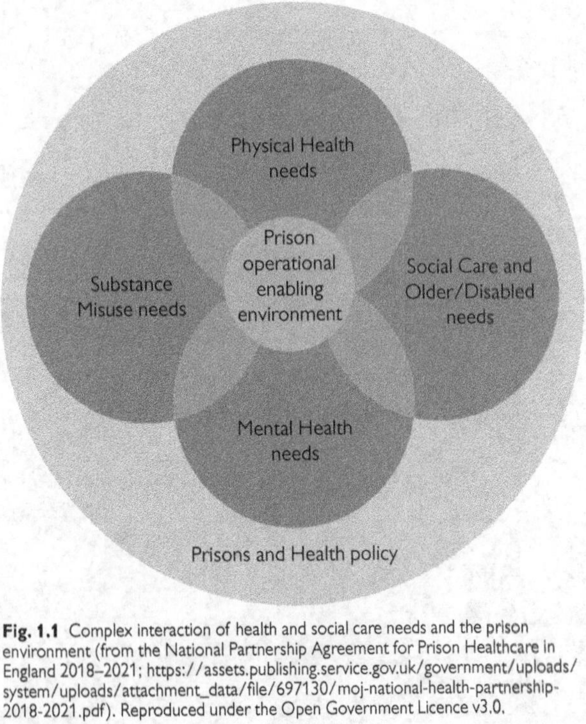

Fig. 1.1 Complex interaction of health and social care needs and the prison environment (from the National Partnership Agreement for Prison Healthcare in England 2018–2021; https://assets.publishing.service.gov.uk/government/uploads/system/uploads/attachment_data/file/697130/moj-national-health-partnership-2018-2021.pdf). Reproduced under the Open Government Licence v3.0.

International standards for prison healthcare

The United Nations (UN) 'Basic Principles for the Treatment of Prisoners'[2] states that 'Prisoners shall have access to the health services available in the country without discrimination on the grounds of their legal situation' (Principle 9). The revised European Prison Rules, adopted on 11 January 2006 by the Committee of Ministers of the Council of Europe,[3] specifically refer to the obligation of prison authorities to safeguard the health of all prisoners (§39) and the need for prison medical services to be organized in close relationship with the general public health administration (§40).

In 2013, the World Health Organization (WHO) and the United Nations Office on Drugs and Crime (UNODC) published a policy brief on the organization of prison health, *Good governance for prison health in the 21st century*,[4] which recognized that people in prison have the same right to health and well-being as any other person, and that the State has a special duty of care to them. Furthermore, it stated that health services in prisons should be at least of equivalent professional, ethical, and technical standards to those in the community. It also recommended that health services in prisons should be integrated into national health policies and systems, including the training and professional development of healthcare staff.

Principles for prison healthcare in the UK

A Health and Social Care Committee report on prison health published in November 2018[5] advised that 'The health of people in prison is a public health issue. Prisons could be an opportunity to address serious health inequalities which are part of the cycle of disadvantage faced by people in prison'. In response, the UK government[6] recognized their 'special duty of care', reaffirmed international standards and human rights, committed to equivalence of care, and undertook to work in partnership to understand and meet the health and social care needs of people in prison.

In the UK, key principles for prison healthcare (Fig. 1.2) which are centred on the '3 Ps' have evolved:

- *Person-centred* care: this considers the needs of the person as a whole, including their wider social needs and impact of imprisonment on their well-being.
- *Patient-led* care: care should be delivered according to the needs of the patient who must be fully informed about and consent to health interventions, including any use of their health information.
- Care is delivered in *partnership*: this includes the wider prison custodial, health, and social care teams as appropriate, working 'through the gate' with organizations supporting people to transition from custody, as well as sharing information appropriately and with medical confidentiality to inform care, and supporting continuity of care.

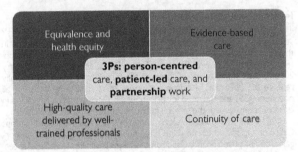

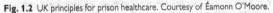

Fig. 1.2 UK principles for prison healthcare. Courtesy of Éamonn O'Moore.

In England, this approach has been reflected in national partnership agreements between the Ministry of Justice, the Department of Health and Social Care, the National Health Service (NHS) in England, His Majesty's Prison and Probation Service (HMPPS), and the UK Health Security Agency (formerly Public Health England (PHE) until April 2021).[7] Furthermore, on 18 July 2018 (International Prisoner Day), the Royal College of General Practitioners (RCGP)[8] published a new position statement on equivalence of care in secure settings stating that the 'aim of ensuring that people detained in secure environments are afforded provision of or access to appropriate services or treatment (based on assessed need and in line with current national or evidence-based guidelines) and that this is considered to be at least consistent in range and quality (availability, accessibility, and acceptability) with that available to the wider community in order to achieve equitable health outcomes'.

The history of prison healthcare in the UK

The UK is one of the few countries in Western Europe where the national health system is responsible for prison healthcare. Other countries where this applies are France, Italy, Norway, Sweden, and Finland. The first public health service in the UK was a prison health service, established in 1774 when a prison surgeon or apothecary was appointed to prevent spread of 'gaol fever' to the population in general—a resonance with more recent concerns that prisons could be a source of coronavirus disease 2019 (COVID-19) for the wider population.[9] The key developments since then are represented in Fig. 1.3 up to the point when the NHS assumed responsibility for commissioning health services in prisons in every part of the UK by April 2013. This is in line with the WHO recommendation that 'health ministries should provide and be accountable for health care services in prisons and advocate healthy prison conditions (rather than Ministries of Justice/Ministry of the Interior)'.[4]

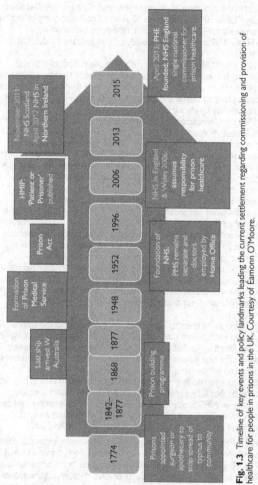

Fig. 1.3 Timeline of key events and policy landmarks leading the current settlement regarding commissioning and provision of healthcare for people in prisons in the UK. Courtesy of Éamonn O'Moore.

Key points in the evolution of prison healthcare in England are described in a report by PHE in 2016 reflecting on 10 years of commissioning by the NHS of prison healthcare in England.[10] This highlighted the following:

- The Home Office historically provided, managed, and funded healthcare in prisons.
- *In 1996*, Her Majesty's Inspectorate of Prisons published a critical report[11] that focused attention on the high level of health needs among people in prison and asked for reform to ensure that they received care according to their needs and equivalent to that provided to people in the community by the NHS.
- *In 1997*, the Department of Health-sponsored Joint Prison Service and NHS Executive Working Group reported their findings in 'The Future Organisation of Prison Healthcare',[12] which recommended that a formal partnership should be created between the NHS and the prison service in order to ensure that 'prisoners should receive the same level of community care within prison as they would receive in the wider community', that is, the principle of equivalence.
- *In September 2002*, the Home Office announced that funding responsibility for healthcare within the prison service would become part of the NHS no later than April 2006.[13] Eighteen NHS primary care trusts, which were responsible for commissioning local NHS services, completed a self-assessment against six criteria for readiness: local leadership, partnership working, modernization plans, finance, workforce, and sharing learning. Regional consultation followed before recommendations were made to government ministers. As a result, three waves of transfer were agreed and the Department of Health took over funding responsibility for prison primary healthcare from April 2003.
- The 'National Partnership Agreement on the Transfer of Responsibility for Prison Health from the Home Office to the Department of Health' was published in April 2003.[14] This set out the high-level agreement between the two government departments and the expected process required to achieve an effective transfer by 2006.
- *In 2006*, commissioning responsibility for prison healthcare in England and Wales was fully transferred to the NHS. In Scotland, a similar process saw NHS Scotland assume responsibility for prison healthcare by *November 2011* and then Northern Ireland completed a similar transfer of responsibility for its prison healthcare by *April 2012*.

1. In 2017, PHE published a peer-reviewed paper on the impact of changes in prison healthcare over the 10-year period of NHS commissioning.[15] It found that English prison healthcare had undergone 'transformation' during this period, leading to increased quality of care through organizational engagement, professionalization of the healthcare workforce, transparency, use of evidence-based guidance, and responsiveness of services. However, the paper recognized that there was still room for improvement, for example, relating to the prison regime and the lack of focus on early/preventive interventions, as well as specific challenges from limited resources.

The review findings support the WHO position on the value of integrated prison and public health systems in improving quality of healthcare. It also recommends future policy needs to take account of the 'whole prison approach', recognizing that healthcare in prisons cannot operate in isolation from the prison regime or the community.

These developments continued to evolve the principle of equivalence, which informed a wide range of policy developments leading to the current position enshrined in the national partnership agreement on prison healthcare.

References

1. Revolving Doors Agency, Public Health England, Home Office. Rebalancing Act: A Resource for Directors of Public Health, Police and Crime Commissioners, the Police Service and Other Health and Justice Commissioners, Service Providers and Users. London: Revolving Doors Agency; 2017.
2. United Nations. Basic principles for the treatment of prisoners. 1990. http://www.ohchr.org/EN/ProfessionalInterest/Pages/BasicPrinciplesTreatmentOfPrisoners.aspx
3. Council of Europe. Recommendation No. R (2006) 2 of the Committee of Ministers to Member States on the European Prison Rules. Strasbourg: Council of Europe; 2006.
4. World Health Organization, Regional Office for Europe. Good Governance for Prison Health in the 21st Century: A Policy Brief on the Organization of Prison Health. Copenhagen: World Health Organization; 2013. https://apps.who.int/iris/handle/10665/326388
5. House of Commons Health and Social Care Committee. Prison health: twelfth report of session 2017–19. October 2018. https://publications.parliament.uk/pa/cm201719/cmselect/cmhealth/963/963.pdf
6. Department of Health and Social Care. Prison health inquiry: government response. The UK government's response to the Health and Social Care Committee's inquiry into prison health. January 2019. https://www.gov.uk/government/publications/prison-health-inquiry-government-response
7. Department of Health. National partnership agreement for prison healthcare in England. April 2018. https://assets.publishing.service.gov.uk/government/uploads/system/uploads/attachment_data/file/697130/moj-national-health-partnership-2018-2021.pdf
8. Royal College of General Practitioners. Equivalence of care in secure environments in the UK: position statement. July 2018. https://www.rcgp.org.uk/representing-you/policy-areas/care-in-secure-environments
9. SAGE EMG Transmission Group. COVID-19 transmission in prison settings. March 2021. https://assets.publishing.service.gov.uk/government/uploads/system/uploads/attachment_data/file/979807/S1166_EMG_transmission_in_prisons.pdf
10. Public Health England. Rapid review of evidence of the impact on health outcomes of NHS commissioned health services for people in secure and detained settings to inform future health interventions and prioritisation in England. October 2016. https://assets.publishing.service.gov.uk/government/uploads/system/uploads/attachment_data/file/565231/Rapid_review_health_outcomes_secure_detained_settings_.pdf
11. Her Majesty's Inspectorate of Prisons. Patient or Prisoner? A New Strategy for Health Care in Prisons. London: Home Office; 1996.
12. Department of Health. The Future Organisation of Prison Healthcare: Report by the Joint Prison Service and NHS Executive Working Group. London: Department of Health; 1999.
13. UK Parliament. House of Commons debates: prison healthcare. March 2003. http://www.publications.parliament.uk/pa/cm200203/cmhansrd/vo030317/text/30317w16.htm
14. Department of Health. National Partnership Agreement on the Transfer of Responsibility for Prison Health from the Home Office to the Department of Health. London: Department of Health; 2003.
15. Leaman J, Richards AA, Emslie L, et al. Improving health in prisons—from evidence to policy to implementation—experiences from the UK. Int J Prison Health, 2017;13(3–4):139–167.

Definition of the specialty

Background

Prison medicine is essentially an emerging specialism within general practice in the UK requiring particular skills in substance misuse, management of blood-borne viruses (BBVs), and a knowledge of how the healthcare being provided interacts with the establishment within which the patient is residing.

Prior to 2006, clinicians working in prisons arose from a variety of clinical backgrounds and were effectively employed by the Home Office rather than the NHS. From an ethical perspective, this raised an important conflict of interest in those clinicians—they were employed by the State and therefore could be considered allied with the custodial regime rather than providing an unbiased service to the patients for whom they were caring. Broadly speaking, once a person has been detained within a secure environment and deprived of their liberty, they no longer have an independent choice about who provides and where they receive their healthcare. This effectively places greater responsibility on both the security and healthcare staff to achieve the required level of care to work in collaboration. It is the case that the punishment of detention or incarceration is only about the deprivation of liberty and *is not* about restriction of access to appropriate healthcare services.

In 1996, Her Majesty's Chief Inspector of Prisons, Sir David Ramsbotham, published his review 'Patient or Prisoner?' in which his terms of reference were 'to consider health care arrangements in Prison Service establishments in England and Wales with a view to ensuring that prisoners are given access to the same quality and range of health care services as the general public receives from the National Health Service'.[1] This report brought to the UK the concept of '*equivalence*' of care and set the scene for what continues to be an evolving area of prison and secure environment medicine.

The responsibility for commissioning healthcare services in prisons in England and Wales transferred to the NHS in 2006 from the Home Office and since then, doctors working in prisons are required to have completed general practitioner (GP) training. This has paved the way for a significant transformation in the quality and consistency of services being delivered to people in prison and has been instrumental in seeing that, in particular, the primary care being delivered in prisons mirrored, where possible, that of primary care in the community.[2]

The principle of 'equivalence' is essentially set out within a number of UN resolutions and European Prison Rules which seek to ensure that the treatment of prisoners is humane. The most famous of these are the 'Nelson Mandela Rules' (NMR)—the 'United Nations Standard Minimum Rules for the Treatment of Prisoners (the Nelson Mandela Rules)', General Assembly resolution 70/175.[3] This document comprises a comprehensive set of 122 rules set out in the Resolution adopted by the General Assembly in 2015, of which rules 24–35 refer directly to the healthcare and treatment of prisoners.

The principle of 'equivalence' had not been formally defined and was open to interpretation by the various accountable organizations. The RCGP Secure Environments Group Position Statement[4] published on 18 July 2018

sets out a working definition and intends to provide clarity on the objectives when considering the provision of 'equivalent' care by all relevant stakeholders, including commissioners, providers, and inspectors.

Being a GP in a prison is a unique opportunity to address the needs of some of society's most vulnerable people and it requires being able to do so without prejudice, just as we would in our community practices. The nature of someone's offence should not alter how they are cared for as a patient, and most people in prison leave at some point and become members of the wider community.

Ultimately, by accepting the principle of providing 'equivalent' care, we are striving to improve the health outcomes of our detained patients and are also committing to the benefits for society as a whole.

Definition

There is no one set of defining features for a GP working in prison. The skills required are many and varied and include having knowledge of the prison system and how it will impact the clinician's ability to deliver care, having the relevant consultation skills when addressing drug-seeking behaviour, safer prescribing in the secure setting, substance misuse treatment, and addressing a high prevalence of mental health issues.

Within the prison setting, the healthcare services have been adapted to serve the increased needs of the patient group although detailed epidemiological data remain an area in need of further development. GPs working in prisons benefit from having an additional set of skills in order to properly address these needs; however, currently there is no requirement for additional training. The RCGP Certificate in the Management of Drug Misuse, Parts I and II, continues to be an important basic additional qualification.

Equally, it must be acknowledged that prison healthcare is a continually evolving and developing area. Clinical information technology (IT) systems have only been available in prisons since around 2010. The improved use of these systems is central to improving the level of care being provided as it will provide the data necessary for a better understanding of the health needs of the population and thereby help us to determine our aims for defining the health outcomes and objectives required to provide 'equivalence' to the community. Future developments within the prison IT system will see connection to the 'NHS Spine' and this will bring much of the functionality available in the wider community, such as electronic referrals, timely transfer of electronic records, access to national screening programmes, and a range of other enhancements.

In summary, prison medicine is an intriguing and engaging strand of general practice that provides engaged GPs with exposure to a range of clinical, practical, and ethical challenges that can only seek to benefit the specialism as a whole.

The very essence of being a GP is about advocacy and addressing an individual's needs on a case-by-case basis—no one case is exactly the same as another. As GPs, both in the community and in secure environments, we work with some of society's most vulnerable people and this requires being able to do so without judgement of any kind.

References

1. Her Majesty's Inspectorate of Prisons. Patient or Prisoner? A New Strategy for Health Care in Prisons. London: Home Office; 1996.
2. National Institute for Health and Care Excellence. Physical health of people in prison, NICE guideline [NG57]. 2016. https://www.nice.org.uk/guidance/ng57
3. United Nations. Nelson Mandela Rules. n.d. http://www.un.org/en/events/mandeladay/mandela_rules.shtml
4. Royal College of General Practitioners—Secure Environments Group. Equivalence of care in secure environments in the UK. July 2018. https://elearning.rcgp.org.uk/pluginfile.php/176185/mod_book/chapter/618/RGCP-secure-group-report-july-2018.pdf

Further reading

Birmingham L, Wilson S, Adshead G. Prison medicine: ethics and equivalence. Br J Psychiatry. 2006;188:4–6.

Jotterand F, Wangmo T. The principle of equivalence reconsidered: assessing the relevance of the principle of equivalence in prison medicine. Am J Bioethics. 2014;14(7):4–12.

Niveau G. Relevance and limits of the principle of 'equivalence of care' in prison medicine. J Med Ethics. 2007;33(10):610–613.

Sparrow N. Health care in secure environments. Br J Gen Pract. 2006;56(530):724–725.

Stürup-Toft S, O'Moore EJ, Plugge EH. Looking behind the bars: emerging health issues for people in prison. Br Med Bull. 2018;125(1):15–23.

United Nations. Basic principles for the treatment of prisoners. 1990. https://www.ohchr.org/EN/ProfessionalInterest/Pages/BasicPrinciplesTreatmentOfPrisoners.aspx

Williamson M. Improving the health and social outcomes of people recently released from prisons in the UK—perspective from primary care. 2006. Sainsbury Centre for Mental Health. http://www.antoniocasella.eu/salute/Williamson_health_care_after_prison_2006.pdf

World Health Organization. Prisons and health. n.d. https://www.who.int/europe/health-topics/prisons-and-health

Prison life and workforce

Daily life in detention settings

All prisons work on timetables, but the schedules will change depending on both the category of the person and the type of prison.
- All people in prison should be able to spend between 30 minutes and 1 hour outside in the open air each day. The time allowed will vary between prisons.
- Physical exercise is important for health maintenance. Many prisons have time set aside for this, but times will vary.

A typical category B prison
- 8 am start:
  - People will be taken to work or education.
  - Those not involved will be returned to their cell by 8.30 am.
- Lunch at midday, followed by afternoon activities.
- After the evening meal there may be a fixed period of association, followed by final evening lockup.
- These times may change slightly on weekends and bank holidays.

Incentives and earned privileges
- A person in prison may earn extra benefits, such as money to spend or extra visiting time.
- The levels are basic, entry, standard, and enhanced.
- Punishment for non-compliance with regulations can downgrade the person's status.

The prison workforce
- For people who are not undertaking full-time education in prison, work will be allocated.
- The jobs will vary depending on the prison. Some examples include:
  - wing cleaner
  - library orderly
  - kitchen worker
  - packing for external companies (e.g. bagging nails/stuffing envelopes).
- People in prison receive money for work which can be spent on items of food or toiletries from the canteen list.

The probation system

The National Probation Service for England and Wales is responsible for the supervision of people who have come out of prison and returned to the community. It also provides reports to the criminal courts to assist them in sentencing. Northern Ireland has a separate probation service, and in Scotland it is managed within local authorities, as part of the social work departments.

All people in prison will be under probation service supervision as part of offender rehabilitation. The service aims to provide a consistent point of contact with people leaving prison during this challenging point of change.

Pre-sentence reports

- After a person has been convicted of an offence, but before sentencing, the judge or magistrate will ask the probation service to produce a report that recommends an appropriate sentence.
- This will cover protection of the public, reducing future reoffending, rehabilitation, and punishment, and will also consider the effect on the person affected by the offence.
- It will also include details about both the physical and mental health of the person who has been convicted.

Roles in prison

- The probation service also assesses people in prison to prepare them for release on licence.
- For people who are deemed high risk, the service also works to reduce the likelihood of reoffending or causing significant harm.

Roles in the community

- Risk assessment.
- Liaising with partner agencies to protect the public and promote rehabilitation.
- Provide support to link people in with the wider health and social care system.

Overview of health needs of people in detention

Introduction

Principles for public health

Health needs within prisons

Overview of health needs of people in detention

Introduction

People in prison generally have poorer health than those in the community. Mental health disorders, including drug and alcohol dependency, are particularly common. Most people in prison are current or former smokers.

The prison environment itself can cause physical and mental health problems. Overcrowding and unsanitary conditions can lead to the spread of infectious diseases. Poor diet and lack of exercise will lead to weight gain and obesity-associated disorders. A lack of purposeful activity, isolation from support networks, and bullying and violence in prisons all negatively impact mental health.

The health needs of people in prison are shaped by the inclusion of highly vulnerable groups. National Institute for Health and Care Excellence (NICE) guidance[1] outlines four major classes of people with special health requirements within prisons:

- People with learning disabilities.
- Older people, and those serving longer sentences.
- People serving short sentences, who may not achieve any sustainable change in their health while in prison.
- Groups with specific health needs (e.g. physical disabilities, history of substance misuse, and pregnant women).

Prison health as public health

- The WHO stated that governments have 'a special duty of care for those in places of detention, which should cover safety, basic needs and recognition of human rights, including the right to health'.[2]
- A whole system approach, from sentencing to release, is needed to reduce the risk of diseases and untreated conditions being introduced back into the community, adding to the burden of disease for the population as a whole.
- A person's time in prison may be the first time they have a settled life with adequate nutrition and a chance to reduce their vulnerability to ill health. Prison healthcare plays an essential role in reducing health inequalities through supporting people in prison to improve their health and well-being and appropriately manage illnesses.

Health needs within prisons

- The WHO has identified four essential components of health services in detention settings:
  - Medical care: providing sufficient care for mental and physical health disorders.
  - Health protection: preventing the transmission of infectious diseases within prisons through provision of hygienic living conditions, testing and treatment for infectious diseases, and managing outbreaks.
  - Health promotion: providing people in prisons with the tools to improve their own health.

- Health resilience: having a whole system approach to health within the prison and linking to the community, recognizing that all staff have a part to play in improving and sustaining the health of people in prison.
- The core of health services should be primary care, as it is in the wider community.
- Every person should have a healthcare assessment at first reception, carried out by a healthcare professional (HCP). This should include the identification of the following:
  - Immediate health and safety issues that may affect the person prior to second-stage assessment.
  - Priority health needs to be addressed at the next clinical opportunity.
  - Relevant information that helps continuity of care (e.g. medicine requirements and relevant clinical records).
- The initial assessment should cover physical health, alcohol and substance misuse, mental health, and self-harm and suicide risk.

Subsequent chapters outline ways that the physician can best treat, manage, and promote health in the prison environment for specific health problems:
- Chronic disease management, see p. 101.
- Infectious diseases, see p. 145.
- Mental health, see p. 175.
- Substance misuse, see p. 203.

Populations that will have specific healthcare requirements are also included:
- Women's health, see p. 241.
- Child and adolescent health, see p. 261.
- Foreign nationals in detention, see p. 293.
- Older people in prison, see p. 315.

References

1. National Institute for Health and Care Excellence. Physical health of people in prison. NICE guideline [NG57]. 2016.
2. World Health Organization, Regional Office for Europe. Prisons and Health. Copenhagen: World Health Organization; 2014. http://www.euro.who.int/__data/assets/pdf_file/0005/249188/Prisons-and-Health.pdf

Ethical considerations in prison healthcare

Basic principles of healthcare ethics in prison

Principles of medical ethics[1] apply for healthcare in prison in the same way as in the community.

Due to the peculiar and ethically challenging environment of detention centres and prisons, international bodies issued additional ethical guidelines specifying for prison healthcare.[2-5] The essence of all these guidelines can be summarized as follows:

- The sole task of healthcare providers in prisons and detention centres is to provide healthcare with undivided loyalty to their patients (including preventive healthcare and recording and reporting violence and ill treatment), acting as their patients' personal caregiver without becoming involved in any medical actions that are not in the scope of their patients' health and well-being.
- Healthcare in prison must include:
  - unrestricted access
  - equivalence and integration with healthcare in the community
  - medical confidentiality and the patient's consent
  - preventive healthcare
  - humanitarian support
  - clinical independence
  - professional competence.

Practical application

For the practical implementation of healthcare ethics in prison, its principles must be made known to, understood, and accepted by non-medical staff, security officers, and prison administrators who often are not familiar with it, in the same way as health professionals working in prison must understand and respect security orders. The mutual understanding of the respective roles, legal and ethical guidelines, and challenges of each profession based on a clearly defined separation of professional tasks is indispensable for both ethical healthcare and for humane detention.

- HCPs caring for imprisoned persons should never become involved in medical interventions ordered by the prison administration for security reasons, such as intimate body searches and drug testing or certifying inmates as being fit for disciplinary punishment. However, inmates sentenced to solitary confinement should be cared for by health professionals on a daily basis.[2,5,6]
- Unrestricted access refers to un-delayed medical examination and consultation upon admission to prison and whenever requested by the patient, free of charge and without pre-selection by non-medical staff and includes unrestricted access to dental, psychiatric, and any other secondary healthcare whenever needed.
- Equivalence and integration of healthcare with the community is a minimum requirement, given that the percentage and severity of many health disorders of imprisoned persons is higher than in the community and given the State's special obligation of care for these persons.

- Medical confidentiality requires that medical examinations and consultations are conducted, as a rule, in the privacy of the medical consultation room without the presence of custodial staff, with the exception of individual cases upon the expressed wish of the HCP for their protection. Confidentiality also needs to be observed by not disclosing any patient-related data from medical files without the express permission of the patient or upon an official order from the court. Any breach of medical confidentiality is ethically justified only in cases of saving the health or life of a person.
- Patients' informed consent or dissent needs to be respected in any medical intervention including the examination on admission, and all the more so for invasive medical procedures. Coercive treatment, justified only in mentally incompetent patients if an immediate danger to health or life of the patient or other persons needs to be averted, should never be conducted in prisons but in psychiatric hospitals.
- Preventive healthcare includes supervision of healthy living conditions, health promotion, and preventive measures in health disorders prevailing in prison such as mental disorders, substance use, and transmissible diseases such as hepatitis B and C, HIV disease, and tuberculosis.
- Humanitarian assistance refers to persons who are particularly vulnerable in prison environments due to their gender, age, mental or physical disabilities, offences, belonging to social, ethnic, religious, or sexual minorities, or dependencies from psychoactive substances. HCPs should identify and support them and, upon their consent, advise the prison administration for their protection and to meet their needs.
- Clinical independence is the assurance that HCPs can exercise healthcare without undue influence by outside parties such as the prison administration and that 'clinical decisions may only be taken by the responsible healthcare professionals and may not be overruled or ignored by non-medical prison staff'.[5] Examples include the decision whether a patient can be appropriately cared for in prison or needs hospital treatment.
- Professional competence for primary healthcare services in prison requires, in addition to continuing medical education-certified training of GPs or family doctors and nurses, a sound knowledge of medical ethics and of health disorders prevailing in prison, such as mental health disorders, drug dependency, and transmissible diseases, and of screening, documentation, and reporting of violence.

Further considerations

Patients in prison cannot choose their healthcare provider and the healthcare provider cannot choose their patients. Therefore, creating a sound patient–physician relationship requires explaining to the patient the doctor's unrestricted clinical independence, medical confidentiality, respect of patient autonomy, and their limitations.

Medical documentation in prison healthcare needs to be as meticulous as in the community, paying special attention to patients' informed consent or dissent, the physician's decision in ethical dilemmas, and the recording and reporting of injuries according to the Istanbul Protocol.[6]

Any medical experimentation that may be detrimental to a prisoner's health is absolutely prohibited. However, prisoners may be allowed, upon their free and informed consent and in accordance with applicable law, to participate in clinical trials accessible in the community if these are expected to produce a direct and significant benefit to their health.

For the management of particularly challenging ethical dilemmas such as the healthcare of hunger strikers, professional guidance should be sought from relevant international recommendations[7] and/or national professional boards or ethics committees.

When prison law or rules come in conflict with medical ethics, physicians should conscientiously object to participating in legal practices which are contrary to the ethical codes of the profession and should work to change the law.[8]

References

1. World Medical Association. International code of medical ethics. October 2022. https://www.wma.net/policies-post/wma-international-code-of-medical-ethics

2. Office of the High Commissioner for Human Rights. Principles of medical ethics relevant to the role of health personnel, particularly physicians, in the protection of prisoners and detainees against torture and other cruel, inhuman or degrading treatment or punishment. 1982. http://www.ohchr.org/EN/ProfessionalInterest/Pages/MedicalEthics.aspx

3. Council of Europe. Recommendation No. R (98) 71 of the Committee of Ministers to Member States concerning the Ethical and Organisational Aspects of Health Care in Prison. Strasbourg: Council of Europe; 1998. https://rm.coe.int/09000016804fb13c

4. Council of Europe. CPT Standards: Substantive Section of the CPT's General Reports. Strasbourg: Council of Europe; 1998. http://www.coe.int/en/web/cpt/resources

5. United Nations. Nelson Mandela Rules. n.d. http://www.un.org/en/events/mandeladay/mandela_rules.shtml

6. Office of the High Commissioner for Human Rights. Istanbul Protocol: Manual on the Effective Investigation and Documentation of Torture and Other Cruel, Inhuman or Degrading Treatment or Punishment. Geneva: United Nations; 2004. www.ohchr.org/Documents/Publications/training8rev1en.pdf

7. World Medical Association. WMA declaration of Malta on hunger strikers. October 2017. https://www.wma.net/policies-post/wma-declaration-of-malta-on-hunger-strikers/

8. World Medical Association. WMA council resolution on the relation of law and ethics. October 2019. https://www.wma.net/policies-post/wma-council-resolution-on-the-relation-of-law-and-ethics/

International standards for prison health

Introduction

In a setting mostly designed for security and discipline, healthcare services in prisons not only play an important role in the health and well-being of people in prison but potentially also the investigation and accountability for torture and cruel, inhuman, or degrading treatment or punishment. International standards for healthcare in prisons give a framework for this role based on a human rights approach.

The United Nations Standard Minimum Rules for the Treatment of Prisoners (1955–2015)

Since 1955, when they were first adopted, the United Nations Standard Minimum Rules for the Treatment of Prisoners (SMR) have been the universally acknowledged minimum standards for the detention of people in prisons and have served as a guide in the development of correctional laws, policies, and practices.

Sixty years later, the SMR underwent revision and in 2015 they were adopted by the UN General Assembly as the United Nations Standard Minimum Rules for the Treatment of Prisoners (the Nelson Mandela Rules) (NMR). The revision included changes in the medical services section, including changes from the terms 'prisoners' to 'patients' and 'medical officer' to 'physician'.

Seven fundamental principles and functions of healthcare in prisons as outlined in the Nelson Mandela Rules

- The provision of healthcare is the State's responsibility.
- Equivalence of care: care should be of the same quality and standard as is afforded to those who are not imprisoned or detained.
- All health facilities, goods, and services must be respectful of medical ethics and confidentiality.
- There must be clinical independence and professionalism.
- People in prisons should have access to the necessary healthcare services free of charge at any time during imprisonment, irrespective of their detention regime.
- Healthcare in prisons is not limited to treating sick patients, but must include prevention of disease, violence, and ill-treatment.
- Continuity of care is essential for individual healthcare and is a public health responsibility.

Diversity of prison population and healthcare needs

Prisons host people of different sexual orientation and identity, different religious and cultural background, different national origin, different age, and people with functional diversities. Based on Article 1 (equality) and Article 2 (non-discrimination) of the Universal Declaration of Human Rights, the NMR state that people in prison should have access to necessary healthcare services 'without discrimination on the ground of their legal status'. The NMR stipulate that 'there shall be no discrimination on the grounds of race, colour, sex, language, religion, political or other opinion, national or social origin, property, birth or any other status'. This principle also applies with regard to healthcare. It does not imply that all people in prison should receive the same treatment; rather, it implies that all people in prison should receive appropriate healthcare based on their needs.

Women in prison

In 2010 the United Nations Rules for the Treatment of Female Prisoners and Non-Custodial Measures for Women Offenders, known as the Bangkok Rules, were adopted by the UN General Assembly (Resolution A/RES/65/229). The Bangkok Rules recommend States to consider alternatives to detention for women and girls. If incarcerated, the rules call for appropriate healthcare for women and girls including the following:

- Initial screening should detect HIV and other sexually transmitted infections (STIs) as well as document the reproductive health history and determine sexual abuse and other forms of violence suffered prior to admission (Rule 6).
- Women who have suffered sexual abuse or violence shall be informed about the possibilities of legal action and assisted if they choose to take such action (Rule 7).
- Children who accompany their mothers to prison shall undergo medical screening, preferably by a child specialist and shall receive appropriate care (Rule 9).
- Gender-specific healthcare services at least equivalent to the community shall be provided; if a male medical practitioner undertakes examinations then a female staff member should be present during the examination (Rule 10), and non-medical staff should in principle not attend examinations, yet, if necessary, it should be female staff (Rule 11).
- Other Rules (Rules 14–18) relate to the specific needs of women and girls with regard to HIV, substance abuse, suicide and self-harm, and preventive healthcare services.

Children in detention

The United Nations Rules for the Protection of Juveniles Deprived of their Liberty were adopted by the UN General Assembly in 1990. The rules refer to persons under the age of 18 and state that deprivation of liberty of a child should be used as a last resort and for the minimum necessary period and should be limited to exceptional cases.

With regard to medical care (Rules 49–55), the Rules stipulate the following:

- Every child shall receive adequate medical care, both preventive and remedial, as medically indicated, and that care should be provided through the services in the community.
- Every child has the right to entry screening for the purpose of health and of recording any sign of ill-treatment prior to admission.
- Medical care should be prompt and appropriate and detect all conditions that might hamper rehabilitation.
- Medical officers should care for the health and well-being of imprisoned children and report all negative health impacts caused by detention to the director and the relevant independent authority.
- Children with mental illness should be treated in a specialist institution under independent management.
- Child detention facilities must adopt professional preventive and rehabilitative programmes that are appropriate with regard to sex and age.
- Children shall be protected from any form of ill-treatment related to healthcare.

Article 37 of the Convention on the Rights of the Child, adopted by the UN General Assembly in 1989, requires that States take all necessary measures to avoid the detention of children. The SMR in 1955 and the NMR of 2015 deliberately exclude any provisions for imprisoned children because they contain the principle that young persons should not be imprisoned. So far, the NMR only relate to children as children of an imprisoned parent. NMR 29 §1(b) states that child-specific healthcare services shall be provided.

The scale and magnitude of children's suffering in prisons remains almost invisible. The UN global study on children deprived of liberty was commissioned in 2014 to examine the scale and conditions of children deprived of liberty, identify good practices in non-custodial solutions, and make recommendations for effective measures to prevent human rights violations against children in detention and reduce the number of children deprived of liberty. The report of the study was submitted to the UN General Assembly in 2019. It shows that detention has a negative impact on both the physical and mental health of children and that children deprived of their liberty have an increased risk of premature mortality compared to their peers in the community.

People in prison with special needs

The UNODC, in 2009, published the *Handbook on Prisoners with Special Needs*. The book aims to support countries in implementing the rule of law and the development of criminal justice reform. It is designed to be used by all actors involved in the criminal justice system. It covers the special needs of eight groups of people in prison:

- People with mental health care needs.
- People with disabilities.
- Ethnic and racial minorities and indigenous peoples.
- Foreign nationals (people who are not a citizen of the country in which they are imprisoned).

- Lesbian, gay, bisexual, and transgender (LGBT) people.
- Older people.
- People with terminal illness.
- People under sentence of death.

Core international standards

See Table 2.1.

Table 2.1 Core international standards for healthcare in prisons (Adopted by UN General Assembly resolutions)

Standard	Target population(s)	Year of adoption/ entry into force
Standard Minimum Rules for the Treatment of Prisoners	All prisoners	1955
International Covenant on Economic, Social and Cultural Rights (Article 12: right to health)	All people	1966/1976
International Covenant on Civil and Political Rights (Article 6, para 1: right to life; Article 7: prohibition of torture or cruel, inhuman, or degrading treatment or punishment; Article 10, para 1: right to humane treatment and respect of dignity for people in prisons)	All people/all prisoners	1966/1976
Declaration on the Protection of All Persons from Being Subjected to Torture and Other Cruel, Inhuman or Degrading Treatment or Punishment	All prisoners	1975
Convention on the Elimination of All Forms of Discrimination against Women	All women	1979
Principles of Medical Ethics	All prisoners	1982
Convention against Torture and Other Cruel, Inhuman or Degrading Treatment or Punishment	All prisoners	1984
Body of Principles for the Protection of All Persons under Any Form of Detention or Imprisonment	All prisoners	1988
Convention on the Rights of the Child	All children	1989/1990
Basic Principles for the Treatment of Prisoners	All prisoners	1990
United Nations Rules for the Protection of Juveniles Deprived of their Liberty	Juvenile prisoners	1990
Convention on the Rights of Persons with Disabilities	All persons with disabilities	2006
Optional Protocol to the Convention against Torture and other Cruel, Inhuman or Degrading Treatment or Punishment	All prisoners	2006

Standard	Target population(s)	Year of adoption/ entry into force
United Nations Rules for the Treatment of Women Prisoners and Non-Custodial Measures for Women Offenders (the Bangkok Rules)	Women prisoners	2011
United Nations Standard Minimum Rules for the Treatment of Prisoners (the Nelson Mandela Rules)	All prisoners	2015

In *italic*: human rights treaties, which are considered as legally binding on the parties involved.

Implementation of standards for healthcare in prisons

A wide range of tools of information, education, and communication as well as international and national monitoring mechanisms are available in order for prison systems to comply with international standards.

Information, education, and communication

Specialist UN agencies such as the UNODC or the WHO but also non-governmental organizations offer special resources for provision of better healthcare in prisons such as manuals, handbooks, or checklists.

In addition to the sources referred to, relevant resources may be found here (without any claim to completeness):

- UNODC. Prison reform (https://www.unodc.org/unodc/en/justice-and-prison-reform/cpcj-prison-reform.html).
- WHO Regional Office for Europe. Prisons and health (https://www.who.int/europe/health-topics/prisons-and-health).
- World Medical Association, Norwegian Medical Association (2001, last update 2014). Doctors working in prison: human rights and ethical dilemma. A web-based course on human rights and ethics for prison doctors. (https://nettkurs.legeforeningen.no/enrol/index.php?id=39).
- International Committee of the Red Cross (2017). *Health Care in Detention: A Practical Guide* (https://shop.icrc.org/health-care-in-detention-a-practical-guide.html?___store=default).
- Penal Reform International. Resources (https://www.penalreform.org/resources/).

Monitoring mechanisms

International, regional, and national mechanisms for independent prison monitoring include the following:

- Special Procedures of the Human Rights Council including the Special Rapporteurs on Torture, Health, and Violence Against Women.
- Other UN Human Rights Bodies such as the Committee against Torture (CAT) and its Subcommittee on Prevention of Torture (SPT) which monitors places of detention in States party to the Optional Protocol to the Convention against Torture and Other Cruel, Inhuman or Degrading Treatment or Punishment (OPCAT).
- On a regional level, in Europe, the European Committee for the Prevention of Torture and Inhuman or Degrading Treatment or Punishment (CPT) monitors places of detention in Member States of the Council of Europe under the relevant European Convention.
- On a national level, States which have ratified the OPCAT are under the obligation to install a National Preventive Mechanism (NPM) to monitor places of detention.

Prison healthcare

- When a state deprives people of their liberty, it must guarantee their right to health and provide them with the best possible care.[1]
- Healthcare in prisons in England is provided by the NHS and people in prison have the same entitlements to such services as any other person.

For some time, the official aim of healthcare in prison has been to give people in prison access to the same quality and range of healthcare services as the general public receives from the NHS: 'equivalence of care'.[2]

- The NHS and the prison service are required to cooperate with each other to provide health services to people in prison.[3,4] The service in England is provided under an agreement between the Ministry of Justice, HMPPS, the UK Health Security Agency, the Department of Health and Social Care, and NHS England.[5] The agreement is administered by a National Prison Healthcare Board consisting of all five organizations and Local Delivery Boards.

- Services are commissioned by NHS England.[6] Commissioning is intended to be undertaken in accordance with 'the principle of equivalence', that is, a service equal to that available to the general population.[7] These services include public health services for adults and children in detained and secure settings in England (pursuant to an agreement with the Secretary of State for Health and Social Care under section 7a of the National Health Service Act 2006.[8] It is important to recognize that equivalence pertains to having the same opportunities to access care of a quality equal to that found in the community, but that the health needs of persons within prisons are likely to differ from those of the general population.

- All NHS bodies, including for this purpose local authorities, and the prison service are under a duty to cooperate with each other with a view to improving the way in which those functions are exercised in relation to securing and maintaining the health of people in prison. The range of services which are directly commissioned for prisons include primary (GP) and secondary (hospital) care services (hospital care), public health (including substance misuse services, under a section 7a agreement with the Department of Health), dental services, ophthalmic (eye care) services, and mental health services.[4]

- Local authorities are under a duty to assess the social care needs of all adults in custody in their area and to commission or provide the care that is needed.[9]

- The health services, and some social care services, are regulated by the Care Quality Commission (CQC) who registers the providers of services and undertakes joint inspections with His Majesty's Inspectorate of Prisons (HMIP).[10] Both the CQC and HMIP have responsibilities under the UK NPM to prevent ill-treatment of people in prison. The NPM is required under international treaty and the OPCAT. Unlike other settings, the CQC does not currently award a rating to prison health and social care services, but it does assess as with other settings whether services are safe, effective, caring, responsive, and well led. Inspection reports are published on the CQC website on a separate page for each prison. CQC's enforcement powers are limited in prison settings but such action can on occasion be taken against registered providers.[11]

- The standard of healthcare service available in prison has been a matter of concern for some time. The House of Commons Health and Social Care Committee has recently stated that 'The Government is failing

in its duty of care towards people detained in England's prisons ....
No one is sentenced to worsened health but that, largely as a result of
overstretched staff, overcrowding and poor facilities, is too often the
outcome'.[12]

- Therefore, recognizing the impact that the prison environment has on
  overall health and well-being, the Committee and the CQC support the
  development of a 'whole system' and a 'whole prison' approach.
- People in prison are owed the same duty of care in relation to medical
  treatment and advice as others. It has been reported that over
  £2 million was awarded in damages for clinical negligence to people
  in prison between 2010 and 2017.[13] Whether or not there has been a
  breach of the standard of care has to be assessed with due regard to
  the constraints of a prison setting. A person in prison may be at fault for
  the purpose of contributory negligence by reason of drug abuse but if
  they have informed the authorities of this history it is unlikely to be an
  operative contributor to an injury resulting from clinical negligence (see,
  e.g. St George v Home Office[14]). The Ministry of Justice is not liable for
  clinical negligence in prisons.[15]
- Deaths in prisons should, largely, be avoidable, and so it is essential
  for any deaths to be reviewed carefully to identify any shortcomings
  in care or lessons to be learned. A death in a prison setting may give
  rise to the need for an inquest which is a full and effective investigation
  into it, if this is likely to be the only way in which the procedural duty
  under Article 2 of the European Convention on Human Rights can be
  fulfilled.[16]
- Article 3 of the European Convention on Human Rights imposes on
  the State a positive obligation to ensure that a person's health and
  well-being are adequately secured by the provision of the requisite
  medical assistance and treatment and a failure to do so may entitle the
  incarcerated person to a remedy for a breach of their human rights.
  The standard of care to be provided should be compatible with human
  dignity but should also take into account the practical demands of
  imprisonment.[17]

References

1. Enggist S, Møller L, Møller G, et al. (eds). Prisons and Health. Copenhagen: WHO Regional Office
   for Europe; 2014. http://www.euro.who.int/__data/assets/pdf_file/0005/249188/Prisons-
   and-Health.pdf
2. HM Prison Service, NHS Executive. The Future Organisation of Prison Health Care. London: HM
   Prison Service; 1999. https://webarchive.nationalarchives.gov.uk/20110504020423/http://www.
   dh.gov.uk/prod_consum_dh/groups/dh_digitalassets/@dh/@en/documents/digitalasset/
   dh_4106031.pdf
3. Legislation.gov.uk. The Prison and Young Offender Institution (Amendment) Rules 2009. 2009.
   https://www.legislation.gov.uk/uksi/2009/3082/contents/made
4. Legislation.gov.uk. National Health Service Act 2006, section 249. 2006. https://www.legislation.
   gov.uk/ukpga/2006/41/section/249
5. HM Government. National Prison Healthcare Board's National Partnership Agreement for 2018–
   21. April 2018. https://assets.publishing.service.gov.uk/government/uploads/system/uploads/
   attachment_data/file/767832/6.4289_MoJ_National_health_partnership_A4-L_v10_web.pdf
6. Legislation.gov.uk. Health and Social Care Act 2012, section 15. 2012. https://www.legislation.
   gov.uk/ukpga/2012/7/section/15
7. NHS England. Health and justice. n.d. https://www.england.nhs.uk/commissioning/health-just/

8. Department of Health and Social Care. Public health commissioning in the NHS 2018 to 2019. 2018. https://www.gov.uk/government/publications/public-health-commissioning-in-the-nhs-2018-to-2019

9. Legislation.gov.uk. Care Act 2014, section 76. 2014. https://www.legislation.gov.uk/ukpga/2014/23/section/76

10. Care Quality Commission. Provider handbook: how the CQC regulates health and social care in prisons, young offender institutions and health care in immigration removal centres. July 2015. https://www.cqc.org.uk/sites/default/files/20150729_provider_handbook_secure_settings_0.pdf

11. Health Select and Social Care Committee. Written evidence from the Care Quality Commission. May 2018. http://data.parliament.uk/writtenevidence/committeeevidence.svc/evidencedocument/health-and-social-care-committee/prison-health/written/83095.html#_ftn2 May 2018

12. Health Select and Social Care Committee. Prison health. HC 963. October 2018. https://publications.parliament.uk/pa/cm201719/cmselect/cmhealth/963/963.pdf

13. Buchan L. Inmates receive payouts of £2m for poor healthcare amid 'unprecedented pressures' in prisons. The Independent, 26 February 2018. https://www.independent.co.uk/news/uk/politics/inmates-prison-healthcare-payouts-nhs-hmp-liverpool-prisons-uk-a8225071.html

14. St George v Home Office [2009] 1 WLR 1670 [2008] EWCA Civ 1068.

15. Razumas v Ministry of Justice [2018] EWHC 215 (QB); [2018] P.I.Q.R. P10.

16. R (Davies) v HM Deputy Coroner for Birmingham [2003] EWCA Civ 1739; R (Middleton) v West Somerset coroner [2004] UKHL10; [2004] 2 AC 182; McGlinchey v UK ECHR (Appln No50390/99).

17. McGlinchey v UK (July 2003) (Appln No 50390/99); Golubar v Croatia (August 2017) Application no. 21951/15.

Prescribing in prisons

Prison pharmacy services

The prison pharmacy service is modelled on community services, with additional clinical pharmacy services and governance to deliver safe medicines optimization in the prison environment. Commissioning structures for prison pharmacy services will vary by geography; this chapter strives to provide a general overview, but may at times refer to policies and processes applicable only to the English prison estate as the primary frame of reference.

There are two key elements of service provision:

- The dispensing of prescriptions and delivery of these to the prison if the pharmacy is outside the prison. Bulk stock is also provided by the dispensing pharmacy if the pharmacy is also a licensed wholesaler.
- Clinical and medicines optimization and governance services provided in the prison by a pharmacy team. This includes:
  - advising and supporting people in prison in taking their medicines
  - delivering medicines reconciliation and medication review clinics
  - development and implementation of medicines policies, procedures, and formularies
  - oversight and management of medicines storage and disposal, including controlled drugs (CDs)
  - training and supporting healthcare staff in medicines use and safety
  - leading the prison medicines management committee which is a multidisciplinary committee that underpins the agreement and implementation of all medicines use and processes in the prison.

The quality of pharmacy services and medicines optimization

In England, prison pharmacy services are commissioned by NHS England with the expectation that providers of the services deliver them to national standards and guidance. These include generic requirements that apply to all sectors of healthcare and pharmacy service provision and bespoke standards for services delivered in prisons. Specific prison standards and guidelines are:

- NICE publications on the physical[1] and mental health services[2] for people in prison
- professional publications for prescribing in prisons[3] and optimizing medicines and safer prescribing in secure environments[4,5]
- expectations from inspecting bodies.[6]
  1. If there is a dispensing pharmacy within the prison (which dispenses medicines for that prison or additional prisons), there will be premises and medicines storage facilities for providing these pharmaceutical supply services that align with those expected for registered pharmacy premises in the community (i.e. standards set and inspected by the General Pharmaceutical Council). HMPPS is responsible for ensuring the structural elements including that temperature control of these premises meets the national standards.

The pharmacy workforce and infrastructure

The composition of the pharmacy team working in a prison depends on what pharmacy services are delivered within the setting and how the healthcare provider chooses to use the skills mix of HCPs in their services. The premises, pharmacy opening hours, and infrastructure in which the pharmacy team works are also dependent on these local factors.

In the dispensary premises, pharmacists, pharmacy technicians, and pharmacy assistants make up the workforce. They deliver the services that are equivalent to those within community pharmacies. As most prison pharmacies are registered with the General Pharmaceutical Council, the pharmacy team work within The Medicines (Pharmacies) (Responsible Pharmacist) Regulations 2008. If patient consultations such as medicines use reviews are provided by the pharmacy staff, these usually happen in a separate room within the main healthcare centre or in a treatment room on a prison wing.

In these prisons and in those where there is no in-house pharmacy, the pharmacy team work within the main healthcare centre or wing treatment rooms to supply or administer over-the-counter and prescribed medicines, deliver patient consultations, advise and train other healthcare staff, and manage the ordering, storage, and receipt of medicines into the prison. These clinical and governance roles are shared and integrated with nurses and medical staff in a similar way to pharmacists and pharmacy technicians working in GP practices and community health centres.

Infrastructure support

As for other healthcare consultations and practices in prison, prison officers and prison governors support the access to and delivery of pharmacy services by:

- supporting the safe transporting of medicines on delivery and as they are moved to prison wings
- supervising the supply and administration of medicines to keep the healthcare staff safe and to detect and minimize the diversion of prescribed medicines
- attending the medicines management committee and influencing the model of medicines management so that this fits in with the prison regime and population risks and needs
- escorting incarcerated people to appointments with the pharmacy team or to medicines administration points on the wings or within the main healthcare centre.

References

1. National Institute for Health and Care Excellence. Physical health of people in prison. NICE guideline [NG57]. 2016. https://www.nice.org.uk/guidance/ng57
2. National Institute for Health and Care Excellence. Mental health of adults in contact with the criminal justice system. NICE guideline [NG66]. 2017. https://www.nice.org.uk/guidance/ng66
3. Royal College of General Practitioners. Safer prescribing in prisons, 2nd ed. https://elearning.rcgp.org.uk/pluginfile.php/176185/mod_book/chapter/620/RCGP-safer-prescribing-in-prisons-guidance-jan-2019.pdf
4. Royal Pharmaceutical Society. Professional standards for optimising medicines for people in secure environments—prisons, young offender institutions and secure training centres (edition 2). February 2017. https://www.rpharms.com/recognition/setting-professional-standards/optimising-medicines-in-secure-environments
5. NHS England. Health and justice mental health services: safer use of mental health medicines. September 2017. https://www.england.nhs.uk/wp-content/uploads/2017/10/health-and-justice-safer-use-of-mental-health-medicines.pdf
6. HM Inspectorate of Prisons. Our expectations. July 2021. https://www.justiceinspectorates.gov.uk/hmiprisons/our-expectations/

The medicines pathway

The lead pharmacist for a prison develops and oversees the provision of a safe and effective medicines pathway that people in prison receive and other HCPs and prison staff work within. The following section describes some key parts of the medicines pathway relevant for practitioners working in prisons.

Medicines reconciliation

Medication reconciliation is the process of creating the most accurate list possible of all medications a patient is taking—including drug name, dosage, frequency, and route—and comparing that list against the admission, transfer, and/or discharge medication, with the goal of providing appropriate and safe continuity of care.[1]

- When a person comes into prison, an initial list of medicines is compiled during reception screening (see Reception and first night screening, p. 82). This is validated via a formal medicines reconciliation completed by nursing or pharmacy staff.
- In England, a national clinical template on the prison clinical system is used to document the process and outcomes of this reconciliation, including any discrepancies between the initial list and the information from community records or the medicines the person has brought in with them.
- The outcomes of the medicines reconciliation inform the clinicians who treat the patient after reception and support the second healthcare assessment (see Second-stage health assessment, p. 88).

Access to critical and urgent medicines

When a person comes into prison, they may not have their medicines with them or the medicines may not be suitable for use. In addition, during their stay in prison, an urgent new medicine (not including those needed in a medical emergency) might need to be accessed when the usual pharmacy service is not available or cannot supply the medicine quickly enough to prevent possible harm from omitted doses.

The pharmacy team supports the patient and clinicians to access these medicines by:

- having a supply of common urgent medicines available for use in an emergency medicines cupboard; this is accessed by authorized staff and the access is recorded by staff removing the medicines and the use and stock held is managed by pharmacy staff
- enabling a prescriber to prescribe on a community NHS prescription form (FP10 in England) that can be taken to a community pharmacy outside the prison; these prison-issued prescriptions do not require the payment of the NHS prescription charge.

Where a pharmacy cannot supply a particular medicine due to a shortage or other delay, the above options can be used or an alternative medicine can be prescribed.

In-possession medication

Since 2003, on the publication by the Department of Health of 'A Pharmacy Service for Prisoners',[2] people entering prison receive an in-possession risk assessment on reception or shortly afterwards. This supports the HCP in deciding if the person is able to have their medicines in their possession for self-administration. The assessment forms part of the prison's in-possession medication policy which is a policy underpinned by national guidance[3] and agreed via the medicines management committee.

The policy works on the principle that people in prison should be able to have their medicines in their possession unless:

• there are safety reasons or individual vulnerabilities which mean they may harm themselves with or divert their medicines
• the medicines they are taking are CDs or other high-risk medicines that are always supplied in the prison under supervision (i.e. not in-possession); examples of medicines not usually held not in-possession include:
  • methadone, buprenorphine, tramadol, and benzodiazepines
  • pregabalin and gabapentin.

The patient is asked to sign a compact that describes their responsibilities in safely managing their in-possession medicines and expectations about their role in making sure any supervised doses are accessed safely. This compact is locally developed and any breach of it results in a clinical medication review and disciplinary action by the prison governor if the breach involves the abuse or diversion of prescribed medicines.

Risk assessment review

As a patient's health is clinically reviewed, or if an incident occurs where patient safety with in-possession medication is a potential risk, the in-possession risk assessment is reviewed and the patient may have their in-possession status changed, preventing them from having in-possession medication. Conversely, if a patient's health improves, their not in-possession status will be reviewed, enabling them to have their medicines in their possession.

Medicines storage in cells

It is not mandatory that every patient having in-possession medication should have a lockable cupboard for storing it in their cells. However, it is recommended for cells which are shared by two or more people.[4]

General issues

It is important to remember the following points about in-possession medication:

• Prescribers and people reviewing patients' care need to:
  • check the current in-possession status is still appropriate for them and if not, change it
  • ensure they prescribe medicines in line with the patient's in-possession status and local in-possession policy; this avoids the risk of delays and errors in supplying the medicines.
• People queuing for not-in-possession medication create challenges for healthcare and prison staff as the sessions need to fit into the prison's daily regimes and also enable the medicines to be supplied and

administered safely. This means that the resulting arrangements for in-possession medication may vary between prisons.

- It is expected that prison officers supervise all not in-possession medicines supply sessions. This enables a partnership approach to the safe supply of these medicines that minimizes the risk of medicines diversion, bullying of patients, and healthcare staff intimidation.
- Once released from prison, a person will be self-administering their medicines as part of their daily lives. Being able to self-administer and manage their medicines while in prison helps them to prepare for managing their health once they are living in the community.
- If a patient is able to have their medicines in-possession but to have 28 days' supply at a time is too high a quantity for them to manage safely, the pharmacy team can supply the medicines packaged as 7-day in-possession packs or monitored dosage systems/compliance aids. This option often means more people can have their medicines in-possession and these needs can continue to be provided for on release into the community.

Medicines storage and supply

Medicines storage in an in-house dispensing pharmacy and within healthcare rooms centrally and on the wings must comply with the General Pharmaceutical Council and professional standards.[5] This includes facilities for storing CDs and medicines that require refrigeration.

In medicines administration points (MAPs) where medicines are supplied to patients, the following requirements are recommended:

- Supplies are made via a gate or hatch that enables the patient to be easily identified and be able to communicate easily with the healthcare staff. The visibility of the patient should be such that the HCP can observe the patient's hands and upper body as the medicine is swallowed.
- The area where the patient stands to receive their medicines is arranged so that they can receive their medicine and have a discussion with the HCP in confidence.
- There is a source of potable water in the MAP room, enabling patients to take their oral medicines with 200 mL of water, and a sink is provided for the HCP to rinse any measuring equipment used to provide liquid medicines.
- A network connection and IT equipment is available in the MAP next to the hatch or gate. The HCP uses the clinical record to record the administration or supply of the medicine or check the record for information about the patient's medicines or care plan.

Medicines supply on release and transfer

- In many cases the transfer of a person between prisons or their release from prison can be planned for in advance. The pharmacy should provide a supply of medicines that will be given to them on their release or handed over to staff in the receiving prison if they are transferred.
- For both released and transferred persons, the expectation in professional standards and NICE guidance is that a minimum of 7 days' supply is provided. This enables the patient to continue taking their

current prescribed medicines until their care can be reviewed by the GP in the community or the new prison.
- In the event that a patient is released unexpectedly, the healthcare team can prescribe on to the NHS community prescription form. This is handed to the patient on release from court and can be taken to any pharmacy in order to receive the medicine without having to pay the NHS prescription charge.

References

1. Royal Pharmaceutical Society. 2013.
2. Department of Health. A Pharmacy Service for Prisoners. London: Department of Health.
3. NPC. 2004.
4. HM Inspectorate of Prisons, Royal Pharmaceutical Society. 2017.
5. Royal Pharmaceutical Society. Safe and secure handling of medicines. 2018. https://www.rpharms.com/recognition/setting-professional-standards/safe-and-secure-handling-of-medicines

Dependence-forming medications

Prescribed medication may be as addictive and sought after as illicit substances.[1] This may be due to a wish for euphoric effects or commonly for sedating and dissociative effects in patients who have experienced trauma. While they can give some emotional numbing and dissociation, this is not a therapeutic effect. In a situation where a person can feel little emotion, they cannot experience any degree of recovery and may well accumulate further harm and trauma in such a state.

Although dependence is a feature of these medicines, it is not a reason to avoid them if clinically indicated. The decision to prescribe or continue dispensing should be made in collaboration with the patient, following the structure of a medicines management plan.

When patients arrive in prison, the GP takes over prescribing responsibility and a medication review should be undertaken ensuring that monitoring is up to date, and that the prescription remains safe and appropriate. There will be instances where this is no longer the case and plans should be made to deal with this. It is important to be aware of the pressures to commence prescriptions for dependence-forming medications and ensure judicious use, always referring to the principles of safe prescribing:

1. Is it indicated?
2. Is it safe?
3. What is the review period or end date?

Please note the suggested detox regimens are for confirmed prescribed medications only. Illicit use is dealt with elsewhere.
The following are the common prescription medications which are dependence forming.

Examples of dependence-forming medications

Opiates

Opiates are the most well-known dependence-forming medication. Short-term courses (e.g. postoperatively) should have a defined period of use. Chronic pain is a more commonly encountered situation. Management of chronic pain is dealt with in Chapter 6 but the basic principles include the following:

- Opiates are not appropriate in chronic pain. Tolerance and dependence will form and other effects can be seen such as hyperalgesia (worsening of pain) and complex hormonal and cognitive effects occur.
- 'Opioids Aware'[2] provides some excellent guidance for clinicians and it should be noted that doses above 120 mg oral morphine equivalent/ day show no evidence of increased clinical benefit but significant increase in risk.
- The pain ladder is frequently cited but was designed for cancer/ palliative care and is not relevant to chronic pain management.[3]

Benzodiazepines

- Benzodiazepines are frequently seen on long-term prescriptions. Both physiological and psychological addiction are seen within weeks and 2–4 weeks of prescribing is advised as a maximum in the *British National Formulary* and only when appropriately indicated.
- Withdrawal symptoms can be psychologically very difficult and there is a risk of seizure with abrupt withdrawal as well as acute mental effects including mood and potentially psychotic effects.
- Long-term use will cause worsening anxiety and often reduces a person's positive coping skills further.
- A gradual reduction is suggested: 2 mg per week for long-term prescriptions (illicit use is covered elsewhere).

Sleeping medications

- Z-drugs are frequently seen as long-term medications. These lose efficacy and are addictive.
- They can cause sleep walking, memory symptoms, and falls and have 'hangover effects', making a person tired or less able to cope the following day.
- Long-term use may worsen sleep disorders. Some studies have shown of evidence of an increased number of cancers and higher risk of death in people who take long-term sleeping medications although causality is unknown. The effect on mortality is seen even in those prescribed less than 18 tablets per year.
- Psychological therapies are recommended for longer-term sleep disorders.

Gabapentinoids

- These are the most sought-after medications in the prison environment.
- They are often used in conjunction with opiates for a euphoric effect. However, these combinations are synergistic in their respiratory depressant effect and the number of deaths from combined opiates and gabapentinoids is increasing year on year.
- Recent consensus statements of experienced prison doctors suggest that a comorbid substance misuse disorder should be a contraindication to their prescription.
- Suggested detox regimen: pregabalin 50–100 mg per week. Gabapentin 300 mg every 4 days.

Mirtazapine

- Mirtazapine 15 mg is frequently used off licence for sleep. This can add to a burden of sedating medication and is not a therapeutic dose for depression.
- Ensure the indication is correct and increase to a therapeutic dose where appropriate.

Issues with dependence-forming medications in the prison setting

Concealment

- Patients may attempt to conceal medication to use illicitly or sell. Prisons should have a robust concealment policy which should be enforced. An example of this would be to have a medication compact that a patient must sign, stating that medication will be taken as intended and if not, will be reviewed and likely stopped.

- If concealment takes place, document this and inform the patient of a plan for reducing or stopping medication. Concealment is a contraindication to safe ongoing prescribing.

Co-prescribing
- A common situation is the co-prescription of multiple sedating drugs. 'Orange Book'[4] guidance suggests that no more than two sedating medications should be prescribed together.
- There is a paucity of evidence for the multiple combinations seen in practice with methadone, chlordiazepoxide (Librium), quetiapine, and gabapentinoids being frequently in the mix, often in addition to illicit use.
- Combinations may also lead to prolongation of the QT interval corrected for heart rate (QTc).
- As part of the patient's medication review this should be considered e.g. if commencing a methadone induction, do not routinely prescribe sleeping medication.

The principle of adverse selection is well understood: those with mental health or substance misuse issues are at higher risk of being prescribed high-dose opiates and combinations of sedating drugs. This is a vulnerable population often seen within prisons.

Special prescribing considerations
There are other special considerations for prescribing in prisons. Substances which are of no consequence in the community may be misused in this environment. Examples include the following:
- Proprietary brands of topical analgesics with strong smells due to menthol or similar compounds e.g. "Deep Heat®" may be used to mask the smell of illicit substances and may be considered a security risk.
- Hyoscine-bromide is frequently smoked for a dissociative/hallucinogenic effect and can cause marked aggression.
- Mebeverine or peppermint oil should be used as first line—hyoscine-bromide is not appropriate in the prison environment.
- Other substances may be used to make hooch (e.g. proprietary brands of skin moisturiser, including those containing oatmeal extract and lactulose) or have value as tradeable commodities (supplemental drinks).

Clinician safety
- These can be emotive consultations. Clear explanations and firm boundaries are essential. Ensuring clinician safety is important. For complex and difficult patients there may be value in a multidisciplinary team (MDT) approach, including use of joint consultations.
- It may be useful to send a letter to the patient after a difficult consultation to reiterate the rationale and plan. Clinicians have a duty to communicate with community prescribers about stopped medications.

References
1. National Institute for Health and Care Excellence. Medicines associated with dependence and withdrawal symptoms: safe prescribing and withdrawal management for adults. April 2022. NICE guideline [NG215]. https://www.nice.org.uk/guidance/ng215

2. Royal College of Anaesthetists, Faculty of Pain Medicine. Opioids aware. n.d. https://fpm.ac.uk/opioids-aware

3. National Institute for Health and Care Excellence. Chronic pain (primary and secondary and secondary) in over 16s: assessment of all chronic pain and management of chronic primary pain. NICE Guideline (NG193). April 2021. https://www.nice.org.uk/guidance/ng193

4. Clinical Guidelines on Drug Misuse and Dependence Update 2017 Independent Expert Working Group. Drug misuse and dependence: UK guidelines on clinical management [the Orange Book]. Department of Health and Social Care; 2017. https://www.gov.uk/government/publications/drug-misuse-and-dependence-uk-guidelines-on-clinical-management

Further reading

British Medical Association. Chronic pain: supporting safer prescribing of analgesics. March 2017. https://www.bma.org.uk/media/2100/analgesics-chronic-pain.pdf

Lader M. Benzodiazepine harm: how can it be reduced? Br J Clin Pharmacol. 2014;77(2):295–301.

Public Health Research Consortium. Prescribing patterns in dependence forming medications. https://www.phrc.online/assets/uploads/files/PHRC_014_Final_Report.pdf

RCGP Resources for Secure Environments https://elearning.rcgp.org.uk/mod/book/view.php?id=13151&chapterid=620

Complications, interactions, and overdose

Complications

The secure environment presents unique and complex challenges that make for demanding and rewarding work for HCPs.

When prescribing for people in prison, HCPs need to carefully consider the risks, not only to the individual, but also to the wider prison community.

- Chronic/persistent pain is prevalent among people in prison, and an over-reliance on medications or illicit drugs may occur in the absence of compassionate, balanced expert support. HCPs play an important role in educating patients about chronic pain and promoting self-care and non-pharmacological therapies, where appropriate.
- HCPs should be alert to the possibility that the patient agenda may not be aligned with that of the HCP. There may be inadvertent consequences from well-intentioned treatment plans. Patients may seek certain medications because they are being bullied, or to trade. A referral to hospital may be an opportunity to collect contraband to smuggle back into the prison, or to attempt an escape.
- While HCPs should adhere to safe prescribing practices in regard to analgesic medication for persistent pain, it is also important that bias does not interfere with effective assessment and management of long-term symptoms and painful conditions.

Interactions

Polypharmacy and polysubstance misuse

A high proportion of people in prison have a recent history of substance misuse and dependence. While in prison, substance misuse often continues; however the pattern of use may change. Conventional drugs (e.g. heroin, crack cocaine, and alcohol) are less readily available. People in prison will often turn to other substances, often in combination, depending on the availability; these might include conventional drugs, prescription medications (diverted or prescribed), psychoactive substances (PSs), hooch (homemade alcohol), and nicotine (including liquid from e-cigarettes or nicotine replacement treatment).

This complex polysubstance misuse increases the risk of harm to the user by increasing the risk of unintended effects, drug interactions, and overdose. When sedating substances are taken in combination the risk of overdose is increased, even if the individual doses are small. When prescribing, the HCP must be aware of the potential risks and interactions medications may have if taken with other substances. For some medications, the potential for harm must be carefully mitigated before prescribing (e.g. strong opioids, gabapentinoids, and benzodiazepines), whereas others might be prescribed but with caution (e.g. co-codamol and zopiclone). See Abuse and diversion of medicines, p. 54, for further principles of safer prescribing.

Psychoactive substances

Previously known as novel psychoactive substances (NPSs), now known simply as psychoactive substances (PSs), the term encompasses an increasingly large number of chemicals that have been manufactured to emulate

the effects of the traditional drugs. They can broadly be categorized into four groups (Table 3.1):
- Synthetic cannabinoids (which mimic cannabis).
- Stimulants (mimic amphetamines and MDMA/Ecstasy).
- Sedatives (opioids and benzodiazepines).
- Hallucinogens/dissociatives (mimic LSD and ketamine).

A single batch of PSs may contain multiple chemicals from the same or different groups, so their effects can be varied and unpredictable. They do not show up in standard urine drug screens, and so have become popular within the prison environment. It is therefore important to understand the potential presentation of patients under the influence of PSs and consider these as potential causes for symptoms suggestive of drug interactions or overdose.

Table 3.1 Categorization of psychoactive substances

Cannabinoids
Signs of intoxication: slurred or incoherent speech, inability to speak, poor coordination, injected sclera, vomiting, sweating, anxiety, agitation, sudden aggressive behaviour
Overdose: psychosis, hypertension, arrhythmias, chest pain, hyperthermia, seizures

Stimulants

Signs of intoxication: enlarged pupils, excitable, pressured speech, hypervigilance, aggressive behaviour
Overdose: vomiting, tachycardia, hypertension, seizures, chest pain, stroke, cardiac arrest

Sedatives

Signs of intoxication: pin-point pupils (opioids), drooping eyelids, falling asleep or appearing vacant, disorientation, slurred speech
Overdose: vomiting, reduced conscious state, respiratory depression, cyanosis, respiratory arrest

Hallucinogens/ dissociatives

Signs of intoxication: altered pupil size, nystagmus, poor coordination, confusion, agitation
Overdose: hyperthermia, seizures, psychosis

Synthetic cannabinoids
- The most popular group of PSs in the prison environment are the synthetic cannabinoid receptor agonists, also known as 'spice'.
- Cannabis contains the chemical THC (a partial cannabinoid receptor agonist) which causes the euphoric effect, although it can also trigger anxiety and paranoia. CBD (cannabidiol) is also naturally found in cannabis and is an anxiolytic so tempers the effects of the THC. Synthetic cannabinoid receptor agonists have a much higher affinity to the cannabinoid receptors in the brain, resulting in a much stronger, longer-lasting effect, without any of the softening effects of CBD.

- Synthetic cannabinoid receptor agonists are used to induce euphoria, relaxation, and an altered mental state; however, they may lead to unwanted effects which include anxiety, paranoia, vomiting, psychosis, cardiac toxicity (hypertension, arrythmia, myocardial infarction), seizures, hyperthermia, and renal failure.
- No two batches of 'spice' are the same. They may contain several different SRCAs, resulting in varied and unpredictable duration of action, time to peak effect, side effects, and dosage.
- They may also be mixed with different PSs, for example, sedatives such as fentanyl, which may increase the risk of overdose.

Fentanyl
- Novel opioids[1] are often derivatives of fentanyl and have caused a large number of drug-related deaths internationally.
- Fentanyl is 1000× stronger than heroin and can cause overdose within a few minutes. Other novel opioids, such as carfentanil, can be even stronger and more deadly.
- It is sometimes found in batches of heroin or spice, often unknown to the user, which poses a serious threat of overdose and death.
- It is not detectable in standard urine drug screens.

Alprazolam
- Alprazolam is a benzodiazepine that is not licensed in the UK but is increasingly used recreationally.
- In its pure form, 1 mg is equivalent to ~20 mg of diazepam. However, purity of street alprazolam is very variable and therefore dosing is unpredictable leading to increased risk of overdose.
- Alprazolam may not be detected on standard urinary drug screens.

Pregabalin and gabapentin
- The gabapentinoids, especially pregabalin, are popular among polydrug users.
- They are abused and can cause dependence.
- They have a high value in the illicit prison economy, so are highly divertible.
- They are used for relaxing and euphoric effects.
- They enhance the effect of opiates.
- In overdose they can cause respiratory depression, reduced conscious level, and death.
- The risk of overdose is greatly increased if used with opiates (prescribed or illicit).
- The effects are not reversed by naloxone.
- It is rarely justifiable to prescribe gabapentinoids in the prison environment.
- They are contraindicated if there is a history of substance misuse.

Intoxication and illicit substance use
- Intoxication is a medical problem and should not simply be treated as a disciplinary issue.

- The effects of intoxicating substances are varied and unpredictable. The peak of symptoms may occur rapidly or develop over several hours.
- An incarcerated person who appears intoxicated should be reviewed by an HCP and managed in a location that allows regular observation. If HCPs are not on site (e.g. some prisons do not have healthcare overnight), the person may need to be taken to hospital for monitoring.
- The prescribed medications should be reviewed, and any sedating medications should be withheld and, if appropriate, stopped.

Drug-induced psychosis

- Substance misuse can cause, or exacerbate, a deterioration in mental health.
- Agitated or psychotic patients should be managed in a quiet, well-lit area.
- If the symptoms persist beyond the acute intoxication, involve the mental health team. The patient may require antipsychotic medications or psychological support.
- Involve the prison substance misuse teams to work on harm reduction and promoting recovery.

Serotonin syndrome

- Serotonin syndrome is drug-induced serotonin toxicity. It can be caused by the overdose of serotonergic medications, or from taking two or more serotonergic drugs at the same time.
- Drugs that are associated with serotonin syndrome include the following:
  - Prescribed medication: antidepressants (selective serotonin reuptake inhibitors (SSRIs), tricyclics, monoamine oxidase inhibitors), opioids (methadone, tramadol), antiemetics (metoclopramide, ondansetron), and triptans.
  - Illicit substances: amphetamine-type substances, Ecstasy, LSD, and other hallucinogens.
- Serotonin syndrome presents with some of, but not always all, the following features:
  - Mental state changes: anxiety, agitation, and delirium.
  - Autonomic hyperactivity: hyperthermia, tachycardia, hypertension, diaphoresis, flushing, vomiting, and diarrhoea.
  - Neuromuscular abnormalities: clonus, hyperreflexia, myoclonus, hypertonicity, and tremor.
- Differential diagnosis includes neuroleptic malignant syndrome, sepsis, malignant hyperthermia, benzodiazepine withdrawal, and alcohol withdrawal.
- Severe cases can lead to stroke, myocardial infarction, rhabdomyolysis, seizures, disseminated intravascular coagulation, renal failure, coma, and death.
- If suspected:
  - Stop all causative drugs.
  - Refer to hospital.
  - Pre-hospital treatment is supportive and may include active cooling, fluid resuscitation, and management of seizures.

QT prolongation
- Many of the medications that are prescribed in prisons can cause QT prolongation (Table 3.2).
- The risk is increased if more than one QT-prolonging medication is used in combination.

Table 3.2 Examples of drugs which prolong QTc

Antipsychotics	Haloperidol, amisulpride, olanzapine, quetiapine
Antidepressants	Citalopram, venlafaxine
Antibiotics	Clarithromycin, ciprofloxacin
Antiarrhythmic	Amiodarone
Opioid agonist therapy	Methadone (at doses >100 mg and at lower doses in combination with other QT-prolonging medications)
Antiemetics	Metoclopramide, domperidone
Illicit substances	Cocaine, amphetamines, probably stimulant PS

For the most up-to-date list of drugs which cause QT prolongation see https://www.crediblemeds.org

QT prolongation is also caused by
- congenital long QT syndrome
- electrolyte abnormalities (decreased potassium, calcium, and magnesium)
- myocardial ischaemia.

When to consider checking electrocardiogram (ECG) measurement of QTc
- Patients arriving in prison on QT-prolonging medications.
- Patients on QT-prolonging medications who have not had an ECG in the last 6 months.
- Prior to starting QT-prolonging medications.
- After commencing QT-prolonging medications.

Reference

1. Advisory Council on the Misuse of Drugs. ACMD advice on 2-benzyl benzimidazole and pi-peridine benzimidazolone opioids. **July 2022**. https://www.gov.uk/government/publications/acmd-advice-on-2-benzyl-benzimidazole-and-piperidine-benzimidazolone-opioids/acmd-advice-on-2-benzyl-benzimidazole-and-piperidine-benzimidazolone-opioids-accessible-version

Further reading

Abdulrahim D, Bowden-Jones O, on behalf of the NEPTUNE Expert Group. Guidance on the man-agement of acute and chronic harms of club drugs and novel psychoactive substances. Novel Psychoactive Treatment UK Network (NEPTUNE); 2015. http://neptune-clinical-guidance.co.uk/wp-content/uploads/2015/03/NEPTUNE-Guidance-March-2015.pdf

Abdulrahim D, Bowden-Jones O, on behalf of the NEPTUNE group. The misuse of synthetic opi-
    oids: harms and clinical management of fentanyl, fentanyl analogues and other novel synthetic
    opioids. Information for clinicians. Novel Psychoactive Treatment UK Network (NEPTUNE);
    2018. http://neptune-clinical-guidance.co.uk/wp-content/uploads/2018/03/The-misuse-
    of-synthetic-opioids.pdf

Medicines and Healthcare products Regulatory Agency. Pregabalin (Lyrica), gabapentin (Neurontin)
    and risk of abuse and dependence: new scheduling requirements from 1 April. April 2019.
    https://www.gov.uk/drug-safety-update/pregabalin-lyrica-gabapentin-neurontin-and-risk-of-
    abuse-and-dependence-new-scheduling-requirements-from-1-april

Medicines and Healthcare products Regulatory Agency. Pregabalin (Lyrica) reports of severe respira-
    tory depression. February 2021. https://www.gov.uk/drug-safety-update/pregabalin-lyrica-repo
    rts-of-severe-respiratory-depression

National Institute for Health and Care Excellence. Chronic pain (primary and secondary) in over
    16s: assessment of all chronic pain and management of chronic primary pain. NICE Guideline
    [NG193]. April 2021. https://www.nice.org.uk/guidance/ng193

National Institute for Health and Care Excellence. Clinical Knowledge Summaries. Epilepsy. Last re-
    vised April 2022. https://cks.nice.org.uk/topics/epilepsy/

National Institute for Health and Care Excellence. Clinical Knowledge Summaries. Poisoning or
    Overdose. Last revised March 2022. https://cks.nice.org.uk/topics/poisoning-or-overdose/

Tracy D, Wood D, Baumeister D. Novel psychoactive substances: types, mechanisms of action, and
    effects. BMJ. 2017;356:i6848.

TripSit wiki contributors. Drug combinations. TripSit wiki; February 2021. https://wiki.tripsit.me/
    wiki/Drug_combinations

Abuse and diversion of medicines

Introduction

Some medications are highly sought after in prison settings where patients may seek to acquire these for personal use/misuse or trading.

Individuals with no intent to divert medication, may also be placed under duress by others and be coerced into giving up their medication under threat or to pay off debts.[1]

It is the responsibility of all prescribers to be aware of and reduce the risk that medication(s) they are prescribing may be causing harm to the individual patient or others.

In the secure environment, additional considerations are needed if high-risk medications are clinically indicated. These include:

- opiate analgesia (including oral and transdermal preparations)
- benzodiazepines
- gabapentinoids
- zopiclone/zolpidem
- sedative antidepressants (mirtazapine, trazodone)
- opioid agonist therapy (methadone, buprenorphine)
- antipsychotics.

In some settings restrictions are in place for emollients/medicines/supplements which include ingredients that can be used in fermentation/distilling to produce hooch.

Emollient containers may be restricted due to the potential to be used as a place to hide contraband items and certain emollients have flammable properties. Confirm local pharmacy protocols before prescribing.

Safer prescribing principles

- Confirm clinical diagnosis and indication in line with relevant guidance before initiating and prescribing.[2]
- Use lower-risk medication as first and second line where possible.
- Review medications for all new patients and consider titrating down to lowest effective dose or switching to safer alternatives.
- High-risk medicines should be prescribed as 'Not in possession' (NIP) and consumption of every dose supervised where possible. When this is not achievable, agree a protocol with operational staff for regular in-cell medication checks to ensure the expected number of tablets is in possession.
- Record intended length of prescription for short-term treatment episodes to prevent these being continued without clinical review.

Always work within an MDT framework. Complex prescribing decisions benefit from an MDT approach, with the input of colleagues from physical health (including physiotherapy), mental health, and substance misuse teams.

Use a patient contract to confirm patient responsibilities

- To take medicines as prescribed.
- To comply with supervision requirements.
- Not to use illicit substances.
- Not to conceal or divert medication.
- To attend appointments for medication reviews.

Monitoring of patients prescribed high-risk medication
- Regular face-to-face review of clinical need (e.g. every 12 weeks).[3]
- After any incident of suspected concealment of medication or intoxication, review in an MDT discussion.
- Review any patient where staff are concerned regarding bullying or vulnerability. Ensure this consultation takes place in a confidential setting away from the wing, ideally face to face or utilizing telemedicine solutions.
- Use near-patient urine testing routinely and/or send away urine samples for toxicology when necessary to monitor for the use of illicit substances and to confirm the presence of the prescribed medication. Consider random checks to confirm compliance (e.g. every 8–12 weeks).

Steps to avoid diversion
- Careful supervision of consumption at the medication hatch. This is a joint responsibility with dispensing staff supported by supervision by the prison staff to maintain the safety of the medication queue and prevent the diversion or concealment of medication.
- Patients found to be diverting or concealing medication may be placed on report by the officer and/or dispensing staff and an incident report will usually be raised.
- Using liquid or dispersible forms can offer reduction in the potential for diversion. However, the cost of these preparations can be prohibitive. Confirm with pharmacist which medications can be dissolved, crushed, or opened but beware that this will likely render them off licence.
- Ensure dispensing policy includes the consumption of a cup of water before and after opioid agonist therapy/gabapentinoids to reduce the risk of concealment in the mouth or regurgitation.

Managing suspected diversion or misuse
Respond to all reports of suspected diversion or intoxication promptly and consistently. Have an agreed MDT response and document this in a local policy.

Use an agreed sequence of actions such as the following:
- Verbal instruction to comply with supervision at the hatch, for example, 'Please open your mouth, lift your tongue, and show me your hands'.
- Verbal intervention/warning if the patient does not comply with the instruction given.
- Standard letters which can be issued by the dispensing team for a first warning and second warning for non-compliance with medication supervision.

If diversion is suspected or the patient is found to be intoxicated
- Offer one warning letter.
- If possible, take a random body fluid sample to confirm the presence of illicit and prescribed substances.
- If behaviour is repeated, begin a safe but rapid non-negotiable reduction.
- Offer the patient the option of booking an appointment to discuss alternative treatments.

If diversion is confirmed/unequivocal

Stop prescription immediately (there is no need to reduce slowly if you have evidence the patient has not been taking the medication).

Medical emergencies

Review patient medications before dispensing/administering following any emergency event, including intoxication or if the patient has any incident relating to illicit substance use, including respiratory depression, collapse, or seizure.

Consider stopping high-risk medication(s) immediately unless doing so would increase the risk of seizures.

See Overdose, p. 352.

Further reading

Clinical Guidelines on Drug Misuse and Dependence Update 2017 Independent Expert Working Group. Drug misuse and dependence: UK guidelines on clinical management [the Orange Book]. Department of Health and Social Care; 2017. https://www.gov.uk/government/publications/drug-misuse-and-dependence-uk-guidelines-on-clinical-management

General Medical Council. Good medical practice. 2013. https://www.gmc-uk.org/ethical-guidance/ethical-guidance-for-doctors/good-medical-practice

Royal College of General Practitioners. Safer prescribing in prisons, 2nd ed. https://elearning.rcgp.org.uk/pluginfile.php/176185/mod_book/chapter/620/RCGP-safer-prescribing-in-prisons-guidance-jan-2019.pdf

Promoting health and well-being in prisons

Stop smoking support

Introduction

April 2018 saw the culmination of a 3-year programme to create an entirely smoke-free prison estate in England and Wales. As part of the programme, healthcare and prison staff were trained to provide stop smoking support which was offered to every person who was incarcerated. The Minimum Service Offer—a de facto service specification—describes the requirements of a prison 'stop smoking' service.[1]

The situation for providing support in prisons was recognized as being different to that in the community for several significant reasons. Firstly, this was a forced abstinence, rather than a choice, so motivations were recognized to be different. Secondly, very many of the cues to smoke and access points for tobacco that people in the community were exposed to would not exist. Finally, electronic cigarettes, which were not initially available in prisons, were becoming more popular and effective in helping people to stop or abstain from smoking.

As the programme rolled out it became apparent that though people's motivations to stop may be different from those in the community, the gold standard of treatments and support remained effective: behavioural support from a trained practitioner, effective nicotine replacement therapy, and access to electronic cigarettes which delivered nicotine consistently.

Management

All people who provide stop smoking support should be trained to a standard equal to that provided by the National Centre for Smoking Cessation and Training.[2] However where a person does not wish to engage in a full course of cessation, stop smoking treatments (nicotine replacement therapy and varenicline) as well as e-cigarettes can be prescribed or recommended.[3]

People assessed as having a high level of nicotine dependence, being at high risk of tobacco-related harm, or who have current medication that may be affected by stopping smoking, or starting smoking cessation treatment, should always be referred to a stop smoking service for treatment.

Dependence

- A person's dependence on nicotine can be assessed by the following shortened Fagerström nicotine dependence scoring system—the higher the score, the greater the level of nicotine dependence:
  - How many cigarettes they smoke per day: 0 points for 10 or less, 1 point for 11–20, 2 points for 21–30, 3 points for 31 or more.
  - How soon after waking they smoke their first cigarette: 3 points for within 5 minutes, 2 points for 6–30 minutes, 1 point for 31–60 minutes, 0 points for after 60 minutes.
- People in the following specific groups may be at high risk of tobacco-related harm:
  - People with mental health problems.
  - People who misuse substances.
  - People with a very long history of tobacco use.
  - People with a smoking-related illness (e.g. lung cancer).

- People with medical conditions exacerbated by smoking:
  - Asthma.
  - Cardiovascular disease.
  - Chronic obstructive pulmonary disease.
  - Type 1 diabetes mellitus.
- Women who are pregnant.
- Most interactions between medicines and smoking are not clinically significant, but there are a small number of medicines that may need increased monitoring or dose adjustment when a person stops smoking.
- Smoking cigarettes (not the nicotine) increases the metabolism of some medicines by stimulating the hepatic enzyme CYP1A2.
- When smoking is stopped, the dose of these drugs may need to be reduced, and the person monitored regularly for adverse effects.[4]

References

1. HM Prison and Probation Service. Prisons minimum service offer for stop smoking service. 2017. https://www.england.nhs.uk/wp-content/uploads/2017/08/smoke-free-mso-national.pdf
2. National Centre for Smoking Cessation and Training. Training resources. http://www.ncsct.co.uk/
3. National Institute for Health and Care Excellence. Clinical Knowledge Summaries. Smoking cessation. Last revised August 2022. https://cks.nice.org.uk/smoking-cessation#!topicsummary
4. Joint Formulary Committee. British National Formulary, 84th ed. London: British Medical Association and Royal Pharmaceutical Society; 2022.

Nutrition and activity in secure settings

Within the prison setting, nutrition and activity have important impacts on people's health and well-being but can receive inadequate attention. The importance of these factors is acknowledged by both the WHO through their statement that '[a]dequate nutrition should be considered one of prisoners' basic human rights' and HMPPS' acknowledgement that 'physical education contributes to the safety, order and control within prisons'.

Nutrition and activity are also of importance to the prison population themselves. As well as the benefits for physical health, imprisoned people highlight a number of wider benefits such as improving self-esteem, reducing stress and depression, forming social bonds, and providing a sense of purpose. Women in particular emphasize the social aspects of activity. It should also be seen as an opportunity for staff to have meaningful interactions with those in their care.

Obesity is a significant issue in prisons. Weight gain following reception into a detention setting is common, particularly among women. Malnutrition is also common and is independent of weight status. Many imprisoned people are likely to enter prison with poor nutritional status, with a high proportion coming from lower socioeconomic groups, whose diets are more likely to be low in micronutrients such as vitamins A–D, iron, iodine, and essential fatty acids, and are more likely to consume high-fat, high-sugar processed foods and snack foods. Added to this, many will have complex health issues, such as alcohol use, associated with nutritional deficiencies.

In prison, mealtimes are the focal point of the day, providing an opportunity for socialization and breaking up the monotony of life inside. They also provide the imprisoned person with some, albeit limited, control in an otherwise controlled environment.

Prisons in England spend around £2 per person per day for catering. The quality and quantity of food provided is highly variable, with examples of good and poor practice seen across the prison estate, with research showing both an excess of calories and salt in many prison catering offers.

Addressing nutrition in prisons

- Improving the nutrition and activity status of people in prison is likely to have many physical, mental, and behavioural health benefits.
- Imprisoned people have limited choice over what, when, where, or how much they eat. It is important therefore that available food not only promotes healthy eating but is also sympathetic to the wants and needs of the people who eat it.
- Specific groups such as children, ethnic minorities, women, and older people will have specific nutritional needs. They may need support and guidance from healthcare teams for these to be adequately met.
- Women's nutritional needs differ considerably from men. Women in prison are particularly interested in food and see it as a health issue. They are unhappy with the diet provided, perceiving it to be a carbohydrate-heavy diet created for imprisoned men rather than women, leading to weight gain and poor nutrition.
- There are some examples of good practice which could be encouraged, where imprisoned people are involved in planning, preparing, and

cooking menus and meals. This develops skills which can be important when they are released.
- The positive impacts of any effective interventions are likely to extend beyond the prison walls, especially for women who are often the primary carers for dependent children; improved nutritional habits developed in prison may influence what is bought and cooked in the family home.
- Health professionals play a key role in supporting the development of improved nutrition for imprisoned people by:
  - promoting healthy eating through personalized advice and more generic educational materials
  - providing advice on the needs of patients with special dietary requirements
  - monitoring the weight of imprisoned people in line with WHO guidance
  - acting as advocates for improvements in the standards of meals in places of detention, for example, through producing health needs assessments.
- Vitamin D supplements are recommended for imprisoned people throughout the year and the supplement is available free of charge through the canteen.

Addressing physical activity in prisons

- The legal minimum provision of physical activity, set out by the Prisons Act 1952, is 1 hour per week for adults and 2 hours per week for children and young people. A specific Prison Service Instruction (PSI 58/2011) focuses on physical education in prisons and effective provision.
- All people in prison should be able to spend 30–60 minutes outside in the open air each day. They should also have access to weekly exercise opportunities. Implementation of these rights is, however, dependent on many factors such as the weather, operational capacity, and security.
- The current legal minimum does not enable imprisoned people to meet the UK government guidelines of at least 150 minutes of moderate-intensity activity a week or 75 minutes of vigorous-intensity activity a week.
- Health professionals have a key role in supporting physical activity opportunities for imprisoned people by:
  - advising on whether people in prison are fit to exercise or undertake other physical activities
  - ensuring there is a referral procedure agreed between healthcare and physical education that includes rehabilitative and healthy lifestyle referrals—this will enable imprisoned people to have access to remedial physical education activity, where identified
  - supporting people in prison to identify and utilize opportunities to exercise, such as signposting to suitable resources and groups
  - advocating for improvements in the provision of opportunities for physical activity within the prison to meet the needs of all imprisoned people.

Reference

1. Ministry of Justice. Physical education (PE) for prisoners: PSI 58/2011. 2011. https://www.gov.uk/government/publications/physical-education-for-prisoners-psi-582011

Further reading

Douglas N, Plugge E, Fitzpatrick R. The impact of imprisonment on health—what do women prisoners say? J Epidemiol Community Health. 2009;63(9):749–754.

Herbert K, Plugge E, Foster C, et al. A systematic review of the prevalence of risk factors for noncommunicable diseases in worldwide prison populations. Lancet. 2012;379(9830):1975–1982.

Nelson M, Erens B, Bates B, et al. (eds). Low Income Diet and Nutrition Survey. London: HM Stationary Office; 2007.

Plugge E, Neale J, Dawes H, et al. Drug using offenders' beliefs and preferences about physical activity: implications for future interventions. Int J Prisoner Health. 2011;7(1):18–27.

Smoyer AB, Kjær Minke L. Food systems in correctional settings: a literature review and case study. 2015. WHO Regional Office for Europe. https://apps.who.int/iris/handle/10665/326323

WHO Europe. 2022. Addressing the noncommunicable disease (NCD) burden in prisons in the WHO European Region: Interventions and policy options.

Sexually transmitted infections

Introduction

There tends to be a higher incidence of STIs and BBVs in the prison population compared to the non-imprisoned population. The causes of this are likely multifactorial and mirror what is observed among marginalized groups and persons with lower socioeconomic opportunities in the community, including a greater likelihood of experiencing risk factors for acquiring infection, as well as lower access to and uptake of testing and treatment services. It should also be noted that sexual contact, be that consensual, coercive, or transactional, can and does occur within prisons, and carries with it varying degrees of risk for STI and BBV transmission.

People arriving at prison or transferring between prisons should all be offered BBV testing in line with the national opt-out testing policy, and assessed for risk of STIs and have access to specialist treatment.

The current national prison reception and second screening templates do not screen for sexual health concerns, so it may be appropriate to amend local templates to ensure people in prison are correctly screened and signposted to sexual health services when clinically appropriate.

Screening

Most patients with STIs have no symptoms so it is important to offer well-informed screening to all. British Association for Sexual Health and HIV guidance advises all symptomatic patients should be offered an appointment in a sexual health clinic within 48 hours of contact (further information is available at http://www.bashhguidelines.org).

The second-stage health assessment appointment is the best time to offer STI and BBV screening if there is good attendance and the following should be considered:

- All asymptomatic female patients should be offered screening with self-take nucleic acid amplification test (NAAT) swabs for *Chlamydia trachomatis* (CT) and *Neisseria gonorrhoeae* (GC) and self-take microscopy, culture, and sensitivity (MCS) swab for *Trichomonas vaginalis* (TV)/bacterial vaginosis (BV)/*Candida*. These should be done 2 weeks after last sexual contact.
- Any symptomatic female patient or asymptomatic female who has anal or oral sex should be seen by the sexual health clinic and screened with vulvovaginal NAATs for CT/GC and post-fornix MCS for TV/BV/*Candida*. An endocervical MCS swab should be done for GC sensitivities if suspicious of GC. Other orifices used should have GC/CT NAAT screening done. Swabs should be repeated 2 weeks after last sexual contact.
- All asymptomatic male patients should be offered screening with first-pass urine for GC/CT. Again, this should be done 2 weeks after last sexual contact.
- Any symptomatic male patients or men who have sex with men (MSM) should be seen by the sexual health clinic to have NAATs to screen for GC/CT as first-pass urine and anal and pharyngeal swabs if those sites

have been used. A urethral MCS should be done if urethral discharge is present.

- All female and male patients should be offered hepatitis B/C and HIV testing, and screened for syphilis at this appointment. If tested, these should be repeated within the following window periods: hepatitis B/C, syphilis—3 months; HIV—1 month.

There should be a low threshold for bringing incarcerated people into the clinic to be examined. Chaotic lifestyles in the community due to drugs/ alcohol and poor mental health of people in prison mean symptoms go under-reported and undertreated. This puts them at increased risk of complications.

Clinical features

- Vaginal/penile discharge.
- Pelvic pain.
- Intermenstrual bleeding.
- Postcoital bleeding.
- Genital ulcers or lumps.
- Deep dyspareunia.
- Dysuria.
- Testicular pain.

Examination

For symptomatic patients:
- External genitalia: lumps, ulcers, inguinal lymph nodes, visible discharge, female genital mutilation, structural abnormalities.
- Speculum: cervical abnormalities, discharge, vaginal wall abnormalities.
- Other sites: for example, perianal or any sites for peripheral manifestations of STIs.

Prevention

As in the community, people in prison require access to devices that reduce the risk of STI and BBV transmission. This includes condoms, dental dams, and lubricants. The distribution and disposal plans for these products will need risk assessing and agreeing with operational colleagues in prisons.

Appropriate contraception should be offered to people at the time of release from prison, as well as signposting to local community sexual health services.

Treatment

Treatment regimens for STIs are generally low risk in overdose and having the medication in possession can encourage compliance and should be encouraged where safe to do so. See Table 4.1.

Table 4.1 Treatment for STIs in the prison setting

Infection	Recommended regimen	Pregnancy risk	Test of cure	Partner notification
Chlamydia and contact	First line: doxycycline 100 mg BD for 7 days Alternate or if compliance concerns: azithromycin 1 g stat follow by 500 mg OD for 2 days *Rectal CT* Female: doxycycline 100 mg BD 7 days MSM: doxycycline 100 mg BD for 14 days while awaiting LGV results	Azithromycin 1 g stat followed by 500 mg OD for 2 days	Only if pregnant or for rectal CT 3 weeks after treatment completed	Yes
Non-specific urethritis and contact	First line: doxycycline 100 mg BD for 7 days Alternate or if compliance concerns: azithromycin 1 g stat follow by 500 mg OD for 2 days		No	Yes
Gonorrhoea and contact: ensure MCS swab have been sent prior to treatment due to the increasing prevalence of drug-resistant GC	Ceftriaxone 1 g IM stat unless sensitivities known and is susceptible to ciprofloxacin then give 500 mg stat orally	Ceftriaxone 1 g stat IM	2 weeks post treatment	Yes. Empirical treatment only for those presenting with 14 days of exposure

Pelvic inflammatory disease: if suspected at first presentation this should be treated immediately. Symptoms: pelvic pain, cervical excitation, adnexal tenderness, bloating, fevers	Doxycycline 100 mg BD for 14 days, plus ceftriaxone 1 g intramuscularly stat, plus metronidazole 400 mg BD for 5–14 days	Refer urgently for specialist treatment	Dependent on swab	Yes
TV: unpublished studies show particularly high prevalence of this in female prisons, presumably due to the high number of sex workers treated	Metronidazole 400 mg BD for 5 days If compliance concerns can use metronidazole 2 g stat If persistent: metronidazole 400 mg BD for 7 days	Metronidazole 400 mg BD for 5 days	Only if symptomatic following treatment	Yes
Genital herpes	Primary outbreak: aciclovir 400 mg TDS for 5 days, lidocaine gel or Diprobase ointment Recurrence: low threshold for in-possession aciclovir course in prison to enable prompt treatment	Discuss with consultant	No	No
Genital warts	Cryotherapy if available; the Histofreezer is a small portable cryotherapy system which can be used without any special storage requirements Podophyllotoxin BD for 3 days a week for up to 4 weeks Imiquimod 5% cream, 3 times weekly for up to 16 weeks		Treatment not always warranted Cryotherapy is safer method	No

(Continued)

Table 4.1 (Contd.)

		Review for resolution of symptoms	
Syphilis	Refer to local genitourinary clinic on diagnosis		Yes
Epididymo-orchitis	Doxycycline 100 mg BD for 14 days	Yes	Yes
Prostatitis	Doxycycline 100 mg BD for 28 days	No	No

BD, twice daily; LGV, lymphogranuloma venereum; OD, once daily; stat, immediately; TDS, three times daily.

Further reading

Fifer H, Saunders J, Soni S, et al. 2018 UK national guideline for the management of infection with Neisseria gonorrhoeae. Int J STD AIDS. 2020;31(1):4–15.

National Institute for Health and Care Excellence. Physical health of people in prisons. NICE guideline [NG57]. November 2016. https://www.nice.org.uk/guidance/ng57

Nwokolo NC, Dragovic B, Patel S, et al. 2015 UK national guideline for the management of infection with Chlamydia trachomatis. Int J STD AIDS. 2016;27(4):251–267. [See also Update 26 September 2018: http://www.bashhguidelines.org/current-guidelines/urethritis-and-cervicitis/chlamydia-2015/?show=1220]

Public Health England. Improving testing rates for blood-borne viruses in prisons and other secure settings. May 2014. https://www.gov.uk/government/publications/improving-testing-rates-for-blood-borne-viruses-in-prisons-and-other-secure-settings

Vaccination programmes in prisons

Vaccination is an important factor in reducing the burden of infectious diseases. Many people enter prison having never received their childhood vaccinations or vaccinations appropriate for them as an adult. People in custody should be offered the same opportunities for immunization as those residing in the community.

Immunization, governance, and training

- Prison vaccination programmes should follow the UK vaccination schedule for adults.
- Staff should be familiar with national and local policies and procedures for safe storage, handling, distribution, and disposal of vaccines.
- For the administration of each vaccination an authorized Patient Group Direction (PGD) or Patient Specific Direction (PSD) should be in place.
- Before running a vaccination programme, staff must have access to locally provided training in immunization and vaccination and be fully competent to plan, schedule, and administer vaccinations as well as to deal with any adverse events.
- Prison staff escorting people to healthcare appointments should be informed of the importance of attendance and given tools to encourage and facilitate vaccination uptake.
- Identifying a lead immunization nurse can assist in promoting and running an effective vaccination programme.

Administration

- All people in prison should be asked about their vaccination history upon prison reception.
- Every effort should be made to communicate and discuss the importance of vaccination and encourage people to attend vaccination appointments. Utilize communication methods such as digital or paper noticeboards, leaflets, and healthcare champions.
- Prior to vaccination it is important to determine the patient's immunization history through questioning and looking at the individual's electronic record.
- Informed consent must be obtained prior to administering a vaccine.
- Following administration, the vaccination must be recorded on the individual's electronic record.
- People in prison are at increased risk of hepatitis B because of the increased prevalence of risky behaviours in this group such as intravenous drug use. Hepatitis B vaccination is recommended and should be offered to all people in prison upon reception. A very rapid schedule should be used with the three doses administered at 0, 7, and 21 days. A fourth dose is recommended 12 months after the first dose to provide longer-term protection.

Information and uncertain vaccination status

Prison offers an opportunity for patients to receive or catch up on childhood and adult immunizations that have been missed.

- Prior to administering any vaccination, a full immunization history should be taken and the individual electronic records checked.
- Access to the 'Green Book'[1] online will ensure up-to-date information is accessed.
- If the patient is unsure about their vaccination history, attempt to access the patient's primary care record or contact the Child Health Office to obtain the history.
- If the immunization history remains unknown, an incomplete or uncertain immunization can be accessed through the UK Health Security Agency website (https://www.gov.uk/government/collections/immunisation).

Encouraging vaccination

- Having an effective recall system in place can ensure patients who are due their vaccinations or who fail to attend their appointment can be identified and contacted. Utilize recall facilities such as flags on patient digital records or registers of vaccine uptake/decline to keep track of patients.
- Offering immunization opportunistically can increase the uptake and ensure patients are offered vaccinations at every healthcare opportunity and optimize the number of vaccines administered.
- Offer vaccines on wing areas to increase uptake, maintaining the cold chain by transporting in cool boxes. Refer to the 'Green Book'[1] for further details on transport and storage of vaccines.

Reference

1. UK Health Security Agency. Immunisation against infectious disease (the Green Book). 2013, last updated 27 November 2020. https://www.gov.uk/government/collections/immunisation-against-infectious-disease-the-green-book

Further reading

UK Health Security Agency. Immunisation. 2013, last updated 30 November 2022. https://www.gov.uk/government/collections/immunisation

UK Health Security Agency. Vaccination of individuals with uncertain or incomplete immunisation status. 2013, last updated 17 March 2022. https://www.gov.uk/government/publications/vaccination-of-individuals-with-uncertain-or-incomplete-immunisation-status

Oral health

Introduction

Oral health is multifaceted and includes the ability to speak, smile, smell, taste, touch, chew, swallow, and convey a range of emotions through facial expressions with confidence and without pain, discomfort, and disease of the craniofacial complex.[1]

Dental surveys of people in prisons in the UK have shown that they are more likely to have experienced oral diseases and have higher levels of untreated oral diseases than the general population.[2] They are also less likely to have visited a dentist especially prior to imprisonment due to service availability and affordability.

Risk factors for poor oral health include poor diet, increased use of alcohol, smoking, and recreational drugs. There may also be differing attitudes and values towards oral health.

Poor oral health can lead not just to pain and infection but also to nutritional compromise and negative impacts upon self-esteem and general health.[3]

The most common oral diseases are dental caries (tooth decay) and periodontal (gum) disease. Mouth cancer is more common in people who smoke, use recreational drugs, and drink alcohol and is therefore likely to be more common in the prison population.

Dental caries and periodontal disease are largely preventable. Dental caries can be prevented by restricting the amount and frequency of consumption of added sugars and optimizing the availability of fluoride in the mouth. Periodontal disease can be prevented by regular removal of dental plaque through tooth brushing. Mouth cancer risks can be reduced by not using tobacco products and keeping alcohol consumption in line with national guidance.[4]

Clinical features of mouth diseases

- Toothache.
- Facial pain.
- Orofacial swelling.
- Raised temperature if infection with systemic effects.
- Fractured teeth.
- Mobile teeth.
- Ulceration.
- Lesions/lumps in the oral cavity including non-healing ulcers.

Investigations

- Radiographs: undertaken by a dentist within the prison setting.
- Blood tests: undertaken by the healthcare team in the prison clinic.
- Biopsy:
  - Can be done on referral to secondary care, or if facilities allow oral surgeons can visit the prison.
  - Ensure to discuss logistics of getting sharp instruments into the prison, and arranging safe and prompt transport of samples back to hospital, with operational staff.
  - Consider referring a non-healing ulcer.

Management

On entry to a secure setting, all incarcerated people should have an assessment of oral health status with triage and referral of those with urgent dental needs. At that dental screening visit, information on prison dental services and how to access these should be provided, as well as information on self-care to promote oral health.

- People with any clinical features of mouth disease should be referred to the dental team.
- All people in prison should have access to a good-quality toothbrush and fluoride toothpaste. Interdental cleaning aids may also be available through the prison canteen list.
- Prescribed medications should be sugar free, particularly methadone.
- Upon discharge, prison leavers should be informed of any ongoing care needs and how to access dental care in the community.

Oral health improvement in prison

As the risk factors for oral diseases are common to other chronic diseases and conditions, oral health should be considered as part of general health improvement programmes in the prison.

- Encourage the kitchen/catering staff to ensure food served in the prison is in line with the 'Eatwell Guide'.[4]
- Provide smoking and tobacco cessation advice to those needing support.
- Incorporate oral health messages within general health promotion.
- Oral health kits should be available in the canteen including toothbrush and fluoride toothpaste.
- The canteen list should include information about the sugar content of products and sugar-free alternative products should be available.

Key messages for self-care

As most oral diseases are preventable, it is important that people in prison are supported to improve and maintain good levels of oral self-care. This includes those who do not have any of their own teeth but who may have soft tissue pathology.

The following messages to support good oral health can be embedded into general health promotion materials and advice. The messages can be given by all prison staff, healthcare staff, and representatives of people in prison:

- Brush your teeth at least twice a day with fluoride toothpaste (1350–1500 parts per million fluoride).
- Brush last thing at night and at least one other time during the day.
- Spit toothpaste out after brushing but do not rinse it away with water or mouthwash as the fluoride is then rinsed away.
- Reduce how much and how often you have food and drinks that have sugar in them because the sugar causes tooth decay. Take extra care not to have sugary food and drinks just before you go to sleep.
- See the prison dentist regularly for check-ups even if you have no teeth or think you have no problems in your mouth. The dentist can help to keep your mouth, teeth, and gums in good health.

It is important to recognize that some people may have particular difficulty in caring for their own oral health, for example, some people with impairments and disabilities and some of the neurodiverse group. These people will need to have oral care as part of their daily care plan to ensure they receive good mouth care every day.

References

1. Glick M, Williams DM, Kleinman DV, et al. A new definition for oral health developed by the FDI World Dental Federation opens the door to a universal definition of oral health. Br Dent J. 2016;221(12):792–793.
2. Heidari E, Dickinson C, Newton T. Oral health of adult prisoners and factors that impact on oral health. Br Dent J. 2014;217(2):69–71.
3. Chapple ILC, Bouchard P, Cagetti MG, et al. Interaction of lifestyle, behaviour or systemic diseases with dental caries and periodontal diseases: consensus report of group 2 of the joint EFP/ORCA workshop on the boundaries between caries and periodontal diseases. J Clin Periodontol. 2017;44(Suppl 18):S39–S51.
4. Department of Health and Social Care. Delivering better oral health: an evidence-based toolkit for prevention. 2012. https://www.gov.uk/government/publications/delivering-better-oral-health-an-evidence-based-toolkit-for-prevention

Gender dysphoria

Introduction

Gender dysphoria describes the distress which arises due to a mismatch between a person's biological sex and their gender identity. It is a uniquely distressing condition with up to 50% of people with gender dysphoria having suicidal ideation or attempting suicide. This coupled with the prison environment can make them an exceedingly vulnerable population.

People experiencing gender dysphoria and those identifying as transgender are entitled to treatment in a non-discriminatory, respectful, and humane manner, in line with the principles of a human rights-based approach to care, and equivalence of healthcare for people in prison.

The key to looking after a patient presenting with gender dysphoria is providing a safe space to explore their thoughts and feelings about gender.

Terminology

- Transman: a transgender individual who identifies as a man.
- Transwoman: a transgender individual who identifies as a woman.
- Cisgender: refers to an individual whose gender identity matches their birth sex.
- Genderfluid: refers to an individual who has fluctuating gender identity, including being agendered or gender neutral.
- Non-binary: refers to a gender identity which is not fixed as male or female.

Ask what pronouns a person prefers; this can be added as an alert on SystmOne (or local patient record system).

Legal and prison aspects

Equality Act 2010

The Equality Act 2010 protects transsexual people (those who have the protected characteristic of gender reassignment) from discrimination and harassment in various areas, such as work or the provision of goods and services.

Gender Recognition Act 2004

- Under the Gender Recognition Act of 2004, transsexual men and women can:
  - apply for and obtain a gender recognition certificate to acknowledge their gender identity
  - get a new birth certificate, driving licence, and passport in their acquired gender
  - marry in their new gender.

The application is completed in conjunction with a gender identity clinic (GIC) and does not require full surgical transition to have taken place.

Prison-specific issues

- In some situations there may be potential secondary gain in prison such as being offered a single cell. This should not, however, bias any assessments or interventions that would be appropriate for patients. The history of gender dysphoria should be assessed as would any other medical condition.
- Healthcare staff may be the safest and most accessible route for this patient group to report complaints or concerns over safety without fear of retaliation.
- Clinicians should have a low threshold for referral to a GIC but should seek to include information regarding the length of sentence, whether there was an 'Imprisonment for Public Protection' sentence, and, if possible, information regarding offending history as this can be very relevant for risk assessment and psychological assessment at the GIC.
- People who are placed on 'basic' as a disciplinary measure should not have items they use to maintain their gender identity removed from them.
- Choice of estate: generally, this will be in line with legal sex (birth certificate) or affirmed gender (gender recognition certificate). A MDT meeting can be used to decide a person's location in other cases, especially where there are complexities such as risks due to the offending history.

Initial appointments

(For practical reasons this is often best achieved over more than one appointment.)

- Explore gender dysphoria history (thoughts and feelings, discussions they have had with friends and family, and how they would like to proceed).
- Concurrent mental health issues (may need stabilization first) including substance misuse and risk.
- Relevant medical history (include smoking status).
- Social history: discussion with families/ partners.
- Offer up-to-date health screening: body mass index (BMI) and blood pressure (BP); cervical screening for transmen who still have a uterus.
- Health promotion: smoking cessation and sexual health screening as appropriate.
- Relevant family history: especially venous thrombosis, cardiovascular disease, and cancer.
- Offer initial bloods: full blood count (FBC), urea and electrolytes (U&E), liver function tests (LFTs) and gamma glutamyl transferase, lipids, fasting glucose/glycated haemoglobin (HbA1c), thyroid function tests (TFTs), sex hormone-binding globulin, follicle-stimulating hormone, luteinizing hormone, vitamin D, prolactin, testosterone, dihydrotestosterone, and oestradiol.

Referrals

There are seven centres in the UK. The average wait time is between 18 and 24 months, at the time of writing.

Prior to consideration of hormonal treatment, people are seen by two psychologists/psychiatrists and may be offered a session of psychotherapy. Clinics offer *triadic therapy*—real-life experience, hormonal therapy of desired gender, and genital reconstruction surgery—but the decision about how far a patient may progress through this is their own. The ultimate aim is to relieve distress and help a person feel comfortable with their body.

Prescribing

The long wait for GIC appointments can leave GPs under pressure to prescribe hormonal therapy. The General Medical Council is clear in its position on this—GPs must prescribe within the scope of their knowledge and competency. The following exceptional circumstances are noted where a bridging script may be considered:

- The patient is already using hormones from an unregulated source.
- The bridging prescriptions are intended to mitigate risk of self-harm or suicide.
- The GP has sought the advice of a gender specialist and prescribed the lowest acceptable dose.

It is important to counsel patients on risks of self-medication. A key point is that fertility is impaired on commencing hormones. Gamete storage should be discussed and encouraged to keep future reproductive choices open.

Hormonal treatments are low risk for trading and abuse and this should be reflected in individual security assessments regarding in-possession medication.

Ongoing care and management

Once a patient has been seen in the GIC, the primary care team should receive clear instructions on prescribing and monitoring. As the intricacies of monitoring are beyond the scope of standard general practice, it is recommended to discuss any concerning results with the GIC. The treatment plan will be individualized but a few general rules are shown below.

Responsibilities of the primary care team

- Ongoing prescribing of endocrine therapy.
- Organizing blood and other diagnostic tests as recommended by the specialist.
- Monitoring tests (should be specified by the specialist).
- Annual medication review.
- Ongoing screening/health promotion/usual GP care.

Specific items of note

- For transmen: testosterone levels of 25–30 nmol/L post injection and 8–12 nmol/L pre injection (low normal male range). Common side effects include polycythaemia, hyperlipidaemia, and exacerbation of certain psychiatric disorders (mania and psychosis).
- For transwomen: oestrogen levels of 350–600 pmol/L (normal female follicular range). Side effects: deep vein thrombosis risk is 2.6% (20× that of people not on treatment), mostly during first 2 years. Raised prolactin in 10–14%. Deranged LFTs—usually mild and just require monitoring. Hypertriglyceridemia, hypertension. Breast cancer—likely

not a particularly increased incidence (there have been only four case reports).
- Name changes: these do not require a gender recognition certificate. There needs to be a written request with a discussion of implications if gender also changes, that is, if pre-treatment they will no longer be called to the correct sex-specific screening programmes (e.g. cervical screening, prostate screening) and blood result ranges may be incorrect. Requests sent to: PCSE.enquiries@nhs.net.

Take-away message

Prison healthcare services can provide important holistic care for patients experiencing gender dysphoria and other gender identity concerns. Life expectancy for patients post transition is the same as the general population and an improvement in mental health conditions is frequently seen.

References

Gender Identity and Research Education Society. Terminology. n.d. http://www.gires.org.uk/terminology

General Medical Council. Trans healthcare and bridging prescriptions. n.d. https://www.gmc-uk.org/ethical-guidance/ethical-hub/trans-healthcare#mental-health-and-bridging-prescriptions

Ministry of Justice. National Offender Management Service Annual offender equalities report: 2016/17. Ministry of Justice Statistics Bulletin. 30 November 2017. https://assets.publishing.service.gov.uk/government/uploads/system/uploads/attachment_data/file/663390/noms-offender-equalities-annual-report-2016-2017.pdf

Ministry of Justice. Review on the care and management of transgender offenders. November 2016. https://assets.publishing.service.gov.uk/government/uploads/system/uploads/attachment_data/file/566828/transgender-review-findings-web.PDF

NHS England. Interim gender dysphoria protocol and service guideline 2013/14. 2013. https://www.england.nhs.uk/wp-content/uploads/2013/10/int-gend-proto.pdf.

NHS UK. Gender dysphoria services: a guide for general practitioners and other healthcare staff. 2012. https://www.nhs.uk/Livewell/Transhealth/Documents/gender-dysphoria-guide-for-gps-and-other-health-care-staff.pdf

Royal College of General Practice. Learning module on gender variance. https://elearning.rcgp.org.uk/course/view.php?id=341

Royal College of General Practice. Guidelines for the care of trans patients in primary care. 2017. http://transiness.co.uk/wp-content/uploads/2013/12/GP-trans-care-guidelines.pdf

United Nations Office on Drugs and Crime. Technical brief: transgender people and HIV in prisons and other closed settings. November 2022. https://www.unodc.org/documents/hiv-aids/publications/Prisons_and_other_closed_settings/22-03088_Transgender_HIV_E_ebook.pdf

World Professional Association of Transgender Health (WPATH). Standards of care for the health of transgender and gender diverse people, version 8. 2022. https://www.tandfonline.com/doi/pdf/10.1080/26895269.2022.2100644

Chapter 5

Conducting consultations

Reception and first night screening

Introduction

- Systematic first night screening is an essential part of delivering safe, effective healthcare in prison.
- Each person newly arriving in prison from police custody, court, or from another secure setting (prison transfer or secure hospital remission) must have a health assessment (usually in reception) in order to identify any:
  - immediate medical needs, including essential medication[1]
  - risks to safety
  - long-term conditions requiring coordinated care planning and management.
- Assessment findings must be clearly documented and followed up with effective communication within the healthcare team and with any necessary external agencies (e.g. community pharmacy and community GP practice) to ensure:
  - safe first night prescribing
  - suitable location for any required monitoring
  - continuity and coordination of care.
- Communication with prison staff will be essential to ensure safe location and monitoring of the patient.
- People returning from a day at court or from hospital should also be seen on arrival in reception, in order to identify and manage any new or emerging issues such as distress due to sentencing, new diagnosis, or treatments that may have been commenced.

First night reception assessment

- Log all new arrivals on reception ledger for systematic screening.
- Provide any required support to facilitate the assessment (e.g. translation service).
- Record patient consent. Record personal details and match to national NHS demographics database and prison number, where possible.
- A qualified nurse or healthcare assistant under the supervision of a nurse must complete the health assessment. Screening questions should cover physical and mental health conditions, risk of self-harm/suicide, risk of keeping medicines in possession, use of alcohol and other substances, problematic use of prescribed medicines, injuries in few days prior to prison, recent and upcoming hospital appointments, mobility aids, social care needs, and special medical diet.
- Infectious disease screening must be done on the first night, including tuberculosis (TB) and COVID-19. If suspected: patient must be isolated, prison team informed, investigations (chest X-ray, sputum for TB, swab for COVID) arranged, follow-up appointments booked, contact tracing initiated, and public health team informed. Refer to local hospital team (TB).
- Identify other relevant health/risk information by checking, for example, Summary Care Record additional information, the patient's electronic health record (EHR) (SystmOne), and collateral information provided by liaison and diversion services, court, or police custody.

- Gather information on prescribed and over-the-counter medicines (patient report, medicines brought in, patient care summary, past medications prescribed in prison). Use collateral sources (e.g. community pharmacy, hospital discharge letter, and community GP summary) to confirm and document specific current medication formulation (e.g. capsule/tablet), administration frequency, and doses in order to minimize disruption to treatment.
- Examine patient: record weight, height, BMI; pulse, BP, respiratory rate, oxygen saturations; temperature. Document injuries on body map. Describe wounds, including dimensions. Ask mental health screening questions, include self-harm/suicidal thoughts/plans. Observe and record the general demeanour, including any agitation, sedation, or alteration in conscious level.
- Clearly document all responses on the patient's EHR. Information within medical records may be used as evidence in coroners' or legal cases.

Immediate first night care and follow-up

- Physical health: refer to GP/advanced nurse practitioner (ANP) in reception if immediate action required (e.g. medicine prescription, suspected infectious disease). Add to GP/ANP or specialist nurse waiting list/book appointment for further, more comprehensive, follow-up of complex or long-term conditions. Advise patient that:
  - a full medicines reconciliation process will be carried out before second assessment in order to confirm details of current prescriptions
  - a medicines review will be planned to assess ongoing clinical need for prescribed medicines.
- Pregnancy: ask women about pregnancy and offer testing. Refer to GP and midwife if pregnant.
- Mental health or possible long sentence: refer to mental health team.
- Learning disabilities, neurodevelopmental disorders: refer to appropriate healthcare team and liaise with prison disability/diversity lead to ensure teams are made aware and further assessments arranged.
- Immediate risk of self-harm/suicide: open ACCT, inform prison team, ensure safe location/observation while in reception area and on transfer to wing, and administer any prescribed medicines under supervision.
- Suspected drug and/or alcohol misuse: urine drug screen (UDS) and refer to substance misuse nurse and GP/ANP in reception for further detailed assessment.
- Suspected drugs concealment: if secreted drugs are suspected on body scanning, there is potential for fatal leaking of packages. A full clinical assessment (including NEWS2) should be done but an internal examination must *not* be done. An emergency escort to a hospital accident and emergency (A&E) department must be recommended. Further investigation will be required at hospital and the patient will need close monitoring. If the patient declines to go to hospital, they should be asked to sign a disclaimer and arrangements made for safe location and monitoring in the prison.

- Physical disabilities: liaise with the prison to ensure a suitable location (e.g. ground floor, shower accessible) and provision of mobility aids (e.g. frame taken to cell); further assessments should be arranged.
- Injuries: perform any essential treatment such as a dressing; refer to GP/ANP for analgesia, antibiotics, etc. If severe, refer to hospital (senior nurse/manager to liaise with prison to arrange escort, senior clinician to liaise with hospital). Add to clinic ledger for follow-up (e.g. triage nurse for removal of sutures/dressing). If outpatient follow-up planned, task/email administration (see below).
- Outstanding secondary care appointments: task/email administration team to make contact with hospital and arrange escort.
- Other medical equipment such as glasses, hearing aid, or a continuous positive airway pressure machine should be taken to the cell.
- Special medical diet: send letter to kitchen. NB: patients may request diets that are not 'medical' and should be advised that catering team (not HCPs) manage such requests.

First night prescribing

- First night prescribing must be based on face-to-face patient assessment by a qualified HCP.
- Prescribers must record confirmed and immediately necessary prescriptions on the patient's EHR. They must either assess the patient directly (in person or via secure approved video call) or be satisfied with a face-to-face screening assessment by a qualified nurse.
- Where a remote prescriber requires clarification about history or examination details, there must be a two-way conversation between the remote and the on-site clinician using a video call, telephone call, or secure messaging. Alternatively, a joint remote consultation (video/telephone call) should be arranged between the remote clinician, the on-site patient, and the on-site HCP. A patient must never be left alone with IT equipment and national telemedicine protocols and policies must be followed.
- If a patient brings in a supply of medicines, details must be checked for patient name, date dispensed, expected/actual remaining doses, and expiry date before prescribing. In certain circumstances it may be necessary to use the patient's own supply for short periods in order to maintain continuity.
- NICE guidance[1] contains a table of critical medicines that may result in harm if doses are omitted (Table 5.1). If a patient presents without medicines in this category, or if they bring inadequately labelled medicines, interim medication should be prescribed and dispensed from emergency stock, where clinical assessment confirms need.
- Non-controlled drugs: following clinical assessment, where medication is required, a prescription should be written and saved in the patient's EHR (drug, dosing regimen, start date, duration, quantity). A drug administration chart should be generated.
- It is good practice for on-site prescribers to print and sign all prescriptions written on the first night. If a medical prescriber is working remotely, it is legal for on-site nursing staff to administer medicines from stock, provided the electronic prescription is part of a treatment plan documented in the patient's EHR.

- Controlled drugs (CDs): CDs may be prescribed on the first night where face-to-face assessment confirms clinical need, such as treatment of opioid or alcohol withdrawal (methadone, buprenorphine, chlordiazepoxide).
- CDs may also be requested for pain (e.g. tramadol, pregabalin) or attention deficit hyperactivity disorder (ADHD) (e.g. lisdexamfetamine). Before prescribing, confirm current prescription, clinical indication, and evidence of medication adherence. Advise the patient of any side effects, risks of dependence, or potential for misuse in the prison context. Refer for a medication review.
- Prescribing and handling of CDs must meet legislative requirements (Misuse of Drugs Act 1971, Misuse of Drugs Regulations 2001) and any breaches must be reported (local incident reporting system, e.g. Datix, to CD Accountable Officer).

Table 5.1 Critical medicines that may result in harm if doses are omitted

Area	Medicine
Cardiovascular system	Anticoagulants
	Nitrates
Respiratory system	Adrenoceptor agonists
	Antimuscarinic bronchodilators
	Adrenaline for allergic emergencies
Central nervous system	Antiepileptic drugs
	Drugs used in psychoses and related disorders
	Drugs used in parkinsonism and related disorders
	Drugs used to treat substance misuse
Infections	As clinically indicated, such as anti-infectives or antiretrovirals
Endocrine system	Corticosteroids
	Drugs used in diabetes
Obstetrics, gynaecology, and urinary tract disorders	Emergency contraceptives
Malignant disease and immunosuppression	Drugs affecting the immune response
	Sex hormones and hormone agonists in malignant disease—depot preparations
Nutrition and blood	Parenteral vitamins B and C
Eye	Corticosteroids and anti-inflammatory preparations
	Glaucoma treatment
	Local anaesthetics
	Mydriatics and cycloplegics

Source: data from UK Medicines Information, National Patient Safety Agency Rapid Response Report. Reducing harm from omitted and delayed medicines in hospital, revised January 2016.

- All CD prescriptions *must* be printed and signed; a 'wet signature' is required for auditing the CD register and CD reconciliation by the pharmacy team.
- Remote prescribers must print and sign the CD script with 'wet ink' at their remote location, at the time of prescribing, and should then scan the hard copy into the patient's EHR (SystmOne Record Attachments) so that it is immediately visible on the patient record. The hard copy of the prescription should be sent to the prison (recorded delivery) or handed to pharmacy by the prescriber when next in the prison, to be reconciled with the CD register.

Immediate management of substance misuse

- When drug or alcohol problems are identified by screening questions, a UDS should be requested and the patient referred to an Integrated Drug Treatment System (IDTS) nurse and GP/ANP for more detailed first night IDTS assessment, care planning, and prescribing. Ideally the UDS sample should be supervised to ensure it belongs to the patient (e.g. collect in assessment room in the presence of HCP/nurse, while behind a privacy screen).
- Advise the patient that UDS results are required prior to prescribing withdrawal treatment but will not be shared with prison staff.
- Check records to confirm details of any opioids or benzodiazepines prescribed while in police custody.
- Explain, agree, and document initial care plan with the patient on the first night. Include prescribing plan, monitoring and follow-up details, and safety-netting advice (i.e. when to ask for help between planned observations and appointments).
- Only prescribe opiate or benzodiazepine withdrawal drug treatment if all of the following criteria are met: (1) history of regular drug use, (2) presence of drug in UDS, and (3) signs and symptoms of withdrawal (see relevant local policies and the 'Orange Book'[2]). See also First night prescribing, p. 84.
- Without UDS, do not initiate opiate or benzodiazepine withdrawal prescriptions but ensure the patient has regular observation for emerging objective signs of withdrawal. Offer symptomatic relief where appropriate. See also First night prescribing, p. 84.
- If there is a clear history of heavy alcohol use and objective evidence of alcohol withdrawal (using the Clinical Institute Withdrawal Assessment—Alcohol, revised (CIWA-Ar) scale), prescribing to support alcohol withdrawal should be initiated on the first night, even in the absence of a UDS. Further requests for a UDS should be made within the first 24 hours in prison to exclude concurrent drug use.
- Book follow-up review appointments with the substance misuse teams and refer to other agencies as required (e.g. psychosocial team).
- Communicate with prison staff to ensure the patient is located for safe substance misuse monitoring.

Summary

A detailed first night assessment is particularly important for identifying and managing immediate risks within the early days of custody. It is also essential for guiding the frequently complex care needs of patients from the point of arrival in prison.

References

1. National Institute for Health and Care Excellence. Physical health of people in prison. NICE guideline [NG57]. November 2016. https://www.nice.org.uk/guidance/ng57
2. Clinical Guidelines on Drug Misuse and Dependence Update 2017 Independent Expert Working Group. Drug misuse and dependence: UK guidelines on clinical management [the Orange Book]. Department of Health and Social Care; 2017. https://www.gov.uk/government/publications/drug-misuse-and-dependence-uk-guidelines-on-clinical-management

Further reading

National Institute for Health and Care Excellence. Mental health of adults in contact with the criminal justice system. NICE guideline [NG66]. March 2017. https://www.nice.org.uk/guidance/ng66
National Institute for Health and Care Excellence. Preventing suicide in community and custodial settings. NICE guideline [NG105]. September 2018. https://www.nice.org.uk/guidance/ng105

Second-stage health assessment

Introduction

- Reception screening on the first night should identify and meet immediate medical need and risk. Offer a further clinical 'second-stage' assessment within the first week to identify physical and mental health conditions and substance misuse requiring more detailed assessment, to offer screening and vaccination, to answer patient questions, and to provide tailored health and well-being advice.
- If second-stage health assessment, national screening programme, or vaccination opportunities are refused, explain the importance and benefits of them and offer further opportunities for uptake.

Second-stage health assessment (secondary screening)

Review of first night information

- Review information provided at first night screening and check that all planned actions are complete or are being followed up:
  - In-possession risk assessment.
  - Medicines reconciliation and allergy/sensitivity.
  - Community GP/other collateral information received.
  - In-house referrals/appointments booked (e.g. substance misuse, mental health, GP, and dressing clinic).
  - Outpatient hospital appointments followed up.
- Check for any new/unaddressed health concerns and for injuries sustained since arrival.

Identify physical health problems—past and current

- Review medical problem list and first night screening notes. Cross-check with problem list recorded in community GP summary. Confirm current health conditions with patient, to ensure prison medical record is complete and accurate.
- Ask about history of TBI (associated with aggressive behaviour, disinhibition, and criminality, particularly if TBI in childhood/young adult). Document number of episodes of TBI and duration of associated loss of consciousness. Ask if loss of consciousness ever lasted longer than 20 minutes. Ask about memory problems and reduced concentration.
- Ask about family history of medical conditions (e.g. asthma, chronic obstructive pulmonary disease (COPD), diabetes, epilepsy, cardiovascular disease, and cancer).
- Ask about details of medical equipment (e.g. hearing aid, glasses), physical disability, mobility aids (frame, wheelchair), and support required for activities of daily living (ADLs).
- Review observations from the first night (BMI, BP, pulse, respiratory rate, oxygen saturations, and temperature). Complete missing data and repeat abnormal observations. Book follow-up appointment if further observations required.
- Complete examination relevant to current medical conditions (e.g. peak expiratory flow rate and blood glucose). Complete urinalysis for every new patient.

- Confirm with patient and document care plans for each current health condition, including any awaited hospital appointments. If additional information is required (e.g. further hospital letters, investigation results), send task/email to administration team to follow up.
- Refer to GP/ANP/specialist nurse for:
  - further detailed assessment and follow-up of long-term conditions (e.g. diabetes, COPD)
  - assessment/treatment of new problems
  - possible secondary care referral.
- Refer to primary care clinical lead if:
  - broken/missing equipment (e.g. hearing aid, walking stick)
  - support with ADLs/referral for social care assessment
  - release due in less than 1 month (referral to discharge planning team).
- Refer to dentist, optometrist, podiatrist, and physiotherapist if needed.

Identify mental health problems—past and current

- Second-assessment mental health screening may be performed by the primary care team or delegated to mental health colleagues.
- Review problem list, first night screening notes, and community GP summary for documented mental health problems. Confirm these with patient.
- If patient reports diagnosis (unconfirmed), for example, 'bipolar', 'schizophrenia', or 'split personality', ask about contact with community mental health team, key/support worker contact details, and past/recent hospital admissions (voluntary/under section). Gather further collateral information to verify self-reported diagnosis.
- Ask about family history mental health problems (e.g. depression).
- If no mental health diagnosis is recorded or volunteered but a mental health problem is suspected from first night responses, patient presentation (eye contact, speech, behaviour), communication from criminal justice agencies (court liaison/diversion services, police), or the community mental health team, use a context-specific screening tool, suitable for preferred gender (e.g. Correctional Mental Health Screen for Men (CMHS-M) or Women (CMHS-W)) to identify possible mental health problem.
- Also use the CMHS-M/CMHS-W if a person has functional impairment associated with a long-term physical health problem (e.g. multiple sclerosis, chronic pain, or heart failure).
- If more than five 'Yes' answers on the CMHS-M, or more than three on the CMHS-W, or other evidence of a likely mental health problem, refer to the mental health team for a more detailed assessment by appropriately trained professionals.
- Refer to GP if diagnosis of uncomplicated anxiety/depression.
- Refer to mental health team if other mental health diagnosis, dual diagnosis, or if history of community mental health team support (e.g. for severe depression).
- If a learning disability or neurodevelopmental disorder is suspected, refer to learning disability lead nurse/mental health team for further assessment and inform prison disability lead to plan joined-up support and avoid inappropriate disciplinary action.

Review of smoking and substance misuse

- If there is a history of smoking, offer referral to a smoking cessation service.
- Review first night screening notes. Check with the patient if they have any previously undisclosed problems with alcohol, drug use, or misuse of prescription medicines; if so, refer to IDTS team.
- If referred to substance misuse team following first night screening, check that the patient has had further detailed alcohol and substance misuse assessment, regular tailored monitoring (e.g. CIWA-Ar, Clinical Institute Withdrawal Assessment—Benzodiazepine (CIWA-B), Clinical Opiate Withdrawal Scale (COWS)/Subjective Opiate Withdrawal Scale (SOWS)), and that they are happy with the current care plan.
- Refer for tailored harm reduction interventions such as in-cell work, group work, alcohol brief intervention, and substance misuse—naloxone training/overdose prevention.
- Refer to other services if housing or employment support is required.

Sexual health and blood-borne virus screening

- Offer sexual health and BBV screening to all patients, at either first night or second-assessment (depends on local policy). Document refusal and offer further opportunities.
- Document date of last sexual health screen.
- Sexual health: offer chlamydia, gonorrhoea, and syphilis screen.
- If high-risk STI, offer appointment with trained practitioner/refer to sexual health service.[1]
- BBVs: offer hepatitis B/C and HIV testing (dry blood spot test, point-of-care test options preferable). Advise patients that if test is positive, counselling, referral, and treatment will be provided.
- Provide tailored advice/information leaflets on STIs/BBVs.
- Offer barrier contraception. Refer to GP/ANP/midwife for contraception, cervical screening, and pregnancy.

Vaccinations

- Check vaccination status, allergies/adverse reactions, and eligibility:
  - Measles, mumps, and rubella (MMR).
  - Meningitis and septicaemia (MenACWY).
  - Tetanus, diphtheria, and polio (Td/IPV).
  - Influenza, pneumococcus, and pertussis.
  - Shingles (>70 years).
  - Human papillomavirus (HPV).
  - Hepatitis A/B.
  - COVID-19.
- If clinically appropriate, obtain informed consent and offer vaccination during second assessment clinic. Alternatively, add to waiting list/book vaccination clinic slot.

National screening programmes and other health checks

- Check screening status and eligibility.* Document date and result last test. Offer/refer if screening due. Document if declined.

- Bowel: all aged 60–74* years, every 2 years (50–74* years in Scotland; 60–74 years in England, Wales, and Northern Ireland).
- Abdominal aortic aneurysm: males aged 64/65 years (and older, if no previous test).
- Breast: females aged 50–70 years, every 3 years (transwomen taking long-term hormone therapy may be at increased risk of developing breast cancer and should be offered breast screening[2]).
- Cervical: people with a uterus aged 25–64 years, every 3 years (25–49 years) or every 5 years (50–64 years).
- Retinal: diabetes (age 12 years onwards), every year or more often if clinically indicated.
- Offer screening for vascular disease and its risk factors to all eligible* patients. This is an important screening opportunity in prisons for a population with higher morbidity and mortality than community peers and who tend to engage less well with community primary care.
- England: NHS Health Check age 40–74 years every 5 years, if there is no pre-existing coronary heart disease, cardiovascular disease, type 2 diabetes mellitus, chronic kidney disease, or dementia. Scotland: Keep Well 40–64 years, higher deprivation areas only.
- Offer an annual health check if individual has a learning disability.

(* Eligibility varies across the four UK nations.)

Provide tailored advice

- Offer tailored patient advice (which is accessible, e.g. first language/easy read) on:
  - healthy eating/diet and exercise
  - alcohol, drugs of addiction, and smoking
  - sexual health.
- Advise how to contact the healthcare team and request appointments (e.g. GP, dentist, optometrist, and access recovery services).
- Advise on access to health promotion and well-being activities.
- Advise on medicine adherence and consequences of abuse/diversion.

Summary

Second-stage health assessment provides a valuable opportunity to identify previously unrecognized medical problems and risk factors, to confirm the patient has access to appropriate medication following medicines reconciliation, to offer in-house referrals and ensure continuity of access to hospital specialists, to offer screening and vaccination, and to offer harm reduction and health promotion advice.

References

1. British Association for Sexual Health and HIV https://www.bashh.org/guidelines
2. NHS England. NHS population screening: information for trans and non-binary people. January 2023. https://www.gov.uk/government/publications/nhs-population-screening-information-for-transgender-people/nhs-population-screening-information-for-trans-people

Further reading

National Institute for Health and Care Excellence. Mental health of adults in contact with the criminal justice system. NICE guideline [NG66]. March 2017. https://www.nice.org.uk/guidance/ng66
National Institute for Health and Care Excellence. Physical health of people in prison. NICE guideline [NG57]. November 2016. https://www.nice.org.uk/guidance/ng57

Determining risk in consultations

General practice has a high degree of uncertainty and many times clinicians are not aware of the risks involved. There are many unknowns, especially in the secure environment. Managing this area is complex but it can be controlled effectively by ensuring awareness of the potential risks.

Consultations require a risk assessment for each interaction, something that should be done prior to any dialogue. Doctors in the community do this daily with minimal thought; however, secure environments have many of the same risks as day-to-day general practice, with added risks due to the patient population and organizational structures.

A four-step clinical risk process is generally used:
1. Identify risks.
2. Assess frequency and severity of risks.
3. Reduce or eliminate risks with long-term planning.
4. Assess whether risks have been eliminated.

This four-step process can be applied to various aspects of the secure environment:

Practitioner
- Assess own physical and mental health.
- Assess own knowledge base, keeping up to date with guidelines,[1] remaining in contact with other professionals in secure environments (British Medical Association (BMA), RCGP, Royal College of Nursing), and carrying out a serious event analysis/audit when appropriate.
- Knowledge of secure environment protocols in the working environment.
- Review room at beginning of consultation; ensure area clear of unnecessary equipment and that the patient will not be situated between yourself and the door. Be aware of emergency bells/alerts.
- Vaccination status, for example, hepatitis B (as per occupational health guidelines).

Patient
- Ensure the full medical history is available (where possible) as well as information on medications taken.
- Knowledge of history of violence, hostage-taking (particularly involving extremist views, misogyny, and homophobia), mental health disorders, historical medical engagement, and addiction issues.
- Be aware that mental health conditions are much more prevalent in prison settings than in the general population (see Mental health in prisons: overview, p. 176).
- Hepatitis B/C and HIV status (including date of last test, viral load, and/or curative treatment).
- Duration of sentence (as this helps in making decisions on short- and long-term healthcare that can be provided).

Team
- Assess knowledge, experience, and expertise of team members.

- Understaffing or recent changes in staff membership can place extra pressures on the healthcare team as a whole, or on other more experienced staff.

Workload/organization
- Clinicians should be aware of their own workload and expectations. Many errors are made due to demands of a system:
  - Lack of clinical time may lead to rushed consultations, the potential for incorrect diagnosis, or prescribing errors. This may also be of detriment to the doctor–patient relationship and cause friction with poor outcomes.
  - Lack of administrative time may lead to prescribing errors, inadequate record keeping, incorrect clinical decisions, and poor continuity of care.

Communication
- Failure of clear communication with the patient can lead to misunderstanding of diagnosis or treatment and can result in confrontation at a later date (sometimes with an unsuspecting colleague). See Managing expectations, p. 101.
- Failure of clear communication with team members may lead to poor medical care and incorrect medication or support decisions.

Strategies for decreasing risk
Practitioner
- Keep up to date and connect with fellow secure environment colleagues (e.g. RCGP Secure Environments Group and consider joining the BMA listserver through the BMA GP Committee prison representative).
- Attend regular clinical update courses.
- Attend supervision sessions to discuss secure environment activities.

Patient
- Ensure that the patient has/had full health checks on coming into prison/coming from previous prison.
- MDT meetings for any patients living with complicated conditions (consider: doctors, nurses, substance misuse, mental health, physiotherapists, and administrative and prison staff).

Teams
- Regular (weekly or more frequent) team meetings.
- Knowledge of the rota for the working days (understand the skills mix of those working to support the service).
- Organize and attend regular teaching sessions, resuscitation refresher, and so on.

Workload/organization
- Arrive on time and assess workload at start of shift.
- Prioritize as things can change rapidly within the secure environment, and complete urgent tasks/work early.

- Flag any issues that may appear to the administrative team—they can consider adding or changing placement of staff if issues arise and are notified early enough.

Communication
- Regular healthcare team meetings to ensure everyone is clear of direction and any issues are handled in a timely manner. Also allow time to discuss experiences and reflect on difficult situations as needed.
- Regular meetings between healthcare and the prison staff.
- Ensure use of language that the patient will understand, and check that they have understood the diagnosis, treatment, and plans going forward.
- Use Language Line or prison-appointed translator when necessary.

Medication errors, especially when a patient is new to the secure environment, can cause issues due to incorrect, under-, or overprescribing. Initial knowledge of medications and prescribing of critical medicines is important (anticoagulants, antiepileptics, drugs affecting immune response, antibiotics/antiretrovirals, etc.).

It is very important to assess patients properly as they come into the secure environment as well as continual assessment of the systems that are in place.

The consultation itself requires
- engaging with the patient
- understanding the patient's ideas/concerns/expectations
- developing a trust to ensure optimal patient care
- awareness of any triggers that may cause aggressive reactions
- confidence in decision-making and clear communication with the patient and colleagues.

Reference
1. Royal College of General Practitioners. Safer prescribing in prisons, 2nd ed. https://elearning. rcgp.org.uk/pluginfile.php/176185/mod_book/chapter/620/RCGP-safer-prescribing-in-pris ons-guidance-jan-2019.pdf

Further reading
Centre for Mental Health. Pathways to unlocking secure mental health care. 2011, https://www. centreformentalhealth.org.uk/sites/default/files/2018-09/Pathways_to_unlocking_secure_men tal_health_care.pdf

World Health Organization. Patient Safety Curriculum Guide. Topic 6: Understanding and managing clinical risk. In: pp. 162–175. Geneva: World Health Organization; 2011. https://www.who.int/ patientsafety/education/curriculum/who_mc_topic-6.pdf

Managing patient expectations

Understanding and managing patient expectations is one of the most important aspects of providing healthcare in the secure environment. This requires building trust and clear pathways of communication.

Managing patient expectations can be difficult as the doctor and patient may have different or even competing expectations. A previous study showed that medications are prescribed more when a doctor and/or a patient expects these to be prescribed. However, it was only three times more likely when a patient was expecting them, but ten times more likely when a doctor thought a patient expected medication to be prescribed. This suggests that doctors need to manage their own expectations before they can objectively and honestly manage those of a patient.[1]

Another study showed patients overestimate the benefits of intervention and underestimate the risks associated with this. Open and clear discussions on risks and benefits help to develop realistic expectations. The more knowledge and understanding a patient has about treatment options, the better the recovery.[2]

Understanding the options and remaining confident in clinical decision-making can help to ensure a better management of expectations for patients. This leads to trust with a cohort of people who traditionally do not trust easily. Honesty and taking time to explain decisions, (based on best practice and clinical guidelines) may not always coincide with a patient's initial expectations but may well lead to longer-term trust and engagement with new pathways of treatment.

Each patient interaction (and initial impression) can have a knock-on effect on future consultations, even with other patients (due to the enclosed nature of secure environments). If an impression comes out that a clinician does not listen and has their own agenda or that they are happy to prescribe sleeping tablets easily, this can translate to the secure environment community with patients discussing their experiences with each other.

Often a clinician may feel that a treatment/advice went well (clinically appropriate treatment) but a patient may feel that their expectations were not met due to non-clinical reasons. It would be advisable to attempt to turn a negative (such as correctly refusing a desired medication) into a positive by listening to the patient's concerns and showing compassion, while building trust.[3]

Issues contributing to problems surrounding expectations

- Lack of information (the patient may not have been informed of options and limited themselves to specific medications as the only option).
- Incorrect information/conflicting treatment advice (the patient may have searched for information and come to an incorrect conclusion, or another clinician may have given conflicting advice for the same condition).
- Time constraints (the clinician may have a busy day with too many clinical cases and not enough time to clearly communicate options and a clinical decision, as well as evidence to support this decision if conflicting with patient expectations).

- Communication (language barriers to patients, explanations using difficult terminology, poor communication between healthcare team members, and poor communication with secure environment staff).

Methods to better manage patient expectations

Availability of information

- Provide opportunities for patients to discuss health concerns and options with healthcare staff (while ensuring that information/advice is of the same quality).
- Provide alternative options for information (leaflets, print off advice during consultation).
- Review information provided regularly and ensure it is up to date, following current guidelines.

Ensure information is correct and consistent

- Have regular team and MDT meetings to discuss medical issues, and ensure current advice is coherent throughout the medical team and prison staff.

Time management

- Ensure there is sufficient time to spend with each patient and discuss ideas, concerns, and expectations (by understanding these, the clinician can better frame their clinical response).
- Ensure there is time to return to difficult consultations and update the notes or produce alternative information that can be given to the patient.
- Use appropriate translation services and ensure there is sufficient time for this.

Communication

- Take time to connect and understand the patient's position.
- Explain, clearly, in easy-to-understand language, your own ideas and advice. Take time to clarify and ensure the patient has understood what you are attempting to convey.
- Use MDT meetings to ensure that all healthcare staff (and prison staff if necessary) are aware of guidelines/protocols and general advice (if the prison staff give the wrong message, this can cause unrealistic expectations).
- Deal with any feedback/complaints in a timely manner, using this to better and clearly communicate decisions made and the evidence that these decisions were based upon.

References

1. Cockburn J, Pit S. Prescribing behaviour in clinical practice: patients' expectations and doctors' perceptions of patients' expectations—a questionnaire study. BMJ. 1997;315(7107):520–523.
2. Hoffman TC, Del Mar C. Patients' expectations of the benefits and harms of treatments, screening, and tests: a systematic review. JAMA Intern Med. 2015;175(2):274–286.
3. Medical Defence Union. Managing patient expectations. 2019. https://www.themdu.com/guidance-and-advice/guides/managing-patient-expectations

Telemedicine

Telemedicine refers to the use of video consultations for the delivery of healthcare services. This section covers the principles of telemedicine in prison settings. It includes information on the basic expectations for equipment, benefits and limitations of use, and example clinical uses.

Principles

- Telemedicine involves delivery of healthcare consultations over an internet-enabled video link.
- Hardware and software used in prisons for telemedicine consultation delivery will need to be approved in advance by prison digital teams/ cyber security teams.
- Telemedicine can be synchronous (real-time live consultations) or asynchronous (store and forward of recorded consultations or photographic images).
- In prison telemedicine consultations the patient will remain in the prison and connect to a healthcare clinician over the video link.
- Video appointments will be facilitated in the prison by a chaperone from the prison healthcare team.

Benefits

- Use of remote video consultations removes the need to transfer patients from prisons to other locations such as hospital sites. This relieves pressure on prison staffing required to accompany patients on external visits and can reduce delays in accessing external and specialist care services for patients.
- The use of remote consultations within prison removes the need for patients having to travel to external hospitals in handcuffs, which can be highly stigmatizing and stressful. By reducing the potential 'security risk' associated with offsite transfer, the patient is also permitted to know the time and date of their appointment in advance. This can improve patient experience and quality of care.
- The presence of a chaperone from the prison healthcare team within the consultation facilitates direct discussion regarding the onward treatment plans with the remote clinician, improving continuity of care.

Equipment

- At its simplest, telemedicine requires a computer or mobile device, a webcam, an internet connection, and secure video consultation software.
- Internet connectivity may be limited in prisons, and so should be assessed in advance of commencing telemedicine consultations. Poor internet connectivity will limit audio and visual capabilities during a consultation, limiting clinical use.
- Telemedicine peripherals can be used to enhance monitoring and assessment during a remote consultation, for example, remote stethoscopes, ECGs, and dermatoscopes. These will likely have to be approved in advance by prison security teams.

- Prison healthcare teams can support clinical evaluation related to consultations using their existing equipment, for example, undertaking blood tests or BP readings.

Uses

See Table 5.2.

Table 5.2 Uses of telemedicine

	Example use	Prison connecting to
Primary care	Management of long-term conditions, e.g. diabetes, asthma, and hypertension	Remote GP or specialist nurse Primary care staff in other prisons
Secondary care	Hepatitis, dermatology, cardiology, rheumatology, surgical follow-up, A&E triage, and maxillofacial assessment	Remote hospital staff
Mental health services	Telepsychiatry, telepsychology, and group therapy	Remote psychiatrist Mental health staff
Mental health secure hospital assessment	Mental health gatekeeping assessment	Remote psychiatrist at forensic hospital
Out-of-hours care	Reception screening and first night prescribing	Remote GP or specialist nurse Primary care staff in other prisons
Acute triage	Emergency care triage	Remote hospital or emergency services staff
'Through the gate' services	Pre-release contact with essential services—community substance misuse, housing assessments, and community mental health teams	Community service providers

Clinical considerations

- Telemedicine will not be appropriate for every patient or consultation. Agreement should be made about who will do the initial triage to a telemedicine appointment—the prison healthcare team or the remote clinician (after referral).
- All patients must give informed consent to participate in a video consultation.
- As with any video consultation, the ability to clearly see and hear the patient will influence clinical outcomes of the consultation. If audio or visual quality is significantly impaired, then the consultation should be rebooked or replaced with a face-to-face visit.

- Telemedicine may be less accessible to some patient groups such as those with a learning disability or autism.
- Prison healthcare staff are able to assist with physical examination during telemedicine consultations where they have received appropriate training (e.g. auscultation, palpation).

Other limitations

- Where hospitals are using different software solutions for their video consultation service, they will have to adopt an approved prison software for delivery of consultations to people in prison.
- Booking clinics that fit both hospital schedules and the prison regime can be challenging.
- People in prison may not be permitted to remain with internet-enabled equipment without a responsible chaperone, dependent on prison service rules.

Chapter 6

Chronic
disease management

General principles of long-term condition management in prisons

Introduction

The secure setting can be viewed by some as detrimental to health due to a transient population with lots of movement disrupting continuity of care plus a lack of control of diet and exercise.[1-3] However, many also argue that the secure setting offers services which individuals may not have previously accessed as well as ample opportunity for education and health promotion.[4,5]

Prevalence

Williams and Greifinger[6] estimate that up to 90% of people living in prison over 50 years of age have at least one moderate or severe health condition, with Hayes et al.[7] reporting more than 50% having three or more. Fazel et al.[8] state that health outcomes are worse in individuals with chronic disease than those of the same age in the community setting.

Munday et al.[9] found the following rates in chronic disease among people in prison:

- Cancer: 8%.
- Cardiovascular disease: 38%.
- Hypertension: 39%.
- Diabetes: 14%.
- Asthma: 7%.
- COPD: 4–18%.

Management

The reception screening process should detect those with long-term conditions. Clinical coding which enables data to be gathered to ensure reviews take place is important for ongoing care planning.

Long-term condition reviews should be carried out at least yearly, and sooner if uncontrolled or otherwise deemed necessary.

Each annual review should include the following:

- Test blood and urine to monitor disease progression and complications.
- Carry out care plans which are shared with the individual.
- Review medication compliance and understanding.
- Assess smoking status and provide cessation advice.
- Ensure invitation for appropriate vaccinations, such as for influenza.
- Obtain BMI and provide weight management and health promotion support, including dietary and lifestyle advice.
- Onward referral to secondary care as appropriate and as per national and local guidelines.

Utilization of long-term condition templates should include a recall function to notify when a further review is due. This aids continuity of care especially at sites with a high turnover, such as remand settings.

Engagement

Enabling the patient to take responsibility for their health is crucial for engagement. Offering NHS health checks in line with the community NHS guidelines is one way to engage those patients that otherwise may not access the prison healthcare services.

NHS health checks aim to detect and intervene in the following long-term conditions:

- Diabetes.
- Heart disease.
- Kidney disease.
- Stroke.
- Dementia.

These checks are offered to those patients who do not have a pre-existing health complaint and aim to detect early signs of disease.[10]

Building good working relationships between people in prison, prison staff, and healthcare staff also helps develop trust and overall engagement.

One way to aid this is by running a patient participation group whereby people representing each wing or house block are invited to a meeting with healthcare staff where issues and suggestions will be discussed. This allows people in prison to have their say in what works well and what doesn't work well, as well as building professional working relationships.

References

1. Booles K. Survey on the quality of diabetes care in prison settings across the UK. J Diabetes Nurs. 2011;15(5):168–176.
2. Ginn S. The challenge of providing prison healthcare. BMJ. 2012;345(7875):26–28.
3. Mills L. A prison based nurse-led specialist diabetes service for detained individuals. Eur Diabetes Nurs. 2014;11(2):53–57.
4. Department of Health, HM Prison Service. Developing and Modernising Primary Care in Prisons. London: Department of Health; 2002.
5. Condon L, Gill H, Harris F. A review of prison health and its implications for primary care nursing in England and Wales: the research evidence. J Clin Nurs. 2007;16(7):1201–1209.
6. Williams B, Ahalt C, Greifinger R. The older prisoner and complex chronic medical care. In: Enggist S, Møller L, Galea G, et al. (eds). Prisons and Health, pp. 165–170. Copenhagen: World Health Organization Regional Office for Europe; 2014. https://www.euro.who.int/__data/assets/pdf_file/0007/249208/Prisons-and-Health,-19-The-older-prisoner-and-complex-chronic-medical-care.pdf
7. Fazel S, Hope T, O'Donnell I, et al. Health of elderly male prisoners: worse than the general population, worse than younger prisoners. Age Ageing. 2001;30(5):403–407.
8. Hayes AJ, Burns A, Turnbull P, et al. The health and social care needs of older male prisoners. Int J Geriatr Psychiatry. 2012;27:1155–1162.
9. Munday D, Leaman J, O'Moore É, et al. The prevalence of non-communicable disease in older people in prison: a systematic review and meta-analysis. Age Ageing. 2019;48(2):204–212.
10. NHS England. NHS health check. 2019. https://www.nhs.uk/conditions/nhs-health-check/

Hypertension

Available research suggests that hypertension is increasingly common in people in prison and may occur earlier than in the community given the phenomenon of 'accelerated ageing' in this cohort and the increased prevalence of risk factors for cardiovascular disease.

Hypertension increases cardiovascular morbidity and mortality two- to fourfold. Reducing the prevalence of modifiable risk factors, promoting early diagnosis, and good treatment adherence is key to prolonging healthy life expectancy.

Significant risk factors

- Family history.
- Ethnicity: more common in people of Black or South Asian origin (over-represented in prisons).
- Age:
  - 'Accelerated ageing' in prisons is common, with early onset of age-related health conditions being more frequent. Hypertension may be seen earlier than in the respective community cohort.
  - As well as this, the prison population itself is ageing, and undiagnosed hypertension in older people in prison may also be seen.
- Lifestyle:
  - Obesity, sedentary lifestyle, inadequate exercise, smoking, heavy alcohol use are more frequently found in patients coming into the secure environment.
  - Inactivity is likely to continue in prison through being locked in a cell for long periods and having limited access to gyms or other exercise opportunities.
  - Limited food choices on prison menu.
  - Boredom resulting in comfort eating.
  - High use of salt by people finding prison food bland.
  - Abuse of anabolic steroids can increase risk.
- Stress: being in prison is inherently stressful, and the links between stress and high BP are well known.

Screening and identification

- Prison reception health check—use this opportunity to check BP.
- NHS health check—should be done in prisons in order to provide healthcare opportunities equivalent to those in the community.
- Opportunistically at healthcare appointments.
- Ambulatory monitoring is ideal for diagnosis but pragmatically is unlikely to be feasible within secure environments. Can be done through hospital services but consider purchasing home BP monitors and providing to patients to use in cells.
- Cell-based BP monitoring reduces the 'white coat' effect and promotes patient independence, but may be difficult to organize. Patients need to be risk assessed for potential misuse including ingestion of batteries.

Treatment pathway

- See NICE guidance.[1]

- Dedicated hypertension clinics have been set up in some secure environments with success, both in streamlining healthcare resources and in providing high-quality patient care. An example of how to set up such a clinic can be found in Box 6.1.

Box 6.1 How to set up a hypertension clinic—an example

- Stream patients identified with hypertension into a hypertension clinic (nurse led).
- Create waiting list on SystmOne for referrals.
- Once diagnosis is established, perform initial check for target organ damage:
  - Bloods for renal function and full lipid profile (non-fasting).
  - Baseline ECG.
  - Baseline early morning urine for albumin:creatinine ratio (send specimen bottle with clinic movement slip).
  - Fundoscopy.
  - Ensure correct Read coding and add to disease register.
- Add recall date to patient's record to ensure regular review.
- Record information onto template (using local clinical commissioning group template works well, plus adds Quality and Outcomes Framework information).

Monitoring

Nurse review
Frequency of reviews determined by stability of BP:
- Treated BP: target clinic reading 18–79 years, less than 140/90 mmHg; 80 years and older, less than 150/90 mmHg.
- Record weight:
  - Discuss diet, advise, and give information leaflets.
  - Refer for weight management as necessary and available.
- Discuss exercise:
  - Advise, encourage, and give suggestions for non-gym or in-cell routines.
  - Refer for remedial gym as necessary and available.
  - Older patients may find a gym intimidating, a remedial gym will have fewer bodybuilders.
- Medication problems: check concordance.
- Annual bloods for renal function and lipids, HbA1c if obesity (BMI >30 kg/m^2).
- Calculate QRISK2 score—if greater than 10% offer statin:
  - Set recall for next review.
  - Refer to GP if BP not responding to treatment.

Doctor review
- Review all patients whose BP is not well controlled.
- Review of medications—treatment as per NICE guidance[1]:
  - Uptitrate anti-hypertensive medication to maximally tolerated doses.

(Continued)

Box 6.1 (*Contd.*)

- Refer:
  - Newly diagnosed patients aged under 40 years to cardiologist (even if no target organ damage).
  - If ambulatory monitoring required.
  - Accelerated (severe) hypertension greater than 180/110 mmHg and papilloedema (same-day referral).
  - Suspected renal artery stenosis, phaeochromocytoma.

Reference

1. National Institute for Health and Care Excellence. Hypertension in adults: diagnosis and management. NICE guideline [NG136]. 2019 (updated March 2022). https://www.nice.org.uk/guidance/ng136

Heart failure

Introduction

The increasing ageing population within prisons, and the notable accelerated ageing among this group, means that cardiovascular diseases are seen in higher proportions and younger ages in people in prison. Early diagnosis and multidisciplinary management is key to improving quality of life and health outcomes.

Risk factors

- The high prevalence of lifestyle risk factors such as smoking, poor diet, sedentary behaviour, and alcohol use in prison populations increases the risk of heart failure.
- HIV infection may also be more prevalent in the prison cohort, and has an associated increase in heart failure risk.

Clinical features

- Exertional dyspnoea and orthopnoea. Orthopnoea may present earlier than in the community due to a lack of supply of pillows in secure environments to enable the patient to be supported upright.
- Fluid retention and nocturnal cough.

Investigations and diagnosis

- ECG and relevant blood tests, including B-type natriuretic peptide, should be performed.
- Echocardiography and chest X-ray is the standard for confirming disease; however, these may be difficult to access in prison. Consider discussing the diagnosis and pragmatic management given the circumstances via telephone with the local cardiologist in the interim if a prompt appointment is unlikely.

Management

- Patient education and self-care:
  - Health literacy in the prison population may be poor and there may be language barriers with foreign nationals. The British Heart Foundation (www.bhf.org.uk) and Easy Health (www.easyhealth.org.uk) have easy-read versions and multiple-language versions of leaflets that can be read through with patients.
- Specialist heart failure nurses may support self-care, improve symptom management, and reduce hospital admissions which require prison staff escorts.

Lifestyle modification
- Smoking: all prisons in England are now smoke free (see Smoking, p. 58).
- Diet and fluid intake: if high levels of salt or fluid consumption are present this should be reduced but patients should not be routinely advised to restrict sodium or fluid intake.
- Stopping any illicit alcohol intake.
- Exercise: gym availability is variable across the prison estate and if it is not possible to access a sufficient standard of gym sessions a remedial

gym referral should be considered. Ideally a cardiac rehabilitation programme supervised by gym staff should be offered.
- Mental health: depression is common in heart failure and in patients in secure environments. Screening and appropriate treatment should be considered.

Medication
- Diuretics: the management of all types of heart failure with fluid overload requires the use of diuretics which patients may be reluctant to use due to embarrassment caused by using toilet facilities in a shared cell, the risk of urinary incontinence without the facility to purchase over-the-counter incontinence pads, and requiring permission to access toilet facilities within education or work during the day. Have an open conversation with the patient about this and consider discussing with workplace, education, and operational staff to raise awareness and negotiate a workaround.
- Medications to improve prognosis: beta blockers, angiotensin-converting enzyme inhibitors, and aldosterone antagonists may be recommended by cardiology specialists; however, polypharmacy can be challenging to manage within prisons. Ensure appropriate support is in place and weigh up the risk/benefits of in-possession medications. Remember: all medication has potential tradeable value in secure environments.

Palliative and end of life care of the patient with heart failure

Recognition—NICE guidelines[1] advise that prognostic tools should not be used to determine when a patient requires palliative care and the decision should be a clinical one made at the point when a patient's symptoms are worsening despite optimal treatment. See also Chapter 13.
- The palliative care management of heart failure may require the use of opiates for symptomatic relief of dyspnoea which will require careful monitoring in the secure environment.
- Increased personal care and nursing needs may be challenging to provide in secure environments and requires close cooperation with social care services and consideration of using appropriate assistance from more able-bodied people in prison.
- Patients may experience pain which is best managed with opiates.
- 'Do not attempt cardiopulmonary resuscitation' (DNACPR) decisions: approximately half of the deaths in people with heart failure are related to sudden cardiac death. This raises the importance of identifying at-risk heart failure patients and engaging in a timely discussion with them about the appropriateness of cardiopulmonary resuscitation (CPR). Discuss with the patient the best way to alert operational prison staff—some are happy to keep DNACPR orders in their cells.
- Advance directives: around 40% of patients will die within 1 year of diagnosis and determining patients' wishes during the terminal stages of the illness is important and can be structured using an advance directive.

- Nausea and decreased appetite are common problems which may result in such low nutritional intake that health is impaired. Access to dietetic advice and appropriate homemade supplements may be restricted and needs to be prioritized to provide an equivalent standard of care to these patients to that provided in the community.

Reference

1. National Institute for Health and Care Excellence. https://www.nice.org.uk/guidance/ng106

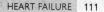

Type 1 diabetes mellitus

Introduction

Diabetes is prevalent in prison, particularly in older people who often experience equivalent morbidity and functional impacts to community peers 10 years older. Although the same disease at a biochemical level, managing diabetes—both type 1 and type 2—in prison can be very different to in the community. Diabetic control on entry to prison is often poor, and health literacy and patients' understanding of their disease can be low. Managing diabetes within the rigid mealtime regimen and restricted dietary options can be challenging. In some cases, diabetes can be misused for secondary gains such as requests for a special diet or even self-harming behaviour.

Clinicians should be aware of the differing needs of the person in prison with diabetes at each stage of their incarceration journey.

First night

- Check blood glucose on reception.
- If patient has their own insulin and knows their regimen, check label to check patient identity and consider repeat prescription. If they do not have their own insulin, write up stock insulin after asking about the dose.
- Issue the patient with a blood glucose monitor, or allow them to have their own if they have it with them.
- If this is not possible, check their blood glucose in 2 hours.
- Advise them how to contact healthcare staff in case of an emergency.
- Check that they are happy with the management of hypoglycaemia and of the symptoms of diabetic ketoacidosis; ask about previous hospital admissions for diabetic-related emergencies.
- Supply the patient with instructions on how to manage a hypoglycaemic event and issue glucose tablets/GlucoGel (formerly known as HypoStop) for acute management of this.
- Book in to see the reception GP or to see the GP or diabetic specialist nurse the following morning if arriving after reception.

During incarceration

- Monitor closely for the first few days: insulin compliance may have been poor or chaotic, and there is a risk of hypoglycaemia if restarting regular doses.
- Risk assess as to whether the patient can keep insulin in their possession. Insulin has street value (e.g. for body building) or can be misused to instigate diabetic ketoacidosis/hypoglycaemic episodes to necessitate a hospital admission. Discuss appropriate medicines management with the prison pharmacist; mitigation could include monitoring their supply to highlight sudden high use or syringes going missing, giving small amounts at a time, or exchanging used needles/syringes for fresh ones.
- Consider keeping extra cereal packs in the officer's office in case of hypoglycaemic episodes out of hours.

- Symptoms of hypoglycaemia and diabetic ketoacidosis can be similar to drug or alcohol withdrawal, or the effects of illicit drug use within prison. Always think about blood glucose when reviewing sudden deterioration in physical or mental state.

Manipulation of insulin, self-harm, and secondary gain

- Sometimes patients can manipulate illness for secondary gain (e.g. meal options) or self-harm.
- A complex Assessment, Care in Custody and Teamwork (ACCT) review should be called if manipulation is suspected.
- A clear clinical care plan needs to be drawn up including how monitoring should be done and what would trigger the use of the Mental Capacity Act 2005. Interventions by the case manager and mental health team should be made to try and influence and amend behaviour.

Value of diabetic treatments

- Glucose tablets are a commodity, which can be used in exchange for contraband (providing extra nutrition, can be cut with amphetamine). Some prisons provide GlucoGel as it is a lot less palatable and sweet. The use and issue of glucose tablet needs to be monitored.
- Insulin is also perceived by some as a commodity as it is considered to have an anabolic effect—bodybuilders take it to increase stamina and improve endurance. This should be considered when risk assessing for in-possession medication.
- If a patient's control is not as you would expect from the medications you are prescribing, it is worth considering whether they are being bullied for their medication.

On release

- Ensure appropriate handover notes are provided to the receiving clinician in the community including current insulin dose and any planned follow-up. If a receiving clinician has not been identified, provide the patient with a discharge summary and guidance on how to register with a GP.
- Ensure the patient is provided with a supply of insulin and an emergency hypoglycaemia kit for release.

References

Booles K. A captive audience: tackling diabetes and obesity in the prison setting. Diabetes Pract. 2013;2(4):142–147.

Condon L, Gill H, Harris F. A review of prison health and its implications for primary care nursing in England and Wales: the research evidence. J Clin Nurs. 2007;16:1201–1209.

Diabetes UK. Diabetes care in prisons. n.d. https://www.diabetes.org.uk/Professionals/Resources/shared-practice/Prisons

Gill GV, MacFarlane IA. Problems of diabetics in prison. BMJ. 1989;298(6668):221–223.

Gulland A. NHS to take over responsibility for prison health services next April. BMJ. 2002;325:736.

Holt RIG, Cockram CS, Flyvbjerg A, et al. (eds). Textbook of Diabetes, 4th ed. Oxford: Wiley-Blackwell; 2010.

Legislation.gov.uk. Mental Capacity Act 2005. 2005. http://www.legislation.gov.uk/ukpga/2005/9/section/1

Marshall T, Simpson S, Stevens A. Use of health services by prison inmates: comparisons with the community. J Epidemiol Community Health. 2001;55:364–365.

Mills LS. Diabetes behind bars: considerations for managing diabetes within the prison setting and after release. Diabetes Primary Care. 2015;17(6):290–295.

The Lancet Diabetes Endocrinology. Diabetes behind bars: challenging inadequate care in prisons. Lancet Diabetes Endocrinol. 2018;6(5):347.

Zammitt NN, Frier BM. Hypoglycemia in type 2 diabetes pathophysiology, frequency, and effects of different treatment modalities. Diabetes Care. 2005;28(12):2948–2961.

Arthritis

Introduction

Joint pain and arthritis are common presentations in prisons. Research has shown that arthritis is more common in the prison population than the general population. Causes for this may include increased rates of homelessness, incidence of trauma, and heavy manual labour; people in prison being less likely to have taken care of their general health and well-being, including an increased incidence of obesity; and an ageing prison population.

Arthritis can be challenging to manage within prisons as prison populations are more likely to suffer with difficult-to-manage pain and have reduced access to some adjunct treatments.

It is also known that prison populations are more likely than the general population to suffer with persistent pain. In part this is because people in prison are more likely to have suffered injuries, trauma, and assaults; however, the psychosocial elements of the perception of pain also need to be considered and addressed. People in prison have a higher incidence of psychiatric illness, chronic stress, and social issues including housing and relationships struggles and a reduced access to social support from friends and family.

Differential diagnosis

See Table 6.1.

History

- Which joints are affected.
- Duration of onset.
- Nature of pain—worse with exercise/worse with something touching it/unable to move the joint at all.
- Stiffness—duration, when does it tend to be worse (e.g. morning, with rest/exercise).
- Swelling or deformity associated with the joints.
- Any associated symptoms—rash/fever/tophi.
- Any previous injury or surgery to the joint.
- Any family history of joint problems.

Examination

- Any swelling/joint effusion/synovitis/deformity present.
- Large or small joints involved.
- Symmetrical joint involvement.
- Changes to skin/nails.
- Crepitus.
- Reduced range of movement.
- Increase in temperature.

Investigation

Beware. Radiological findings often do not correlate well with the clinical picture and impairment of function. Many asymptomatic adults will have radiographic evidence of degenerative changes. But equally, some patients may have a major symptom burden from arthritis with relatively mild radiographic changes—this can be especially true in the acute phase of inflammatory arthritis.

Table 6.1 Differential diagnosis of arthritis

	Degenerative: Osteoarthritis	Inflammatory: Psoriatic Rheumatoid Ankylosing spondylitis	Infectious: Septic joint Reactive	Metabolic: Gout Pseudogout
Age of onset	Middle age	Can start in younger years	Any	Middle age
Duration of onset	Gradual	Sudden	Sudden	Sudden flare
Stiffness	<30 mins	>30 mins	Severely reduced range of movement	Severely reduced range of movement
Pain	Worse with exercise	Improves with exercise	Severe	Severe
Swelling	Seen in flare	Common	Common + systemic symptoms	Seen in flare + erythema
Deformity	Bony swelling, Heberden's/ Bouchard's nodes	Synovitis Rheumatoid arthritis—symmetrical		Metatarsophalangeal joint swelling Tophi
Risk factors	Injury/surgery to joint Obesity	Family history Autoimmune conditions	Injury/surgery to joint Intravenous drug use Infections, e.g. STI/ gastrointestinal/hepatitis	Obesity Alcohol intake Diuretics
Investigations	Clinical diagnosis Joint aspirate sometimes needed in flare	X-ray for erosions Ultrasound scan for synovitis Bloods—inflammatory markers	Bloods—infective markers Joint aspirate	Bloods—urate Joint aspirate
Management	Exercise Lifestyle changes Analgesia Steroid injections Surgery	Disease-modifying antirheumatic drugs	Medical emergency Admission Intravenous antibiotics	Analgesia Lifestyle changes Allopurinol

Management in the prison environment

Management can be challenging in a custodial environment:

- Long-term opiate use can cause hyperalgesia, increasing the patients' experience of pain. Within the prison population long-term opiate use is common: either illicit use or prescribed for chronic pain.
- There is limited access to non-pharmacological interventions such as rubefacients or heat/ice packs (rubefacients and capsaicin are not permitted in many custodial environments due to security risks—they can be used to put off sniffer dogs, and can be used as a weapon if applied to the eyes) and low-impact exercise such as cycling/swimming/ Pilates.
- Addressing the psychosocial aspects of pain as well as the physical pain is essential but challenging for the patient and within the custodial environment.
- Lifestyle—weight management.
- Medical intervention such as analgesia and steroid injections.
- Physiotherapy, transcutaneous electrical nerve stimulation, and use of mobility aids. Be aware that these may be used as weapons—discuss with security.
- Complementary therapy.
- Secondary care referral for consideration of specialist medication/ surgery.
- In extreme circumstances, social care may be required to support patients and assist with ADLs.

The role of medications is limited. Exercise is one of the most evidence-based interventions in arthritis. Consider remedial gym. Exercise is not just time in the gym, it is all the time the person is active throughout the day.

- A sense of purpose (e.g. work) can help with the experience of pain.
- Patients often self-medicate for pain with illicit drugs. Emergent pain can occur as these re-detoxed. Investigate and manage to aid drug recovery.
- Beware of secondary gains as a barrier to improvement (e.g. signed off work, increased healthcare attention, access to desirable/tradable medications, etc.).
- Early and frank discussions about realistic goals are vital. It is unlikely that chronic pain will be totally relieved. The most important thing is to maximize function and well-being.
- Referral to pain teams and pain psychology can be very beneficial.

Septic arthritis

> This is a clinical emergency. If suspected, then refer for same-day assessment in secondary care.

Septic arthritis may be more common in prisons as a result of trauma (possibly without adequate medical attention), intravenous (IV) drug use, and self-neglect/homelessness.

Osteoarthritis

- The most common form of arthritis seen in prisons, often described as 'wear and tear arthritis'.
- Generally found in those older than 45 years.
- Most commonly seen in the hands, hips, knees, and spine.
- Diagnosis is clinical. Imaging is generally not needed unless needed to rule out alternative diagnoses.

Management

- Simple analgesia.
- Weight loss.
- Physiotherapy.
- Steroid injections.
- Surgical interventions.
- There may be a place for adjuncts such as acupuncture.

Guidance advises against using opiate-based analgesia on a long-term basis. The use of short courses of opioid analgesics needs to take into account the risks of previous illicit drug use, diversion/trading, and dependence. Gabapentinoid medications do not have an indication in the treatment of osteoarthritis.

Guidance for neuropathic pain is moving towards offering amitriptyline/nortriptyline and duloxetine.

Crystal arthropathies

These include gout and pseudogout.

Gout

Gout is a disorder of purine metabolism causing hyperuricaemia and the formation of urate crystals within a joint and surrounding soft tissue.

Risk factors

- High-purine diet.
- Renal impairment.
- Diabetes.
- Hypertension.
- Obesity.
- Dehydration.
- Increasing age.

Typically first presents with flares of acute, severe pain affecting the first metatarsophalangeal joint.

Diagnosis is clinical and supported by blood tests. In unclear cases when a septic joint is queried, joint fluid aspiration is helpful.

Management

- Reduce urate levels via allopurinol and dietary changes.
- Manage the above-listed risk factors.
- In an acute phase, anti-inflammatory medication is often needed to control the pain.

In a secure setting, it is often challenging to make meaningful dietary changes due to the limits and restrictions the catering teams face.

Pseudogout

- Pseudogout is part of a crystal deposition condition where calcium pyrophosphate crystals are deposited into and around a joint.
- Pseudogout is the acute phase, presenting with acute joint pain which lasts for ~10 days. It most commonly affects the knees. It can be an oligo- or multi-arthropathy.
- Calcium pyrophosphate deposition can also be asymptomatic and found incidentally on imaging. In its chronic form these deposits can cause a chronic arthritis and it can also be found in combination with osteoarthritis.
- Management is to reduce risk factors such as non-steroidal anti-inflammatory drug (NSAID) use and dehydration and pain management.
- Both the acute and chronic forms can cause progressive and permanent damage to a joint and its function.

Rheumatoid arthritis and spondyloarthropathies

Inflammatory arthritis is less common in custodial environments but important to pick up on.

Acute presentation

- Rheumatology should see suspected inflammatory arthritis cases within 3 weeks (within 3 days if small joints of hands/feet affected, or more than one joint affected). Consider calling rheumatology to discuss.
- Check inflammatory markers but beware they cannot exclude inflammatory arthritis.
- Consider analgesia—NSAIDs if tolerated. Avoid steroids unless on advice of rheumatology.

If an inflammatory arthritis is confirmed then patients are usually started on disease-modifying antirheumatic drugs (can cause immunosuppression as well as more specific side effects such as myelosuppression, liver damage, and rashes). Blood monitoring is generally required.

If patients are not well managed on disease-modifying antirheumatic drugs then biologics may be considered.

Pain management

Introduction

- Pain is defined as an unpleasant, personal, sensory, and emotional experience which may or may not be associated with tissue damage. It is influenced by biological, psychological, and social factors and can adversely impact physical and psychological well-being, sleep, and social functioning. It is a common problem in prisons.
- Recommendations in this chapter are in line with national guidance (see RCGP 'Safer Prescribing in Prisons',[1] NHS England 'Pain Management Formulary for Prisons',[2] and Scottish Intercollegiate Guidelines Network[3] and NICE[4-7] guidelines).
- Comprehensive record-keeping is an essential component of pain management in the prison setting.
- *Acute pain* (lasting <12 weeks) usually associated with tissue injury; intensity related to severity of tissue damage.
- *Persistent pain* (lasting >3 months) more complex, frequently presents without ongoing tissue damage. WHO classification:
  - *Chronic primary pain*: not explained by underlying condition; associated with significant emotional distress or functional disability (e.g. fibromyalgia, complex regional pain syndrome).
  - *Chronic secondary pain*: pain with clear underlying disease/cause (e.g. osteoarthritis, rheumatoid arthritis, surgery, injury) persists beyond successful disease treatment.
- Risk factors for persistent pain include physical trauma, adverse life experiences, mental health disorders, and substance misuse, which are common among prison residents.
- Pain, well controlled in the community, may reportedly be heightened in prison due to poor beds, thin mattresses, limited movement/exercise, lack of meaningful activity or distraction, weight gain from unhealthy menu/canteen choices, anxiety, depression, and poor sleep.
- Medication is usually effective for acute pain but less beneficial in persistent pain; however, patients frequently come into prison on long-term, high-dose, dependence-forming analgesia, at risk of serious side effects, including respiratory depression and death.

Acute pain management

Injuries and acutely painful medical conditions arising in prison

- Injuries frequently occur in prison due to football, weights, fights, slips, falls off top bunk, burns, and deliberate self-harm.
- Painful medical conditions (e.g. acute back pain, torticollis, dental pain) are also common.
- Emergency nurse must attend, assess injuries/acute pain, and refer to GP/ANP if needed.
- History:
  - Injuries: document reported mechanism of injury. Use body map. Be aware residents may not report facts if under pressure (e.g. after assault).
  - Painful medical condition: document SOCRATES (Site, Onset, Characteristics, Radiation, Associated symptoms, Timing, Exacerbating/relieving factors, Severity). Be aware of red flag symptoms.

- Examination: site(s) and appearance of painful body part/injury (use body map, include dimensions); pain intensity (use subjective pain intensity assessment, e.g. numerical pain rating scale, rate 0–10); and functional impairment.
- Management: provide immediate, adequate pain relief. Inform manager/HCP in charge if an emergency escort is required to transfer a patient to hospital for further assessment, investigation, or treatment (e.g. suspected fracture, tendon rupture or tear, red flag symptoms/ signs acute back pain, or medical or surgical emergency). Be aware that delays to treatment may result in complaints and litigation; clear documentation and timely referral are essential.
- Pharmacological: follow the NHS England 'Pain Management Formulary for Prisons',[2] and RCGP 'Safer Prescribing in Prisons'[1] guidelines.
- Check in-possession risk assessment score. Prescribe in-possession if possible. Use longer-acting analgesia if supervised consumption indicated due to individual patient risk or drug-specific risk (opioid). Do not withhold adequate pain relief if the patient has a history of opioid dependence but caution must be applied where the patient is already prescribed a strong OST (see below).

Take a step-wise approach
- Simple analgesia: first-line full-dose paracetamol. Use PGD for small quantities, if governance arrangements in place.
- Add in NSAIDs at lowest effective dose for shortest time unless contraindicated (ibuprofen, naproxen) or COX-2 inhibitors (in line with clinical commissioning group formulary). Do not prescribe diclofenac (except intramuscularly, very short course for severe acute pain).
- Add in a weak opioid, for example, codeine 15 mg, 30 mg (4-hourly as needed, maximum 240 mg/24 hours). Avoid initial use of combination medications (e.g. co-codamol) to allow better dose titration. Before initiating opioids and at every analgesia review, discuss risk of dependence/withdrawal and expectations for step-down and stopping.
- Be aware of the risk of opioid misuse and bullying in prison. Tablets are less easily diverted than capsules. Avoid oxycodone, transdermal, or fast-acting opioids (e.g. fentanyl lollipops).
- Avoid strong opioids unless there is a clear clinical indication (e.g. early days postoperatively, prior to change of burns dressing). Prescribe as morphine and review requirements very frequently, tapering as soon as pain improves.
- Do not prescribe nefopam, rubefacients, or capsaicin.
- Non-pharmacological: use adjuncts (e.g. ice, immobilization). Provide advice to support self-management (physical and psychological tips— verbal, leaflets, in-cell TV, yoga)—avoid using jargon.

Continuing acute pain management initiated in the community
- When patients come into prison with analgesia started in the community, ongoing adequate analgesia must be provided while mitigating prison-specific risks and constraints.

Risks
- Prescribing: self-harm/overdose; misuse/diversion (e.g. opioid central nervous system (CNS) depressant effect/illicit opioid masking; rubefacients conceal illicit drug odour, e.g. cannabis); bullying (e.g. opioid value in 'prison economy'); weapon-making (e.g. capsaicin irritant).
- Non-pharmacological: weapon-making (e.g. splints/crutches); concealing drugs/weapons in cavities (e.g. crutch/wheelchair) or between fabric layers (e.g. strapping, splint); self-harm (ligature risk from fabric, safety pins).

Constraints
- Regime/staffing: restricts supervised consumption.
- Regime: restricts exercise, gym.
- Security/staffing: restricts escorts/hospital outpatient appointment attendance.
- Assessment: clearly document reported history and examination (as described earlier in this section). Take account of notes by other professionals (hospital discharge letter/forensic medical examiner notes in escort documents). Contact hospital/police custody if no/inadequate information.
- Management: document management plan. Continue analgesia started in hospital or prescribe safer equivalent. Explain reasons for choice (see previous bulleted risks/constraints). Offer reassurance. Set expectations:
  - Benefits/limitations, expected time to recovery.
  - Side effects, risk dependency (opioid), risks of long-term prescribing (NSAID, opioid).
  - Supervised consumption, switch to liquid/rapid taper if misuse medicines.
  - Regular review, step-down, and stop.
- Task/email administration team regarding outstanding hospital appointments. Book/add patient to waiting list for in-house appointments (e.g. triage, dressing clinic, physiotherapy, and medication review).

Prescribing for acute pain in patients on opioid substitution therapies
- Use step-wise analgesia approach (as above) in addition to maintenance OSTs.
- If opioid analgesia is required, discuss with IDTS team/MDT. Consider short-term use of additional opioid. Only consider pain management with increased methadone if IDTS/MDT agree to twice-daily dosing (once-daily methadone is less effective).

Management of persistent (chronic) pain
- In reception, advise patient that, if community prescribing is confirmed, a comprehensive pain assessment will be booked to offer a tailored multifaceted approach to analgesia, and to review prescribing safety and suitability.

- Explain importance of concordance, supervised consumption, management of misuse, and local policies relating to dependence-forming medicines and tapering (e.g. pregabalin).
- *Initial appointment*:
  - Take time to listen, observe, and allow the patient to describe their problems. Assess and clearly document severity, impact, type of pain (see Acute pain management, p. 124), and effect of life on pain and pain on life—functional impact: ADLs, disability, work, sleep, emotional well-being, and relationships.
  - Start to build a collaborative and supportive relationship with the patient, characterized by respect, compassion, and empathy. Beware of creating dysfunctional relational dynamics or triggering traumatic memories.
- *Planning care*:
  - Review diagnosis and share subjective/objective assessment. Discuss any disparities with patient.
  - Share aims, expectations, and options for managing persistent pain. Advise that pain will be reduced but not go away. Explain that you will be working as part of an MDT but avoid saying 'I don't make the decisions' or 'I'm just doing what I'm told'.
- *Non-pharmacological care*: mainstay of treatment. Refer to appropriate team(s) to address specific factors influencing pain:
  - Physiotherapy: exercise—supervised group, remedial gym, in-cell; advice to remain as active as possible; acupuncture.
  - Substance misuse support: one-to-one and group/peer support.
  - Mental health/psychological support: acceptance and commitment therapy or cognitive behavioural therapy (CBT) (if available).
  - Chaplaincy: spiritual support, address stressors (e.g. upcoming court, parole hearing, relationship breakdown, problems on wing).
  - Offer further information and self-management support such as The Pain Toolkit (https://www.paintoolkit.org/) and Live Well with Pain (https://livewellwithpain.co.uk/).
- *Pharmacological care*: follow national guidelines for individual conditions (e.g. rheumatoid arthritis/osteoarthritis); follow the NHS England 'Pain Management Formulary for Prisons',[2] RCGP 'Safer Prescribing in Prisons',[1] and NICE guidance NG193.[7]
  - Explain that medicines have limited benefits; side effects including respiratory depression and drug-related death, especially if coexisting respiratory disease or renal or hepatic impairment; long-term prescribing risks including dependence, tolerance, reduced testosterone levels, and low bone density (opioids); and risk of bullying/diversion/misuse by others.
  - If medication is no longer indicated or unsafe, plan to stop or switch to safer alternative (e.g. for pregabalin, switch to duloxetine or amitriptyline for neuropathic pain). *Do not stop dependence-forming medicines abruptly.*
  - If planning taper, agree initial dose reduction/rate (e.g. 50–75 mg pregabalin/week, 300 mg gabapentin/4 days). Agree parameters/flexibility/review interval. Discuss patient at MDT meeting.

- Be aware that initial attempts to address prescribing may be met with distress and resistance, expressed as threats of violence, self-harm, or litigation. If this is the case, plan paired multiprofessional working and reflective supervision going forward.
- *Ongoing care:*
  - Review aims and outcomes at, for example, 8 weeks, 12 weeks after initial appointment, and on transfer/release.
  - Communicate changes to pain management with community GP and outside agencies such as the community drug service (provide details of medication reduced/stopped and multiprofessional input offered).

Summary

Steps to successful management of pain in prisons:

- Assess acute pain early and provide adequate analgesia.
- Set expectations of analgesia (benefits, side effects, dependence risk, stop if ineffective, and consequences of misuse) on initial prescription and at every review.
- Form a collaborative supportive relationship with the patient.
- Carry out well-documented shared individualized care planning.
- Ensure multidisciplinary discussion to support prescribing decisions.
- Ensure multiprofessional input to address complex influences on pain.

References

1. Royal College of General Practitioners. Safer prescribing in prisons, 2nd ed. 2019. https://elearn ing.rcgp.org.uk/pluginfile.php/176185/mod_book/chapter/620/RCGP-safer-prescribing-in-pris ons-guidance-jan-2019.pdf
2. NHS England. Pain management formulary for prisons: the formulary for acute, persistent and neuropathic pain, 2nd ed. October 2017 https://www.england.nhs.uk/wp-content/uploads/2017/11/prison-pain-management-formulary.pdf
3. Scottish Intercollegiate Guidelines Network. Management of chronic pain. SIGN guideline 136. 2019. https://www.sign.ac.uk/our-guidelines/management-of-chronic-pain/
4. National Institute for Health and Care Excellence. Neuropathic pain in adults: pharmacological management in non-specialist settings. Clinical guideline [CG173]. 2013 (updated 2020). https://www.nice.org.uk/guidance/cg173
5. National Institute for Health and Care Excellence. Low back pain and sciatica in over 16s: assessment and management. NICE guideline [NG59]. 2016 (updated 2020). https://www.nice.org.uk/guidance/ng59
6. National Institute for Health and Care Excellence. Back pain (low without radiculopathy): red flags. https://cks.nice.org.uk/topics/back-pain-low-without-radiculopathy/diagnosis/assessm ent/#red-flags
7. National Institute for Health and Care Excellence. Chronic pain (primary and secondary) in over 16s: assessment of all chronic pain and management of chronic primary pain. NICE guideline [NG193]. 2021. https://www.nice.org.uk/guidance/NG193

Further reading

Croft M. Prevalence of chronic non-cancer pain in a UK prison environment. Br J Pain. 2015;9(2):96–108.
Faculty of Pain Medicine. Core standards for pain management services in the UK. 2021. https://fpm.ac.uk/standards-publications-workforce/core-standards
Ford K, Bellis MA, Hughes K, et al. Adverse childhood experiences: a retrospective study to understand their associations with lifetime mental health diagnosis, self-harm or suicide attempt, and current low mental wellbeing in a male Welsh prison population. Health Justice. 2020;8:13.
Prison Reform Trust. Bromley Briefings. Winter 2021. http://www.prisonreformtrust.org.uk/Publi cations/Factfile

Public Health England. Managing persisting pain in secure settings. 2013. https://www.gov.uk/gov ernment/publications/managing-persistent-pain-in-secure-settings

Raja SN, Carr DB, Cohen M, et al. The revised International Association for the Study of Pain definition of pain: concepts, challenges, and compromises. Pain. 2020;161(9):1976–1982.

Royal College of General Practitioners. Top ten tips: dependence forming medicines. https://www.rcgp.org.uk/clinical-and-research/resources/a-to-z-clinical-resources/dependence-forming-medications.aspx

Treede RD, Rief W. Chronic pain as a symptom or a disease: the IASP Classification of Chronic Pain for the International Classification of Diseases (ICD-11). Pain. 2019;160(1):19–27.

Tyler N, Miles HL, Karadag B, et al. An updated picture of the mental health needs of male and female prisoners in the UK: prevalence, comorbidity, and gender differences. Soc Psychiatry Psychiatr Epidemiol. 2019;54(9):1143–1152.

Chest pain

Introduction

Patients can often present with chest pain for a variety of causes ranging from benign to life-threatening. It is therefore important to be able to assess chest pain accurately to ensure rapid treatment of life-threatening presentations and avoidance of unnecessary hospital admission for less serious presentations. History taking is of paramount importance when dealing with a chest pain to differentiate the cause.[1] Causes of chest pain can range from acute coronary syndrome, stable angina, pericarditis, thoracic aortic aneurysm dissection, and arrhythmias, to pulmonary emboli, pneumonia, tension pneumothorax, asthma, to musculoskeletal causes, gastroenterological causes, cancers, or non-specific chest pain for which no cause is ever found—which accounts for ~16% of chest pain presenting to primary care.[2]

One of the many challenges in assessing people in prison complaining of chest pain is the vulnerability of the presenting patient. The prison population have significantly poorer health outcomes and many have at least one physical health complaint and often suffer from psychiatric disorders, which can lead to atypical presentations.[3]

Emergency healthcare within prisons is logistically complex due to security issues, for example, if a patient presents with chest pain at night, there are fewer custodial staff compared to during the day, meaning cell access is limited to emergency situations only. Custodial officers are required to accompany patients to hospital, thus reducing further the number of custodial staff within the prison leading to potential conflicts with the need to maintain prison security. Ambulance access to the prison also requires communication and organization between healthcare staff and prison officers to ensure that security processes are adhered to.

> Challenges should be pre-empted by healthcare staff ensuring that when attending a patient with chest pain, staff have all of the equipment required to conduct a thorough examination in a prepared 'emergency grab bag', along with oxygen, a defibrillator, and an ECG machine, where possible. An early request to call an ambulance is vital to allow for all staff to prepare adequately for its arrival in the prison.

Clinical features

Cardiac chest pain is often an acute onset of central chest pain or pain described as a tight band or pressure around the chest. See Table 6.2.

Assessment

Doorstep assessment—how unwell does the patient look?
- A thorough history, including time of onset, duration, previous episodes, exacerbating and relieving factors; family history.
- Clinical observations and NEWS 2 score.
- Inspection and palpation of the chest.
- Auscultation of all lung fields and heart sounds.

Table 6.2 History and observations for chest pain

	History	Observation/examination
Cardiac (myocardial infarction)	Dull pain/ache radiating to jaw, arms, or back	The patient may present as pale or grey looking; sweating, nausea, or vomiting may also be present
Cardiac (angina)	Pain/pressure across the chest as a 'tight band' associated with exercise or exertion	There may be no physical findings
Musculoskeletal	'Sharp' pain, localized in nature, preceded by trauma/ injury/exertion	Chest wall tenderness, bruising, crepitus
Pulmonary embolism	Sudden onset of pain associated with breathlessness, haemoptysis	Cyanosis, raised jugular venous pressure, pleural rub, tachycardia, low peripheral oxygen saturations, tachypnoea
Pneumonia	Coughing with at least one of sputum, wheeze dyspnoea, or pleuritic chest pain	Coarse crepitations on auscultation, loss of air entry, tachypnoea, cyanosis, tachycardia, low peripheral oxygen saturations

- Inspection of lower legs and ankles to check for oedema, swelling, and/ or tenderness.
- Raised jugular venous pressure.
- Consider an abdominal assessment.[4]

Investigations

- Clinical observations: include conscious level; respiratory rate; manual pulse check to determine the rate, rhythm and regularity; BP; peripheral oxygen saturations; temperature; and blood glucose.
- ECG: this does not give a definitive diagnosis.

If an acute cardiac cause is suspected, and the patient has current chest pain or has had chest pain within the last 12 hours, and has an abnormal ECG or ECG is unavailable, then an emergency admission to hospital via ambulance should be arranged.

- IV access should be obtained as soon as practicable with a wide-bore cannula.
- Administer 400–800 mcg glyceryl trinitrate sublingually providing the BP is greater than 90 mmHg.
- Administer 300 mg aspirin if available and if not contraindicated.

If a cardiac cause is suspected, and the patient is currently pain free but has had chest pain within 12 hours and has a normal ECG, or if the last episode of chest pain was 12–72 hours ago, the patient should be referred for same-day assessment.

If recent acute cardiac syndrome is suspected but the last episode of chest pain was more than 72 hours ago, complete clinical assessment, ECG, and troponin T levels (taking into account the lapsed time between the chest pain and taking the blood sample), and use clinical judgement around referral and its urgency.[1]

References

1. ICE. Chest pain. Last revised in August 2022. https://cks.nice.org.uk/topics/chest-pain/
2. NICE CKS. 2020. https://cks.nice.org.uk/topics/chest-pain/
3. Harel et al. 2018. https://rm.coe.int/drug-situation-and-policy-by-yossi-harel-fisch-sonia-hizi-iris-yogev-a/168075f0e0
4. Innes. 2018. https://shop.elsevier.com/books/macleods-clinical-examination/innes/978-0-7020-6993-2

Chronic obstructive pulmonary disease

Introduction

- COPD is a lung disease characterized by chronic obstruction of lung airflow that interferes with normal breathing and is not fully reversible.
- Patients may refer to 'chronic bronchitis' or 'emphysema' which are synonymous terms with COPD.
- COPD is not simply a 'smoker's cough' but an underdiagnosed, life-threatening lung disease.
- The risk of COPD is greater within prisons due to the high prevalence of smoking among the population. The recent move to smoke-free prisons will reduce exposure, but smoking prior to incarceration is still likely to remain.

Investigations

- Identify patients with features of COPD and refer for spirometry.
- Features:
  - Older than 35 years *and* smoker or ex-smoker 20 pack years smoker *and* exertional breathlessness/chronic. Be aware that in prison settings some patients may present earlier than 35 years old with symptoms, given the high prevalence of risk factors and phenomenon of accelerated ageing in this population.
  - Cough/regular sputum production/frequent 'winter bronchitis'/wheeze *and* do not have clinical features of asthma (lower threshold if smoking cannabis, crack, or heroin).
- No evidence for 'screening' if individuals have not got symptoms.

Diagnosis and assessment

- Spirometry (if possible with reversibility).
- Medical Research Council (MRC) dyspnoea score (Table 6.3).
- BMI, smoking history for tobacco (and other inhaled drugs, e.g. crack, heroin, and cannabis), and pulse oximetry, preferably using template to record observations.
- Chest X-ray will confirm the diagnosis but may be difficult to organize. If unlikely to be undertaken promptly, discuss pragmatic diagnosis and management with a local respiratory physician.

Table 6.3 MRC dyspnoea score

1	Breathless only with strenuous exercise
2	Short of breath when hurrying on the level or up a slight hill
3	Slower than most people of the same age on a level surface or have to stop when walking at own pace on the level
4	Stop for breath walking 100 m or After walking for a few minutes at own pace on the level
5	Too breathless to leave the house

Used with the permission of the Medical Research Council.

Exacerbation

- Patient will implement self-management plan.
- 'Traffic light' management plans as seen in the community can be used in secure settings with some modifications (e.g. call medical staff urgently rather than an ambulance).
- Aim to discuss plans within first week of admission.
- Rescue pack medication, steroid, and/or suitable antibiotic as per local policy should be kept in the patient's cell. Consider holding named patient back-up packs in the pharmacy in case the patient forgets to re-order and experiences exacerbation out of hours.
- In the event that a patient does not have a self-management plan and rescue pack in their possession and there is no doctor on site to prescribe a rescue pack, then a suitably qualified registered nurse may give this under a PGD. This action must be followed up by referral to the GP at the next available clinic or referral to A&E if condition does not improve.

Management

See Box 6.2.

Box 6.2 Management of COPD: shared nurse/GP care

Nurse review

- Minimum of annually.
- MRC dyspnoea score (Table 6.3).
- Forced expiratory volume in the first second.
- Documentation of BMI.
- Pulse oximetry.
- Review of inhaler technique.
- Smoking cessation advice and support.
- Give local self-management plan and rescue pack (GP to prescribe) if MRC dyspnoea score is 3 or above, or at risk of exacerbation.[1]
- Review spirometry.
- Referral for pulmonary rehabilitation if MRC dyspnoea score is 3 or more but consider for scores of 1 and 2 if patient will benefit.
- Review at 12 months, unless the COPD is severe (forced expiratory volume in the first second <50% predicted) in which case it should be set at 6 months.

Doctor review

- Review of symptom control.
- Medication review in line with clinical commissioning group guidelines.
- Blood test and chest X-ray as indicated to rule out other diagnosis and malignancy.
- Need for any onward referrals to secondary care; chest physician where management needs specialist input (e.g. frequent exacerbation, need for supplemental oxygen, and need for respiratory support).
- Liaison with secondary care after admissions for exacerbation to ensure continuity of care.

Further resources

All care should be given in line with NICE clinical guideline CG101[1] and be governed by the principles in NICE guideline NG57.[2]

References

1. National Institute for Health and Care Excellence. Chronic obstructive pulmonary disease in over 16s: diagnosis and management. Clinical guideline [CG101]. 2010. https://www.nice.org.uk/ Guidance/CG101
2. National Institute for Health and Care Excellence. Physical health of people in prisons. NICE guideline [NG57]. 2016. https://www.nice.org.uk/guidance/ng57

Pneumonia and lung disease associated with drug use

Introduction

Respiratory disease is one of the leading causes of death in the UK. WHO statistics show in 2019 there were 46,766 UK deaths attributed to respiratory disease.[1] Pulmonary disease accounts for a significant number of illicit drug-related morbidities.[2] Many people in custodial settings will have used illicit substances prior to arriving in prison and will continue to do so while detained. HM Prison and Probation Service reports that positive random drug tests have increased by 50% between 2012/2013 and 2017/2018.[3] The emergence of synthetic cannabinoids has also further increased the substance misuse issues within prison settings.

Research evidence has suggested that inhalation can be 40% deeper when smoking cannabinoids compared to tobacco smoke,[2] putting individuals at greater risk of developing respiratory disease.

Pneumonia, usually caused by a bacterial infection, can also be caused by aspiration of foreign bodies or harmful substances. This can result from inhalation of adulterants along with the substances being taken and also be due to the neurological side effects of the substance used. Fungi can also be a causative agent for pneumonia from the inhalation of spores from mould, animal droppings, and soil. Individuals who use substances and those in prison are more likely to have weakened immune systems and poorer lifestyle choices, increasing the risk of disease compared to the general population.[4,5]

COPD is a common condition in middle- to older-aged adults with a history of smoking. Within the prison population, high percentages of individuals are reported to smoke prior to prison and continue to do so while in prison.[5,6] When the smoking ban was enforced within prisons, this led to some individuals smoking nicotine patches, which are much more potent than tobacco, quickening the onset of respiratory disease.[7,8]

Crack cocaine use is linked to the most common respiratory complications due to how it is prepared and taken. Individuals who smoke crack cocaine can develop crack lung, which most often occurs 48 hours after smoking crack. This is as a result of inflammation and scaring in the alveoli, leading to alveoli haemorrhage. A high proportion of crack users will report respiratory symptoms which usually improve following a period of abstinence.[2] Damage to the alveoli limits its ability to kill bacteria, therefore increasing the risk of complications such as pneumonia.[9]

Findings on clinical examination

- Shortness of breath.
- Hypoxaemia.
- Tachypnoea/bradypnoea.
- Wheeze.
- Fever.
- Pleuritic chest pain.
- Haemoptysis.
- Melanoptysis.

Investigations

- Peripheral oxygen saturations.
- Chest X-ray.
- Pulmonary function testing—spirometry where available.
- Sputum sampling—MCS where possible.

Management

- All new arrivals in prison and other detention settings should be screened in reception by a registered healthcare professional to determine their medical history, current state of health, smoking status, and drug use status.[10]
- Identify indication and risks of respiratory disease from history taking and examination.
- Undertake long-term condition reviews for asthma and COPD, supporting continued engagement in management of conditions and referral to specialist respiratory services when poorly controlled/ recurrent exacerbations occur.
- Ensure pneumococcus vaccine has been given to those in at-risk groups.[11]
- See local antibiotic formulary for prescribing guidance upon clinical diagnosis of pneumonia.
- Seek specialist management guidance from microbiology team if atypical pneumonia is suspected, or if poor response to initial antibiotic therapy.
- Drug use cessation: refer to substance misuse team upon arrival.
- Smoking cessation: access to electronic cigarettes promoted as harm reduction and smoking cessation support. All new arrivals to be offered e-cigarettes by prison service until person can be seen by a stop smoking advisor. E-cigarettes are also available for purchase in the prison canteen.[12]

References

1. World Health Organization. Non-communicable diseases: mortality. 2021. https://www.who.int/data/gho/data/indicators/indicator-details/GHO/number-of-deaths-attributed-to-non-communicable-diseases-by-type-of-disease-and-sex
2. Mégarbane B, Chevillard L. The large spectrum of pulmonary complications following illicit drug use: features and mechanisms. Chem Biol Interact. 2013;206:444–451.
3. HM Prison and Probation Service. Prison drugs strategy. 2019. https://assets.publishing.service.gov.uk/government/uploads/system/uploads/attachment_data/file/792125/prison-drugs-strategy.pdf
4. Plugge E, Elwood Martin R, Hayton P. Non communicable diseases and prisoners. World Health Organization; 2012. https://www.euro.who.int/__data/assets/pdf_file/0007/249199/Prisons-and-Health,-10-Noncommunicable-diseases-and-prisoners.pdf
5. Wright NMJ, Hearty P, Allgar V. Prison primary care and non-communicable diseases: a data-linkage survey of prevalence and associated risk factors. BJGP Open. 2019;3(2):bjgpopen19X101643.
6. NHS Digital. Statistics on smoking. England: 2017. 2017. https://files.digital.nhs.uk/publication/d/i/smok-eng-2017-rep.pdf
7. Morrissey H, Ball P, Boland M, et al. Constituents of smoke from cigarettes made from diverted nicotine replacement therapy patches. Drug Alcohol Rev. 2016;35:206–211.
8. Lardi C, Vogt S, Pollak S, et al. Complex suicide with homemade nicotine patches. Forensic Sci Int. 2014;236:e14–e18.
9. Akwe JA. Pulmonary effects of cocaine use. J Lung Pulm Respir Res. 2017;4(2):54–58.

10. Department of Health. Drug Misuse and Dependence: UK Guidelines on Clinical Management. London: Department of Health; 2017.
11. UK Health Security Agency. Pneumococcal: the green book, chapter 25. June 2022. https://www.gov.uk/government/publications/pneumococcal-the-green-book-chapter-25
12. NHS England. Minimum offer for stop smoking services and support in custody. 2017. https://www.england.nhs.uk/wp-content/uploads/2017/08/smoke-free-mso-national.pdf

Fractures

Trauma is common in the secure environment but often presents late. Poor engagement with healthcare before incarceration, educational and language barriers, and limited collateral history can complicate the assessment. Within custody there are obstacles to access such as segregation and transfers, which conspire against prompt treatment. When transfer to secondary care is indicated urgently, there is often pressure on GPs to delay. Physical therapy is commonly in short supply, and security concerns over some types of orthotics restrict their supply. Finally, patients can become frustrated and sabotage their treatment, for instance, by taking off casts prematurely.

Risk management

Robust pathways should be developed to treat high-risk injuries. Consider reviewing all elective X-ray referrals to identify those that should be fast tracked, particularly if the service relies on locums who may not foresee delays in imaging or management. Commissioners should be alerted to the inevitable delays when relying solely on external imaging, and where possible this should be performed on site. Some injuries can be prevented. For instance, HCPs should inform prison staff of people who are at risk of seizures, so they can be allocated to bottom bunks.

Red flags

Frontline staff must identify high-risk injuries that lead to irreversible harm if not treated early, and red flags such as neurovascular compromise or poor pain control that signal the need for immediate transfer. They also need training in the early management of suspected fractures, given that delays in transfer are common. Review the procurement of medical equipment such as casts, splints, and aircast boots. Particular injuries that require prompt treatment include those involving the hands, legs, and face:

Hands

- Fight bites: deep space infections can develop rapidly from puncture wounds that are easily missed. Start broad-spectrum antibiotics according to local policy. Have a low threshold for referral for surgical exploration, especially if a joint is involved or there is tracking infection.
- Ulnar collateral ligament injury of the thumb: gamekeeper's or skier's thumb is in prison more commonly caused by assault. Stress in flexion and extension and refer urgently for repair if unstable.
- Volar plate avulsion injuries: commonly arise from hyperextension. These can be simply buddy-strapped to prevent further hyperextension.
- Mallet finger: commonly a result of stubbing. Test for distal interphalangeal joint extension. Have a low threshold for immediate X-ray to exclude fracture/dislocation. These need mallet splints for 6 weeks to prevent disability.
- Metacarpal fractures rarely need referral, unless there is finger rotation, a greater than 70° angulation, or joint involvement, in which case an urgent lateral X-ray is needed. Otherwise, buddy-strap and place in a high sling for 24 hours. See Fig. 6.1.

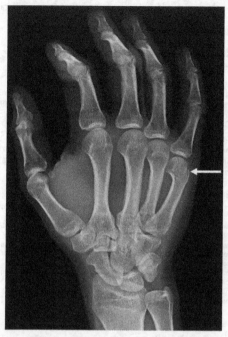

Fig. 6.1 Boxer's fracture. Reprinted from Abujudeh H. *Emergency Radiology*. Oxford: Oxford University Press; 2016, with permission from Oxford University Press.

- Scaphoid fracture: typically arises from a fall onto the outstretched hand. Consider if there is tenderness in the anatomical snuffbox or scaphoid tubercle. If the X-ray is positive, immobilize in a scaphoid cast if tolerated, or splint, ideally the Futuro type if allowed by security. If negative, splinting is required until a mandatory reassessment after 10–14 days. If still painful, a repeat X-ray is indicated: if this is negative, an MRI scan is the most sensitive test to exclude fracture, and if negative no follow-up is needed.

Legs
- Ilizarov frames: remember venous thromboembolism prophylaxis should be given until fully weight bearing. Liaise with orthopaedics about wound care to prevent deep infection.
- Foot and ankle fractures: use the Ottawa rules which state that an X-ray is indicated if there is pain and any one of the following:

- An inability to take four steps both immediately and in the trauma room.
- Bone tenderness at the base of the fifth metatarsal.
- Bone tenderness at the navicular bone.
- Bone tenderness over the posterior aspects of the medial or lateral malleolus.

Face

- Mandibular fractures: a history of assault may not always be given for fear of reprisal. Check for bony tenderness and malocclusion, and note that fractures in the region of the teeth must be considered compound: have a low threshold for immediate transfer.
- Orbital fractures: black eyes are common but always check for orbital floor or 'blowout fracture'. Double vision on vertical gaze or loss of sensation in the upper cheek and upper gums (trigeminal V2 distribution) warrants immediate referral.

Further reading

National Institute for Health and Care Excellence. Bites—human and animal. 2021. https://cks.nice.org.uk/bites-human-and-animal#!scenario

Patient. Mandibular fractures and dislocations. 2016. https://patient.info/doctor/mandibular-fractures-and-dislocations#nav-1

Royal College of Emergency Medicine. Evidence-based flowchart for the management of suspected scaphoid fractures. 2013. https://rcem.ac.uk/wp-content/uploads/2021/10/Suspected_Scaphoid_Fractures_Flowchart_Sept2013.pdf

The British Society for Surgery of the Hand. Skier's thumb. n.d. http://www.bssh.ac.uk/patients/conditions/32/skiers_thumb

The British Society for Surgery of the Hand. Mallet finger injury. n.d. http://www.bssh.ac.uk/patients/conditions/28/mallet_finger_injury

Infectious diseases

Management of tuberculosis in prisons

Introduction

- Tuberculosis (TB) is an infection of the lungs and/or other organs (including bones and nervous system) usually caused by *Mycobacterium tuberculosis* (occasionally by other species such as *M. bovis* or *M. africanum*).
- Airborne droplet transmission occurs from persons with pulmonary TB.[1] Initial infection may be eliminated, remain as latent TB infection (LTBI), or progress to active TB over the following weeks or months.
- Prison populations in both low- and high-income countries are high-risk groups for TB with infection and disease rates three to more than 80 times higher compared to national averages.[2] The number of TB cases in prisons in the WHO European Regions is declining (15,461 in 2014 compared to 12,116 in 2016), but the rate in 2016 was still 25 higher than the general population.[3]
- A disproportionate number of people in prison arise from population groups with a higher prevalence of risk factors for TB including alcohol and drug addiction, mental illness, homelessness, and prior imprisonment.
- Poor nutritional status (linked to drug use) and higher prevalence of BBV infections (particularly HIV) commonly accelerate progression from LTBI to TB disease.
- Prison settings facilitate respiratory transmission of TB due to confined spaces, reduced ventilation, overcrowding, and security considerations given precedence over infection control.

Early detection and diagnosis

- On entry to prison, all people should be questioned regarding prior/current TB, and screened to detect active pulmonary TB using clinical signs and symptoms (Table 7.1). If symptomatic:
  - Urgently isolate in a single cell/room and assess medically.
  - Initiate diagnostic tests (Table 7.2)—collect sputum samples; request urgent chest X-ray.
  - Consult TB specialist.
- People presenting with TB symptoms later during imprisonment are isolated and assessed as above.
- In addition to entry screening, consider undertaking periodic active screening of the entire prison population to detect active TB. Use digital chest X-ray and/or sputum samples for culture.
- Screening for LTBI in asymptomatic people in prison with risk factors for prior exposure or rapid progression to TB disease is indicated.

Table 7.1 Clinical signs and symptoms of TB

General	Pulmonary
Fever, night sweats	Cough lasting >3 weeks
Poor appetite, weight loss	Productive cough (might be bloody)
Tiredness, lack of energy	Shortness of breath, chest pains

Table 7.2 Diagnostic tests for active TB disease (pulmonary)

Test	Use
Chest X-ray	Screening for TB, follow up with sputum culture
Sputum smear microscopy	Rapid detection of highly infectious cases. Follow up with culture. Consider PCR for rapid identification
Liquid culture (sputum) and DST	Active TB disease diagnosis. Confirm drug sensitivities
PCR (sputum)	Active disease diagnosis, drug resistance (rifampicin). Less sensitive but faster than culture

DST, drug susceptibility testing; PCR, polymerase chain reaction (molecular amplification).

Treatment and case management

- Confirmed TB cases should be placed on clinical hold (and unfit for court) in isolation until treatment concordance has been established for more than 2 weeks and no longer infectious. A surgical mask should be worn by the patient when briefly leaving isolation.
- Treatment should be by a TB specialist, taking into consideration bacterial drug resistance and patient characteristics. HIV testing should be offered to all TB patients.
- TB (including LTBI) treatment should always be given by directly observed therapy and never in-possession. Regular assessment of adherence and treatment response is essential to ensure patients are recovering and remaining non-infectious.
- Patients with risk factors for multiple drug-resistant (MDR) TB (prior TB treatment/non-compliance, prior residence in countries with high incidence of MDR-TB, HIV infection, and known contact of MDR-TB) require hospital admission for isolation and specialist treatment.
- Newly diagnosed pulmonary TB cases should be notified to the local public health team and close contacts with the case when infectious should be assessed for symptoms and offered testing for LTBI using interferon-gamma release assay (IGRA) blood tests. Close contacts include those sharing the same cell, educational classes, religious groups, gym, and work, and prison staff.

Discharge and transfer

- Prison healthcare staff should plan drug supply and adherence continuity and clinical follow-up of people released from prison (with TB disease or LTBI) by community TB services—including transfer of medical notes. Clear communication is required.
- Careful planning and transfer of medications also applies to people transferred to other prisons (or court hearings).

References

1. Hawker J, Begg N, Blair I, et al. Communicable Disease Control and Health Protection Handbook, 3rd ed. Chichester: Wiley-Blackwell; 2012.
2. Dara M, Chadha SS, Melchers NV, et al. Time to act to prevent and control tuberculosis among inmates. Int J Tuberc Lung Dis. 2013:17(1):4–5.
3. World Health Organization Regional Office for Europe. The global burden of tuberculosis in prisons. In: Good practices in the prevention and care of tuberculosis and drug resistant tuberculosis in correctional facilities, pp. 3–7. Copenhagen: World Health Organization; 2018. https://www.euro.who.int/__data/assets/pdf_file/0003/360543/TB-prisons-9789289052917-eng.PDF

HIV care in prisons

The people most at risk of HIV infection in a country are often those within the walls of secure environments. People who use drugs (and their sexual partners), commercial sex workers and those trafficked for sex, and migrants from high-prevalence countries make up a vast proportion of the population of prisons and immigration removal centres (IRCs).

HIV is a treatable condition, and if taken in an appropriate regimen, antiretroviral treatments can reduce the risk of transmission to effectively zero. Despite this, stigma surrounding HIV is rife within prisons—both among those detained and staff. As well as stigma, there are many structural barriers to testing and treatment such as lack of access to care within prisons, poor knowledge of the signs of HIV infection, and unavailability of operational staff to facilitate access to external appointments.

HIV care is not just about highly complex and specialized treatment regimens. Healthcare staff in prisons play a vital role in preventing the spread of HIV, delivering holistic care for the health and well-being of people living with HIV infection, and challenging stigma.

Health promotion and harm reduction

Conditions within prisons are a catalyst for the spread of HIV. Widespread drug use coupled with a lack of access to clean equipment ('works') for injecting and snorting means that works are often regularly shared between many people. Tattooing and piercings using unsterile equipment is common practice. Be frank about the fact that sexual relationships and sexual violence do occur in prisons, and condoms are a rare commodity.

- Challenge stigma and misinformation whenever you hear it, and promote the use of person-centred language:
  - HIV infection, not AIDS virus (AIDS is a diagnosis, not an infection, and cannot be transmitted).
  - People living with HIV, not HIV patient/person/carrier.
  - Never use the word infected—contracted, acquired, and diagnosed with are more appropriate terms.
- Talk to patients about new tattoos or piercings, particularly about safe practice in terms of handwashing, single use and safe disposal of sterile equipment.
- Offer condoms to everyone, without asking if they need them. Never ration supplies of condoms, or insist on proof of use.
- If clean works are not freely available within the establishment, link the patient in with an expert drug and alcohol worker who can support them in using drugs as safely as possible.

Testing

Opt-out BBV testing has been in place throughout prisons and IRCs in England since 2014 and this approach has vastly increased the uptake of testing. In 2018/2019, 57,635 people in prisons were tested for HIV and 665 infections identified; however, this still only equates to test coverage of 34% of the total prison population in England.

- Everyone within a prison should at least be offered a test for HIV as part of a general BBV screen, especially new transfers and arrivals.

- Use an opt-out approach to offer testing—'We test everyone for BBVs, is that OK with you?' Challenge poor practice among staff and keep asking patients who decline, exploring their reasons why (see Reception and first night screening, p. 82).
- Repeat testing will be required for people who are at ongoing risk of HIV.
- It is the job of the testing clinician to deliver the results of the HIV test. If a patient has a positive test, tell them face to face and as soon as possible. Staff from drugs and alcohol services or local HIV services will be able to provide help to you and the patient during this consultation, either on the phone or by attending the appointment in person.
- BBV testing should sit alongside TB and STI testing (see Management of tuberculosis in prisons, p. 146, and Sexually transmitted infections, p. 64).

Care

HIV care will be overseen by a HIV specialist. Be aware of the local pathways for rapid referral. In-reach services may be available to facilitate initiation and monitoring of HIV treatment.

- Your patient's right to confidentiality must be strictly enforced. Make this explicit to operational staff who may be present during consultations.
- Continuity of care is absolutely critical for managing patients living with HIV. Patients should have a reliable, continuous supply of antiretrovirals and support from HIV specialists. Plan ahead and prepare for potential interruptions due to transfers between wings or prisons, attendance of court dates or other external appointments, or security lock downs.
- Ensure attendance of external appointments with a HIV specialist is prioritized when allocating escorts.
- Discuss with the patient and pharmacy the best way of ensuring that the patient can reliably access their medication. Ensure patients leave prison with a sufficient supply of medication.
- Drug interactions between antiretrovirals and other medications are common. The HIV specialist team will be able to support you in co-prescribing for other conditions, and there are a wealth of resources online (e.g. https://www.hiv-druginteractions.org/).
- Be mindful that some antiretrovirals have street value for recreational use. In-possession medication may still be the safest and most appropriate option for patients, despite this.
- A often have side effects which make sharing a cell inappropriate (e.g. diarrhoea and vomiting).
- Management of side effects antiretrovirals.
- Ensure patients have access to drug and alcohol support (see Substance misuse, p. 203).
- Peer support available in prisons for people living with HIV?
- The close living arrangements and difficulties in maintaining hygiene mean that infectious diseases spread quickly within prisons. People living with HIV will be more susceptible to these. As well as following recommendations from the patient's HIV team on preventative vaccinations, discuss appropriate nutrition, cleaning, and personal

hygiene with your patient (see Nutrition and activity in secure settings, p. 60).

Further reading

British HIV Association. Current guidelines. n.d. https://www.bhiva.org/guidelines

British HIV Association. Standards of care for people living with HIV 2018. 2018. https://www.bhiva.org/standards-of-care-2018

Enggist S, Møller L, Galea G, et al. (eds). Prisons and Health. Copenhagen: World Health Organization Regional Office for Europe; 2014. https://www.euro.who.int/__data/assets/pdf_file/0005/249188/Prisons-and-Health.pdf

UK Health Security Agency. HIV in the United Kingdom. Last updated February 2021, https://www.gov.uk/government/publications/hiv-in-the-united-kingdom

Chickenpox and shingles

Introduction

Chickenpox is a highly infectious disease caused by the varicella zoster virus (VZV). Transmission is via respiratory droplet spread or direct personal contact with an average incubation period of 7–21 days.

- The infectious period is between 48 hours prior to the onset of the rash until crusting of lesions.
- Chickenpox commonly presents as mild disease in children, but can cause more serious illness in adults, especially pregnant women and immunocompromised individuals. Chickenpox outbreaks occurring in custodial settings present particular infection prevention and control challenges, with high levels of occupancy, vulnerable individuals, and social mixing in close quarters.[1]

Chickenpox outbreaks are more common and problematic in immigration detention settings or in prisons with higher numbers of foreign-born people in prison due to the higher susceptibility to chickenpox among foreign-born and detainee populations because:

- people from rural tropical and subtropical regions are less likely than those from temperate zones to contract chickenpox as children, resulting in susceptibility in adulthood (sixfold higher susceptibility than Western European adults)
- infants and children, the group most likely to be diagnosed with chickenpox, are located in some prisons and places of detention
- increased prevalence of vulnerability to serious illness resulting from chickenpox in some detention populations (e.g. people living with HIV or AIDS, pregnant women, and immunosuppressed people).

Shingles, or herpes zoster, is infectious; however, it is less infectious than chickenpox. It is caused by reactivation of previous VZV infection, which can lie dormant in nerve cells. Shingles is more common in the elderly and the immunosuppressed and presents with blisters in a localized area of skin supplied by the nerve in which the virus has been dormant.[1]

Clinical features of chickenpox

- See Fig. 7.1.
- Vesicular rash starting on the face and scalp, spreading to the trunk and limbs.
- Rash may be preceded by fever and malaise.
- Usually self-limiting.
- Complications in adults include pneumonia, hepatitis, and encephalitis. These may be more common in adults in detention settings due to underlying health issues and co-infection with hepatitis B/C or HIV.

Disease transmission

- Chickenpox is highly infectious. Shingles is also infectious, in terms of spreading the VZV, but less so. Humans are the only reservoir of infection.
- The infectious period for chickenpox is between 48 hours prior to the onset of the rash until crusting of lesions. For shingles (where the rash is

on an exposed site), the infectious period is from the onset of the rash until crusting of lesions.
- Chickenpox can be transmitted directly by person-to-person contact or by airborne droplet spread from a case.
- Spread can also occur from a shingles case if the lesion is on an exposed site and there is direct contact of the blister fluid with a susceptible person.
- Articles of clothing, bed linen, or furniture recently contaminated with discharges from vesicles or mucous membranes may also spread infection.
- *Significant exposure definition*—where all of the following three criteria are met, exposure to VZV is considered to be significant:
  1. Type of infection in the case (chickenpox vs shingles). The case must be clinically assessed by a doctor and chickenpox or shingles must be a probable diagnosis.

(a)

(b)

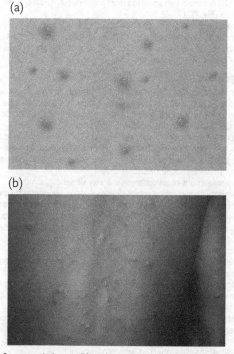

Fig. 7.1 Stage two chickenpox (blisters) presenting on (a) white skin and (b) dark brown skin. Images from https://www.nhs.uk/conditions/chickenpox/ © Crown Copyright. See plate section.

2. Timing of the exposure in relation to the onset of rash in the case: the exposure must take place during the period of communicability, that is, from 48 hours before the development of the rash until it has crusted over for chickenpox, or from rash onset to crusting of lesions for shingles.
3. Closeness and duration of contact with the case: being in the same room for 15 minutes or more with a case of chickenpox, or face-to face contact with a case of chickenpox, or direct contact with a shingles rash on an exposed part of the body when the lesions have not yet crusted over.

Investigations

- Usually clinical diagnosis but this may be unreliable especially in immigration detention settings so confirmatory diagnostic testing is recommended.[1]
- For public health and infection control management, laboratory confirmation via polymerase chain reaction (PCR) may be appropriate. VZV DNA should be requested from a sample of fluid from the base of a vesicle (Fig. 7.2).
- VZV antibody test (immunoglobulin G/M) on a blood sample is not recommended for diagnosis of chickenpox because of the timing of appearance of the antibody and the difficulty in interpreting results if test is not done at the correct time.

Management

- A suspected case of chickenpox or shingles should be isolated while awaiting prompt medical assessment of diagnosis and should be notified immediately to the local health protection team (HPT) based on clinical suspicion alone (without awaiting confirmatory tests).
- Isolation of cases should continue until the lesions have crusted over.
- Following discussion with the HPT, vulnerable contacts who are susceptible and have had significant exposure, may be offered varicella zoster immunoglobulin (VZIG).
- The management of an outbreak will vary depending on the circumstances and may warrant closure and/or restriction following advice from the HPT. A single case does not usually warrant closure to admissions. But a confirmed outbreak will require closure of part of, or quarantine of, the whole prison/centre for 21 days from onset of symptoms in the last case.
- Probable/confirmed cases should be cared for by immune/immunized healthcare and detention staff. Ideally, all staff in higher-risk settings should have their immune status checked prior to employment and offered vaccination if non-immune and if they have no contraindications—this is to prevent infection of and transmission by staff working in detention settings.
- Aciclovir may be considered in an immunocompetent adult who presents within 24 hours of rash onset, particularly for those with severe chickenpox or at increased risk of complications. If serious complications are suspected, admit to hospital.[2]

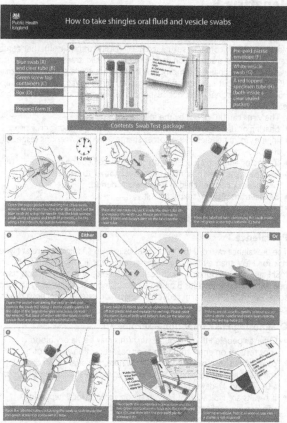

Fig. 7.2 How to take chickenpox oral fluid and vesicle swabs. Reproduced from Guidance on Infection Control for Chickenpox and Shingles in Prisons, Immigration Removal Centres and other Prescribed Places of Detention. Public Health England, 2017, under the Open Government Licence v3.0. See plate section.

References

1. Public Health England. Guidance on infection control for chickenpox and shingles in prisons, immigration removal centers and other prescribed places of detention, 4th ed. August 2017. https://assets.publishing.service.gov.uk/government/uploads/system/uploads/attachment_data/file/648640/guidance_on_infection_control_for_chickenpox_and_shingles_in_prisons.pdf

2. National Institute for Health and Care Excellence. Clinical knowledge summaries: chickenpox. 2022. https://cks.nice.org.uk/chickenpox

Hepatitis B

Transmission

Hepatitis B virus (HBV) is highly transmissible via body fluids. Routes include blood-to-blood contact, sexual contact (easily transmitted), horizontal early childhood transmission, and mother-to-child transmission (vertical transmission; globally common). It is many times more transmissible than HCV and HIV but can be prevented entirely through vaccination (although ~5–15% of vaccinees will not respond). Survives out of the body for at least 7 days.

The virus can be spread by the following routes:

- Sharing or use of contaminated equipment during injecting drug use.
- Injuries from needlesticks or other sharps, including weapons (especially if blood-stained).
- Tattooing and body piercing with contaminated equipment.
- Vertical transmission from an infectious mother to her fetus during pregnancy or to her child in the perinatal period.
- Sexual transmission/sexual assault.
- Receipt of infectious blood (via transfusion) or infectious blood products (e.g. clotting factors).

Prevalence

The prevalence rate of HBV in UK prisons is ~1.6%.[1] Migrants are at higher risk for HBV than almost any other group; people who inject drugs and MSM are also important. *Note*: cell, household, and sexual contacts of people who have hepatitis B must be tested, and vaccinated, as a matter of some urgency. Offer harm reduction advice and refer to infectious disease gastroenterology or hepatology service.

Diagnosing HBV infection—serology

- Offer all people HBV opt-out testing (this may be via dry blood spot testing) on entry to prison at or near reception as part of comprehensive screening for BBVs. To note, the offer of vaccination should not await serology results and the vaccine should be offered on a 0-, 7-, and 21-day schedule.[2]
- If results are indicative of HBV infection, refer to local hepatology services for confirmation of diagnosis, further investigation, and treatment as a matter of priority.
- Ensure that people living with HBV have access to appropriate counselling and information on how to prevent further spread of infection.

Prevention

- *Note*: vaccinate all people in prison using the accelerated schedule unless they are known to have HBV (in which case, confirm serologically and refer to secondary care) or to be immune.
- For those living with HIV, consider the following when reviewing need for HBV vaccination:
  - For patients with CD4 cell counts greater than 500 cells/μL, or where compliance for a full course is doubtful, consider an ultra-rapid

vaccination course (three standard dose administrations over 3 weeks).[3]
- For patients whose HIV status is unknown on reception, give the first dose but also monitor to check the CD4 cell count and to assess for treatment needs that may not be immediately obvious.
- All staff in prisons should be vaccinated. Vaccinations are outlined in the 'Green Book'.[2]

Post-exposure prophylaxis

In the event of exposure to a person living with hepatitis B (e.g. a bite, unsterile tattoo, or sharing of injecting equipment), the exposed person should be assessed as to whether post-exposure prophylaxis in the form of vaccination and/or immunoglobulin is required.
- Determine whether a significant exposure has occurred:
  - Penetrating skin injury (needle-stick or human bite (saliva likely to contain blood)).
  - Exposure of mucous membranes or contamination of an open wound to blood/saliva/other bodily fluids containing visible blood.
- Immediately wash area with copious amount of water and soap.
- Encourage free bleeding.
- Do not scrub, suck, or use antiseptics.
- Next step: refer to A&E or manage in-house if possible.

Patient advice

- Reassure patients that HBV is a controllable infection; that there are well-tolerated treatments but that many people don't need them.
- Advise against alcohol, or to minimize use, while they have the infection, which is likely to be lifelong.
- If diagnosed in adulthood, there is a 95% chance of clearing HBV within 6 months.
- Advise your patient that they need monitoring for as long as they have the infection.
- Arrange testing for HIV and hepatitis C virus (HCV) if this has not already been done.
- Recommend a sexual health screen.
- Refer to a specialist.

Tests needed

A 'liver screen' may be ordered by secondary care:
- HIV.
- HCV.
- Hepatitis A virus (HAV).
- HBV viral load and full serology.
- Hepatitis D virus (HDV).
- U&E, FBC, LFTs.
- Alpha-fetoprotein (at all fibrosis levels).
- Immunoglobulins.
- Autoantibodies.
- Ferritin.
- HbA1C.

- Lipids.
- Caeruloplasmin plus alpha-1 antitrypsin (if <40 years).
- Coagulation (if cirrhosis).

A FibroScan (increasingly done within prison) assesses for fibrosis/presence of cirrhosis. Ultrasound is used to check for the presence of hepatocellular carcinoma (HCC) and structural abnormalities. Secondary care may request an oesophagogastroduodenoscopy if patient is cirrhotic.

Treatment

The British Association for the Study of the Liver (BASL) recommends using European Association for the Study of the Liver. guidance.[4] If indicated, treatment should be initiated by a secondary care team. Tenofovir-DF (TDF) or entecavir are first-line drugs, with high barriers to resistance. Tenofovir-AF (TAF) is used instead of TDF if osteoporosis or chronic kidney disease contraindicate TDF. Interferon is another option in a few patients. Patients with decompensated cirrhosis need to be under a transplant team.[5]

Note: *lifelong monitoring* of liver enzymes for evidence of hepatitis, HBV viral load, which can prompt the need for treatment, and liver ultrasounds and alpha-fetoprotein for HCC monitoring, is *always* indicated for people with a positive hepatitis B surface antigen.

Long-term effects

Extrahepatic manifestations are polyarteritis nodosa and glomerular disease. Mortality derives from cirrhosis and HCC.

References

1. European Centre for Disease Prevention and Control. Systematic review on hepatitis B and C prevalence in the EU/EEA. 2016. https://ecdc.europa.eu/en/publications-data/systematic-review-hepatitis-b-and-c-prevalence-eueea

2. UK Health Security Agency. Hepatitis B: the green book, chapter 18. February 2022. https://www.gov.uk/government/publications/hepatitis-b-the-green-book-chapter-18

3. Brook G, Bhagani S, Kulasegaram R, et al. United Kingdom national guideline on the management of the viral hepatitides A, B and C 2015. Int J STD AIDS. 2016;27(7):501–525.

4. European Association for the Study of the Liver. Clinical practice guidelines on the management of hepatitis B virus infection. J Hepatol. 2017;67(2):370–398.

5. National Institute for Health and Care Excellence. Hepatitis B (chronic): diagnosis and management. Clinical guideline [CG165]. 2013 (updated October 2017). https://www.nice.org.uk/guidance/cg165

Hepatitis C

Transmission

HCV is highly infectious via blood. Routes include injecting drug use, prison tattoos, and rarely sexual contact (especially anal sex). There is a 10% risk of vertical transmission and there are no effective measures to reduce this, so pre-conceptual treatment is the best prevention of mother-to-child transmission. The virus can survive out of the body for 12 weeks, such as in tattoo ink. In general, there is a 20–25% chance of clearing each HCV infection (will occur within 6 months of infection) but reinfection can occur, even after treatment. There is currently no effective vaccine for HCV.

Prevalence

According to public health sentinel laboratory reports, the prevalence rate of HCV in English prisons is ~5.5%, which is about ten times higher than the background population. There are six genotypes of HCV: genotypes 1 and 3 are the most common in the UK with G3 accounting for up to 50% of HCV infections in the North of England, G1 is more common in the South.

Note: 90% of HCV infection arises among people who inject drugs: the remainder is found among immigrant populations.

Diagnosing HCV infection—serology

- All new arrivals in prisons need to be offered BBV opt-out testing, ideally via dry blood spot testing on entry to prison. This will give antibody results for HBV, HCV, and HIV and must include testing for the presence of each virus to confirm chronic infection.
- People who have been exposed to HCV will have a positive HCV antibody, which persists after treatment or spontaneous clearance.
- It is therefore essential to carry out a test to detect viral RNA in the blood before referring for treatment. If venous blood is sent for BBV screening, laboratory services should be commissioned to provide reflex PCR testing of antibody-positive serology results to avoid delays in diagnosis of patients requiring referral for further assessment and treatment.

Prevention

- All prison residents should be made aware of the risks of sharing drug paraphernalia, including snorting tubes and crack pipes, razors, toothbrushes and to avoid prison tattoos. Hair clippers should be sterilized using a dilute solution of bleach. Free condoms and water-based lubricant should be available to reduce the risk of sexual transmission.
- Recommend vaccination for hepatitis A and hepatitis B to reduce the risk of severe acute hepatitis in those already diagnosed with HCV infection.

Treatment and monitoring

Reassure patients that HCV is usually a curable infection; that there are well-tolerated non-interferon-based treatments which last 8–12 weeks. If patient has a short sentence, they can have the necessary tests done while in the prison with a view to treatment following release. Patients can also choose to defer their treatment until in their home environment if on short sentences or on remand. There is currently some debate over whether it is appropriate to start treatment in a patient who will be released in the middle of the course because of the risk of treatment abandonment. Where good discharge and follow-up arrangements are in place, it may be appropriate to commence treatment in patients with short sentences in order to drive the elimination agenda.

'Folk-memory' of HCV treatment

There is a received idea around HCV treatment that relates to historic interferon-based treatment that could cause debilitating side effects. Any fears about this should be ameliorated by explaining that new, well-tolerated, short-course, oral treatment regimens are now used.

Tests needed

It is increasingly common to save time by limiting the number of tests before commencing HCV treatment. A viral load (measured by PCR) and genotype are required. Unless a pangenotypic treatment regimen is provided, the treatment regimen varies depending upon genotype—usually 8–12 weeks.

FBC, U&E, LFTs, and TFTs are the basic tests, with a clotting screen and alpha-fetoprotein where cirrhosis is suspected. It is essential to check other BBVs: HIV and hepatitis B status and offer vaccination against hepatitis A (and B if not already completed).

A FibroScan (increasingly done within prison) and, if cirrhosis is present, an ultrasound to check for HCC are required. Cirrhosis should be managed in line with NICE guidance.

Note: liver biopsy is virtually never required before HCV treatment (this used to put many patients off accessing treatment).

Treatment

Active injecting is no longer considered a barrier to treatment: indeed, it is important that those patients actively spreading HCV are treated as a priority. Excessive alcohol reduces concordance with treatment, so is a caution for referral.

Note: the direct-acting antivirals have revolutionized treatment. Anecdotally, patients involved in trials for the direct-acting antivirals complained that they were on the placebo arm of their trial: they were reassured that there wasn't a placebo arm—they just weren't getting side effects.

Sustained virological response rates—effectively cure rates—are over 95%, and up to 99% depending on the genotype. Interferon is no longer used in the treatment of HCV, so side effects are now minimal: tiredness, nausea, and headaches. Ribavirin may be required in patients with cirrhosis, so blood monitoring as recommended by the local operational delivery network may still be required.

There are numerous drug interactions affecting the direct-acting antivirals, so it is important that prescribers use an interaction checker (such as https://www.hep-druginteractions.org/) if prescribing anything to a patient in treatment.

As every prison should have a treatment pathway for HCV, the use of clinical hold is not mandated, but it is essential that there is good communication to avoid breaks in treatment for patients being transferred within the prison estate.

Note: female patients are advised not to conceive for 6 months after treatment due to the risk of teratogenesis. Male patients are advised to ensure that they do not father a child during the same duration after treatment. This is especially important where ribavirin is used.

Note: it is *essential* that patients entering treatment understand that they cannot be considered cured until their blood tests are negative for viral RNA 3 months post treatment (sustained virological response). Where the patient is not cirrhotic, he/she can be discharged from care on receipt of a negative PCR test at 3 months after completing treatment. The patient should be offered harm minimization advice as reinfection can occur. If cirrhotic, they should be referred for appropriate surveillance.

> When planning transfer back to the community, it is essential to maintain good discharge planning, referral between operational delivery networks, and links with the usual primary care provider in the community.

Long-term effects

Extrahepatic manifestations include depression, autoimmune disorders, joint problems, and, rarely, lymphoma. Mortality comes from cirrhosis and HCC. It is thought that the risk of HCC is dramatically reduced by successful treatment of HCV, but a small, persistent increase in risk has not been excluded.

Outbreak management in prisons

Introduction

The main aims of outbreak management in prison settings are to protect public health by identifying the source and to implement control measures to prevent further spread or recurrence of the infection. This is achieved by reviewing the situation and placing further control measures and possibly further investigations in place for the protection of the prison community, both residents and staff, to control the outbreak. Having agreement on the approach to take, including roles and responsibilities of relevant partner organizations, is key to ensuring a swift and effective response.

Prison settings are considered a 'high-risk setting'

These settings are challenging because:

- the transmission of infection is very high in closed settings with a vulnerable population
- regular transfers between the community and prison setting, increasing the chances of infection from the community to the prison and vice versa, can easily introduce infectious agents into such settings[1]
- community prevalence of infection is introduced into the prison by staff entering the prison
- risk of complications and deaths is also much higher in this vulnerable population, with a lower baseline health status for many, meaning that outbreaks can spread quickly and have a severe impact

Examples of common outbreaks in the prisons are influenza, invasive group A *Streptococcus*, and viral gastroenteritis (or 'diarrhoea, vomiting, and temperature').

Definition of outbreak

An outbreak is defined as an incident in which two or more people experience a similar infectious illness or health-related issue linked in time and place. This can be:

- a greater than expected rate of infection/ill health compared with the usual background rate for the place and time where the outbreak has occurred (e.g. group A streptococcal infections)
- a single case for certain rare diseases such as diphtheria, botulism, rabies, viral haemorrhagic fever (such as Ebola virus), or polio.[1]

Response

An outbreak response should include the steps summarized and detailed below:

Incident notified and reviewed

- If a notifiable communicable disease is suspected or confirmed in the prison or place of detention, the governor or prison healthcare team should contact their local HPT.[2]
- The HPT, prison healthcare staff, and prison operational staff work together to assess the nature of the outbreak within 24 hours of notification.
- The HPT will assess the situation and call for an outbreak control team (OCT).

An outbreak control team is established

An OCT is established as detailed in Table 7.3. The OCT meet regularly to monitor the situation until the outbreak is declared 'over'.

Table 7.3 Typical outbreak control team members and their roles and responsibilities

Organization	Representative	Role and responsibility
Health protection team	Consultant in communicable disease control	Chairs the meeting and makes final decisions on recommendations from the OCT. Has overall responsible for the outbreak
	Public health practitioners/specialist	Support the prison team during process and usually point of contact for the prison
	Epidemiologist	Uses the data provided by the prison team and helps in following transmission within the prison with epidemiological tools, e.g. epidemiological curves
	Local microbiology team	Responsible for testing the samples from the prisons and ensuring that the prison healthcare team receive the results via a systematic and agreed process
	Administrative support	Arrange meetings, take minutes
Prison representatives	Prison governor and their operational team	Provide operational situation updates and agree on feasible recommendations based on operational issues. The governor is responsible for ensuring overall implementation of the recommendations from the OCT
	Prison healthcare team GP, head of healthcare, nurses in the prison	Ensure that residents in the prison receive appropriate medical care Inform the OCT about cases of infections with the prison and other investigations. For example: Date of onset of symptoms; Ensure necessary samples are obtained from cases and contacts
National health and justice team	Consultant in public health	Expert advice based on latest national guidance with a view to ensure that nationally uniform guidance is provided

(Continued)

Table 7.3 (Contd.)

Organization	Representative	Role and responsibility
Regional health and justice lead	Health and justice lead	Local advice based on local knowledge and support to the prison
Regional NHS commissioners	Lead NHS commissioners	Agree to the healthcare arrangements, if currently these are not available, and they agree that aspect of the service is required to control outbreak and seek further support for its implementation (outside the meeting)
Local authorities	Director of public health or their representative	Provide support to the prison as per requirement, e.g. local authorities have supported outbreak testing in prisons during COVID 19 outbreak; support infection prevention and control audit in the prison if required; in agreement with the HPT chair in cases can also chair the meetings
Communication	Press office representatives from UK Health Security Agency, local authority, and Ministry of Justice	Ministry of Justice leads on communication, and UK Health Security Agency
Ad hoc	Examples: infection prevention control services, acute trust representatives, ambulance, or fire service	Depending on the particular outbreak, other services may also be invited to support the outbreak

Review of current situation in the prisons should consider
Information about the cases
- Prison staff (usually the governor) describe the layout of the affected wings in the prison to enable the members of the OCT to understand the possible points of contact and possible route of transmission of the infection.
- Prison healthcare team provides an update of:
  - the number of confirmed cases of the infectious disease in the prison, potential cases, and contacts among residents
  - the location of the cases in the wings
  - the potential source of infection
  - any further information if any of them work in communal areas of the prison.

- Prison staff provide information about cases of infection among staff including:
  - the numbers of confirmed cases, potential and probable cases, and their contacts
  - the areas in the prison where the staff worked while they were infectious—this will vary depending on the disease
  - if there is a potential source of infection.
- The prison healthcare team usually send the details of the diagnosed cases to the HPT before the OCT. The epidemiological scientists prepare an epidemiolocal graph which illustrates transmission of the infection within the prison (Fig. 7.3).
- Based on the above information, the OCT forms a preliminary hypothesis which directs further investigation and control measures.

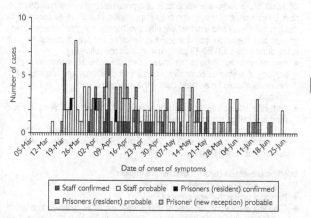

Fig. 7.3 Cases of COVID-19 by date of onset of symptoms or date of positive test result for asymptomatic people in prison and staff linked to a prison during an outbreak. Probable cases were individuals reporting one or more typical COVID-19 symptom (i.e. fever or temperature >37.8°C, new continuous cough, or anosmia). Confirmed cases were individuals with a positive SARS-CoV-2 test result. New reception is a resident in the reverse cohorting unit. Graph provided by Paul Coleman and Roger Gajraj (UK Health Security Agency). See plate section.

Risk assessment
- Based on the information received about the cases in the prison, a risk assessment is jointly agreed by all participants. It is important to remember that balancing risk is a key part of the managing the outbreak. The risk assessment usually determines:
  - whether the cases constitute an outbreak
  - severity—whether the outbreak is severe, moderate, or mild; points to consider include hospitalization and deaths
  - whether this has spread across or controlled within specific wing/s.

Control measures to prevent spread of infection
- Microbiological investigations are discussed with the OCT.
- If the team agrees that further investigations are required to understand the extent of transmission, then the following should be considered:
  - Confirm the type of investigation (e.g. laboratory tests and whole-genome sequencing).
  - Agree on who would be carrying out this investigation (usually prison healthcare team) and which laboratory.
  - Transportation of sample delivery and process of receiving test results are also discussed and agreed.

Cohorting of prison population
Cohorting is a public health strategy implemented during the COVID-19 pandemic for the care of large numbers of people who have symptoms of infection, or who are vulnerable and present heightened risk of infection, by gathering all those who are symptomatic into one area (or multiple designated areas) and establishing effective barrier control between these groups and the wider population.[3] Examples of cohorting arrangement in place during the COVID-19 pandemic include the following:
- *Reverse cohorting units*: to minimize the risk to other residents during periods of sustained community transmission, all new and transferred residents should be isolated during the incubation period of the infection.
- *Protective isolation units*: measures to isolate those who are symptomatic (and any cell or room sharers) and close contacts.
- *Shielding unit*: cohorting strategies should consider arrangements to protect those at risk of severe illness from infectious diseases, defined as vulnerable or clinically vulnerable.

Infection prevention control measures are in place
These would include considering the following:
- Personal protective equipment (PPE).
- Cleaning *and* decontamination, that is, cleaning of wings/cells and touch points including waste disposal.
- Personal hygiene arrangements are in place.
- Laundry.
- Use of communal facilities.

Ensure safe transition into the community
All individuals should be seen by healthcare services as part of normal preparations for release. Persons cannot be detained beyond their tariff. If an individual is being released from prison while they are infectious or the prison is in outbreak mode, then local public health teams must be made aware of any cases or close contacts of known cases who are returning to the community (particularly those with no fixed abode) before completing a full period of protective isolation. Probation services and approved premises/hostels should also be advised to facilitate appropriate self-isolation if the person is infectious. Community guidance on how to deal with an infectious disease will be applicable once a person leaves the prescribed place of detention.[1]

Communication
- Minutes of meeting to be documented and agreed by all members of the OCT.
- Communication format and content to be agreed for staff, prison residents, and visitors.
- Media interest in the prison outbreak to be discussed with the appropriate communication teams.

End of an outbreak
- An infectious disease outbreak in the prison and other complex settings is declared over after two incubation periods from the last symptomatic person or last positive diagnosis.
- This should be noted appropriately and all OCT members informed.

References

1. Public Health England. Multi-agency contingency plan for disease outbreaks in prisons. 2013 (updated January 2017). https://www.gov.uk/government/publications/multi-agency-contingency-plan-for-disease-outbreaks-in-prisons
2. Public Health England. List of reportable diseases to be notified to PHE Health Protection Teams by prison and other detention centre healthcare teams. March 2020. https://assets.publishing.service.gov.uk/govern-ment/uploads/system/uploads/attachment_data/file/880073/Reportable_diseases_prisons_to_HPTs_March_2020.pdf
3. Ministry of Justice, UK Health Security Agency. Preventing and controlling outbreaks of COVID-19 in prisons and places of detention. September 2022. https://www.gov.uk/government/publications/covid-19-prisons-and-other-prescribed-places-of-detention-guidance/covid-19-prisons-and-other-prescribed-places-of-detention-guidance

Infection control

Introduction

- Prisons and other places of detention are high-risk settings for transmission of infectious diseases due to the higher prevalence of infections in incarcerated populations and often overcrowded conditions in poorly designed or maintained environments.
- Disease amplification can occur due to environmental and behavioural issues including poor ventilation, overcrowding, and risk behaviours (e.g. injecting drug use), posing a risk in prison and to the wider community.
- Globally, more than 30 million people move between their communities and prisons annually. So poor infection control in prisons is a threat to wider public health (Fig. 7.4).
- Standard precautions are the basic level of infection control precautions that must be used, as a minimum, in the care of all patients. Compliance with standard precautions reduces the risk of transmission of blood-borne and other pathogens from both identified and unknown sources of infection (human, environmental, and airborne).

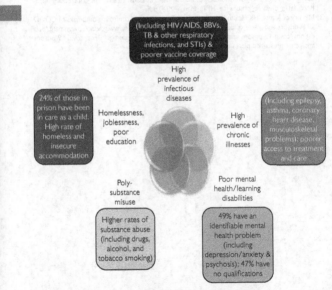

High prevalence of infectious diseases
(Including HIV/AIDS, BBVs, TB & other respiratory infections, and STIs) & poorer vaccine coverage

Homelessness, joblessness, poor education
24% of those in prison have been in care as a child. High rate of homeless and insecure accommodation

High prevalence of chronic illnesses
(Including epilepsy, asthma, coronary heart disease, musculoskeletal problems); poorer access to treatment and care

Poly-substance misuse
Higher rates of substance abuse (including drugs, alcohol, and tobacco smoking)

Poor mental health/learning disabilities
49% have an identifiable mental health problem (including depression/anxiety & psychosis); 47% have no qualifications

Fig. 7.4 Interacting factors that cause challenges for infection control in prisons. Courtesy of EJ O'Moore, 2021.

Challenges for implementation

- Hand hygiene: prisons can often lack sufficient hand washing areas where clinical care is provided. Alcohol-based hand gels are usually prohibited due to potential for abuse. Non-alcohol hand gel can be used except when hands are contaminated with blood or body fluids, when hands should be washed in soap and water.
- Soap and soap dispensers may be damaged or stolen in prison environments, impacting access to means to decontaminate hands for staff and prison residents. People in prison should be provided with appropriate basic hygiene products as well as having access to prison shops to purchase materials
- PPE: prison staff can be exposed to a range of infection threats including BBVs (e.g. through sharp injuries from hidden needles in cell searches or sharps or splash attacks), respiratory infections (e.g. COVID-19, TB, or influenza), or infections due to contaminated surfaces or fomites. Appropriate PPE recommended for specific health threats should be available to healthcare and prison staff and they should receive training in correct use of particular equipment for specific health threats (e.g. appropriate use of FFP3 respirators for aerosol-generating procedures). PPE may also be required by people in prison who undertake specialist cleaning roles—they also require training in appropriate use.
- Safe handling of sharps: sharps containers complying with UN3291 and BS7320 specifications should be available at all sites where sharp instruments are used. Prisons may wish to consider making appropriately secured sharps containers available for use by people in prison to safely dispose of needles and other paraphernalia used for injecting or tattooing or body piercing or for weapons amnesties.
- Safe handling of laundry: all prisons should follow guidelines on safe collection, handling, or disposal of laundry including any materials known to be or potentially contaminated with body fluids. People in prison may wash their own clothes in buckets or sinks to ensure they don't lose their clothes so appropriate cleaning products and drying spaces are required to enable them to clean and dry clothing adequately.
- Clinical equipment: healthcare teams should follow standard advice on decontaminating and sterilizing clinical equipment and ensure such equipment is appropriately secured to avoid misuse or loss.
- Clinical isolation and cohorting: for many infectious diseases, patients require isolation to protect against transmission of infection. This can be in single-cell accommodation or in a healthcare unit depending on need. For some high-risk infectious diseases (e.g. MDR-TB), respiratory isolation with negative pressure may be required—these facilities are scarce in most prison systems so patients may require transfer to a community-based hospital setting. Where isolation facilities are exceeded, systems of cohorting patients may be implemented. Ideally, patients should only be cohorted if there is a confirmed diagnosis but circumstances may require cohorting on the basis of clinical suspicion with signs and symptoms consistent with specific infection.

- Transport: vehicles can be a source of transmission of infectious diseases and therefore should be routinely cleaned with appropriate products to decontaminate them.
- Barbering: all people in prison performing haircuts and barbering should be trained in infection control including cleaning and decontamination of equipment and blood and body fluid spillages. People should be encouraged to hold their own hair clippers or clipper guards for personal use.
- Prevention of sexually transmitted diseases: people in prison should be able to access condoms/dental dams confidentially to minimize the risk of STIs (see Sexually transmitted infections, p. 64) and have access to genitourinary medicine services for diagnosis and treatment of STIs as well as appropriate vaccinations (e.g. HPV vaccine, hepatitis B vaccine).
- Vaccine-preventable diseases: all people in prison should be offered immunization in accordance with the UK/national immunization schedule for adults and children, including catch-up vaccinations for those with unknown or incomplete vaccination status. Some vaccines (e.g. hepatitis B) are recommended for people in prison due to the risk of BBV infection in prison settings.
- BBV testing: due to the high prevalence of infection and high-risk behaviours, all people in prison should be offered testing for hepatitis B, hepatitis C, and HIV upon reception to prisons and during their sentence especially if known to be engaging in high-risk activities.
- Tattooing: encourage conversations around safe tattooing practice (e.g. involving handwashing and site cleaning, obtaining sterile equipment, and safe disposal after use).
- Sharing of razor blades: people in prison should be provided with appropriate shaving equipment including disposable single-use razors which are not shared to minimize the risk of BBV transmission.
- Food safety and hygiene: many people in prison work in kitchens as food handlers and should be appropriately trained in food safety and hygiene. Food handlers should report any symptoms of nausea, vomiting, diarrhoea, or fever to avoid transmission of food-borne infections. Such individuals should be excluded from work until 48 hours symptom free and ideally have appropriate diagnostic tests for infection to support work on preventing or managing food-borne outbreaks. People in prison with open sores on their hands/arms must be prohibited from working until their wounds have healed, or can be covered, or when 48 hours free from symptoms.
- Chlorine-based/bleach disinfectant tablets should be made available for use in disinfecting and deep cleaning areas following a gastrointestinal outbreak as well as for other infection control purposes.
- Identification of infectious disease: people should be asked on reception about symptoms of infectious disease such as TB and at-risk factors for hepatitis B, hepatitis C, and HIV.

Chapter 8

Mental health

Mental health in prisons: overview

- Mental illness is much more common in people in prison than in the general population.
- Depression, psychosis, and substance misuse have the strongest evidence of an increased prevalence compared to people in the community.

Prevalence of mental health problems

Many epidemiological studies have consistently identified that the prevalence of certain mental health problems is considerably higher in people in prison than in the general population. The evidence is strongest for major depression and psychotic illnesses, with one in seven people in prison suffering from at least one of these conditions. The rates for these disorders is two to four times higher compared to the general population.[1] Substance misuse has also been identified as having a much higher prevalence in this population, with high comorbidity with mental illness. Comorbidity has been linked to negative outcomes including poorer prognosis and a greater likelihood of reoffending on release. A number of studies have also suggested higher rates of a range of other diagnoses, including personality disorders (PDs), ADHD, and learning disability, although methodological issues, such as reliance on self-report, mean that overestimates are commonly reported.[2] A recent systematic review found prevalence rates of TBI ranging from 10% to 100%, with an average rate of 46%, but noted that the level of evidence was poor and it was not possible to draw conclusions about the impact on criminality.[3]

Prison mental health services

Prison mental health services should aim to provide a similar level of care to that available in the community. Most mental illness can be treated within prison, but there is usually the option to transfer people to hospital for treatment if necessary. Mental health assessment and treatment takes place within a range of contexts within prison, including screening at first arrival (or reception) to prison, prison primary care services, secondary care services (including 'mental health in-reach' teams in England and Wales), and inpatient services within a dedicated healthcare area. People who are unable to be successfully treated within the prison may need to be transferred to a mental health hospital for a period of further assessment and/or treatment under provisions of the Mental Health Act or similar mental health law outside England and Wales.

Levels of care

Most prisons will screen new arrivals using a standardized questionnaire, which aims to identify relevant health conditions and initiate or continue treatment, including ensuring that medications are correctly prescribed. Screening also seeks to triage those at risk of self-harm or suicide, so that preventative and supportive mechanisms can be considered. Some prisons will provide specialized areas for new arrivals identified to be at high risk, in an attempt to make the experience less stressful. People can move frequently between prisons during a single sentence and should be screened at each new prison.

Several tiers of healthcare exist in most prisons, although the exact nature of services varies between institutions. Primary care services are often led by a combination of GPs and nurses, who provide more basic interventions, such as prescribing, health education, and simple crisis intervention. Secondary care services aim to offer an equivalent level of support that community mental health teams provide and those people in prison who have been under such community teams will usually be referred to secondary care. Secondary care services have access to a wider range of multidisciplinary professionals, including psychiatrists and psychologists.

Some prisons will not have their own inpatient facility, although all will have access through inter-prison transfer. Advantages of inpatient admission include closer observation, reduced access to substances of misuse, and better supervision of medication. At all levels of care, there should be liaison between the relevant health practitioners to ensure that the mental and physical health needs of people in prison are met. The decision to escalate to an inpatient admission or referral elsewhere will usually be taken by the specialist mental health team.

References

1. Fazel S, Danesh J. Serious mental disorder in 23000 prisoners: a systematic review of 62 surveys. Lancet. 2002;359(9306):545–550.
2. Fazel S, Hayes AJ, Bartellas K, et al. Mental health of prisoners: prevalence, adverse outcomes, and interventions. Lancet Psychiatry. 2016;3(9):871–881.
3. Durand E, Chevignard M, Ruet A, et al. History of traumatic brain injury in prison populations: a systematic review. Ann Phys Rehabil Med. 2017;60(2):95–101.

Mental health assessment

The assessment of the mental health needs of people in prison encompasses a wide range of settings and should be a continuous process throughout incarceration, and liaison with community services, if required on release, should be considered. A whole person and life-course approach should be adopted that views healthcare needs in the context of their previous history, rather than just viewing symptoms in isolation.[1]

Screening

Key questions to ask:
- Known psychiatric diagnoses.
- Previous contact with mental health services.
- Substance use history.
- Previous self-harm and suicide attempts.
- Current suicidal thoughts and intent.
- Use of psychiatric medications, including adherence.

The screening process usually starts at reception, where health is routinely screened as part of the admission process on a person's arrival at a new prison. A range of brief screening tools exist to identify people who may require further mental health assessment.[2] A wide range of factors will usually be considered, including known diagnoses and currently prescribed medication, previous use of alcohol and other substances, and risks of self-harm and suicide. The period immediately following reception can be a particularly vulnerable one for a number of reasons. Adjustment to the new environment can be challenging, especially if it is the individual's first time in prison. Withdrawal from drugs or alcohol can be a significant concern. It is essential to ensure that medications are correctly prescribed, as this can be easily overlooked or incomplete, resulting in an increased risk of withdrawal effects and relapse. The risk of suicide is higher during the first days of any prison stay. The overall risk of suicide has been estimated to be four to seven times that of the general population in European countries. Self-injurious behaviour has been reported to be present in around 5% of males and 20% of females in prison over a 1-year period in England and Wales. Those identified as a concern should undergo a second-stage mental health assessment within 7 days.[3]

Emergency situations

Guidelines from the BMA recommend that healthcare staff should only be involved in restraint when this is for the purposes of safeguarding a person's health and not for security reasons.[4] Rapid tranquilization should only be used in areas where CPR is available. The UK's Quality Network for Prison Mental Health Services states that providers should have a clear policy on rapid tranquilization, which includes guidelines on issues of consent.[5] Rapid tranquilization cannot be administered against someone's will under mental health legislation in many circumstances and its use will usually be reserved for cases where serious harm is likely to result without its use.

Assessment during a period of incarceration

Concerns can be raised from a variety of sources to initiate a specialist assessment of a person's mental health. Prison officers may become alerted to unusual behaviour or people in prison can usually request an appointment themselves. Depending on factors such as the medical history, apparent level of need, and services available, the assessment can be undertaken by a variety of health professionals in a range of settings. Assessments can take place in outpatient clinics, on the wings, in segregation units, or in the inpatient healthcare unit.

Conducting the assessment

All assessments should follow the core principles of mental health assessment and cover elements relevant to the prison context:
- Comprehensive history and mental state examination.
- Single or shared cell.
- Location within the prison—ordinary location, healthcare, or segregation unit.
- Collateral history, such as a prison officer or healthcare nurse.
- Occupation on the wings, such as work or education.
- Criminal history (especially if considering referring someone for hospital transfer, as this may determine the required level of security).
- Risk assessment for suicidality, including previous history and current risk factors.
- Consider the need to initiate or continue a suicide risk management plan (currently known in the UK as the Assessment, Care in Custody and Teamwork (ACCT) procedures).

Practical considerations

It is important to maximize confidentiality wherever possible, but this may be challenging due to the limited availability of suitable consulting spaces or the need for officers to accompany a person identified as being high risk. It is usually preferable to ask an officer to wait outside during a consultation, if security risk allows. Alternatively, it may be better to arrange for a consultation to take place in a more appropriate environment, such as the healthcare unit, where confidentiality can be established. There can be periodic restrictions on the movement of individuals around the prison, which may interfere with scheduled appointment times. Some people may have communication difficulties related to language differences, a learning disability, or sensory impairment. It is important to facilitate communication during a consultation, for example, by ensuring a relevant interpreter is present or available over the telephone, using easily comprehensible terminology, and utilizing sensory aids. It is essential to guarantee the safety of all concerned when carrying out an assessment, making sure that the whereabouts of staff are known at all times, the environment is suitable, and there is access to summon help if required.

Management

A range of therapeutic options are available in most prisons, although these may be subject to a series of limitations. The range of medications available may be more limited than those available in community pharmacies, with deliberate prohibitions or restrictions of drugs liable to be diverted or mis-used. These restricted medications can include benzodiazepines, pregabalin, amitriptyline, and quetiapine. Medications can be administered in a range of ways, from dispensing reasonable quantities for someone to keep in their possession, to administering oro-dispersible medication at the dispensary hatch, with visual confirmation of its consumption. Prescribers must be alert to the possibility of medications being diverted from their intended use and choose the method of administration accordingly. Careful atten-tion should be paid to the administration regimen, for example, prescribing medication not in-possession for individuals subject to ACCT procedures, considering the side effect profile, timing of administration, and possible pregnancy in women.

GPs should be careful to ensure that the relevant prescribed medications are continued on arrival in prison. A referral to the mental health team for a review of medication could be considered if the prescribed medication is ineffective despite adequate dosing, if there are concerns about the ap-propriateness of the indication, presence of intolerable side effects, or if there is polypharmacy of psychiatric medications. Alternatives should be considered for restricted medications, such as using antihistamines instead of benzodiazepines or z-hypnotics for insomnia.

Plan for a safe transition to the community on release, by ensuring a 'to take out' supply and informing the community mental health team and registered GP/primary care physician. This is important as high-quality observational studies have shown that antipsychotics, medications for sub-stance use disorders, and psychostimulants, if appropriately prescribed, re-duce violent reoffending rates,[6] and therefore can potentially help break the cycle of reoffending.

A number of psychological interventions are often available, but these can vary significantly between prisons. The evidence base for such interven-tions for mental health problems is limited with effect sizes typically smaller than if they were administered in the community and also than medica-tions. Individual psychological assessment and treatment may be available, although there may be long waiting lists for intensive support. Most prisons will offer some form of group therapies, focusing on common problems, such as hearing voices, managing anger, and overcoming addictions. These groups can be quicker to access, but may not be acceptable to some indi-viduals, and have been shown to be equally effective in prison to individual therapy based on trial research.[7] It is important to consider the expected date of release when planning treatment, to ensure that there is adequate time available for an individual to engage with a treatment plan. Prisoners with an established pattern of drug use and at minimum an 18-month sentence should be considered for a therapeutic community specifically for substance misuse.[3] Referral can also be considered to attend groups sessions or for individual psychotherapy. People with shorter sentences can also be encouraged to access such support if appropriate, with follow-up in the community.

Compulsory treatment and transfer to hospital

Prisons, including their healthcare units, are not recognized as hospitals for the purposes of mental health legislation in England and Wales.

Medication cannot be given to an individual in prison without their consent under the Mental Health Act, although professionals can use the mental capacity legislation and common law in extreme circumstances to involuntarily treat individuals lacking mental capacity.[8]

If an individual in prison appears to be deteriorating or seriously ill, especially if refusing treatment, then he or she can be referred for transfer to hospital for further assessment and treatment. Transfer may also be necessary if the person requires treatment that cannot be administered safely in prison, such as clozapine (for treatment-resistant schizophrenia) or electroconvulsive therapy (for severe depression where conventional treatments have not succeeded or are not possible).

The referral process involves identifying the appropriate service from the local area where the person's GP is located. The service will usually then send one or more mental health professionals to assess the individual to determine if they appear to be suffering from a recognized and treatable mental disorder, if the condition cannot be managed in prison, and if the severity is sufficient to warrant a transfer to hospital. Once a transfer has been agreed and a bed identified, in the UK, it is necessary to apply to the Ministry of Justice for a warrant. The level of security can range from a medium- or high-secure hospital to a psychiatric intensive care unit or even a general ward, depending on the perceived risk of aggression and escape.

Triage questions

- Is common mental illness present, such as anxiety or depression?
  - Consider referral to primary mental healthcare.
- Is a more serious mental illness present that would warrant treatment by a community mental health team in the community?
  - Consider referral to specialist mental health team.
- Is a serious mental illness present that cannot be adequately managed in an ordinary location?
  - Consider transfer to prison inpatient healthcare unit (if one is present).
- Is a serious mental illness present where there are significant risks and/or treatment is being refused?
  - Consider referral for transfer to an external psychiatric hospital, and at the appropriate level of security.

References

1. Forrester A, Till A, Simpson A, et al. Mental illness and the provision of mental health services in prisons. Br Med Bull. 2018;127(1):101–109.
2. Martin MS, Colman I, Simpson AI, et al. Mental health screening tools in correctional institutions: a systematic review. BMC Psychiatry. 2013;13(1):275.
3. National Institute for Health and Care Excellence. Mental health of adults in contact with the criminal justice system. NICE guideline [NG66]. March 2017. https://www.nice.org.uk/guida nce/ng66
4. BMA. The medical role in restraint and control: custodial settings. 2009.
5. Georgiou M, Stone H, Davies S. Standards for Prison Mental Health Services—fourth edition. Quality Network for Prison Mental Health Services; 2017. https://www.rcpsych.ac.uk/docs/default-source/improving-care/ccqi/quality-networks/prison-quality-network-prison/prison-qn-standards/prisons-standards-4th-edition.pdf?sfvrsn=465c58de_2

6. Chang Z, Lichtenstein P, Langstrom N, et al. Association between prescription of major psychotropic medications and violent reoffending after prison release. JAMA. 2016;316(17):1798–1807.
7. Yoon IA, Slade K, Fazel S. Outcomes of psychological therapies for prisoners with mental health problems: a systematic review and meta-analysis. J Consult Clin Psychol. 2017;85(8):783–802.
8. NHS. The Mental Capacity Act 2019. https://www.nhs.uk/conditions/social-care-and-support-guide/making-decisions-for-someone-else/mental-capacity-act/

Depression

Depression

Introduction

Depression is a common mental illness characterized by low mood, accompanied by a range of cognitive and biological symptoms. The prevalence of major depression in the prison population is higher than in the general population. The prevalence is estimated to be 10% in males and 14% in females in prison, which appears stable in most high-income countries over the course of four decades.[1] Incarceration is also linked with increased severity of existing mood disorders.[2] There is some evidence that mood disorders, especially bipolar disorders, are associated with an increased risk of recidivism.[3] Comorbidities are common in people in prison with depression, including anxiety disorders, substance misuse, and physical medical illnesses.

Clinical features

General features
- Low mood.
- Sleep disturbance.
- Anergia.
- Apathy.
- Hopelessness.
- Suicidality.
- Psychomotor retardation.
- Flat affect.

Features to consider in the prison context
- Sleep may be disturbed for other reasons, such as a noisy environment.
- Psychological trauma may underlie symptoms, especially in female patients.
- Withdrawal or detoxification from substances immediately following incarceration may present with mood-related symptoms.
- Presentation may represent acute adjustment to the prison environment, especially if it is the first experience of incarceration.
- Key symptoms that will assist diagnostically include anhedonia and social isolation, and gathering informant history will be important as some people may exaggerate their symptoms in order to be prescribed certain medications.

Investigations

- Exclude physical causes (e.g. TFTs, UDS).
- Confirm the status of comorbid physical health (e.g. diabetes control).
- Diagnostic instruments and indicators of severity have limitations in the prison context, due to lack of item relevance and limited resources to administer them. They should be used and interpreted with caution.

Management

- For mild depression, non-pharmacological approaches may include relaxation groups, ensuring access to physical exercise, and encouraging structured activities.
- Antidepressants are not recommended for mild depression.

- Antidepressants should be considered in moderate to severe depression.
- Selective serotonin reuptake inhibitor medications should be the first choice, unless contraindicated.[4]
- CBT-based group or individual therapy can also be considered, if available.
- If there is a risk of suicidality, then medications that are dangerous in overdose (such as tricyclic antidepressants) should be avoided and medication prescribed as not in-possession.
- Treat comorbidities and implement a substance withdrawal protocol if necessary.
- Consider a transfer to hospital if the risks cannot safely be managed in prison such as self-neglect, suicidality, and dehydration.

References

1. Fazel S, Hayes AJ, Bartellas K, et al. Mental health of prisoners: prevalence, adverse outcomes, and interventions. Lancet Psychiatry. 2016;3(9):871–881.
2. Schnittker J, Massoglia M, Uggen C. Out and down: incarceration and psychiatric disorders. J Health Soc Behav. 2012;53(4):448–464.
3. Chang Z, Larsson H, Lichtenstein P, et al. Psychiatric disorders and violent reoffending: a national cohort study of convicted prisoners in Sweden. Lancet Psychiatry. 2015;2(10):891–900.
4. National Institute for Health and Care Excellence. Depression in adults: treatment and management. NICE guideline [NG222]. June 2022. https://www.nice.org.uk/guidance/ng222

Psychosis and schizophrenia

Introduction

A wide range of mental disorders may present with psychotic symptoms in prison. These include schizophrenia and other schizophrenia-spectrum disorders and affective psychoses, such as psychotic depression and mania. Schizophrenia-spectrum disorders are characterized by perceptual disturbances, usually auditory hallucinations, and delusions, which are frequently bizarre. Affective psychoses will more typically present with mood-congruent symptoms. PDs, previous psychological trauma, and the effect of substances can all present with, or contribute to, hallucinations. Auditory hallucinations are particularly common in the prison population and it requires careful history taking and mental examination to determine the most likely cause—internal voices are typically not part of a severe mental illness. Visual hallucinations are likely to be caused by illicit drugs, and are rare in schizophrenia. Classically, the Schneiderian first-rank symptoms are important for a diagnosis of schizophrenia. The overall prevalence of psychotic disorders has been estimated to be around 4% in people in prison, with no significant difference between men and women.[1]

Clinical features

- Delusions—including thought alienation, passivity, and ideas of reference.
- Hallucinations—most typically third person, externally located auditory hallucinations, including running commentary and thought echo.
- Thought disorder.
- Negative symptoms, including avolition, diminished emotional expression, and blunted affect.

Features specific to the prison environment

- Behavioural disturbance may lead to administrative segregation, which may further exacerbate psychosis.
- Drugs available on the wings may precipitate or exacerbate psychosis, these can include illegal drugs, PSs, and diverted prescribed medications.
- Psychotic features may be manufactured or exaggerated for secondary gain, including a lighter sentence, to avoid deportation, for prison privileges, or to obtain a transfer to hospital.
- Hearing voices (especially inside one's head) is very common in incarcerated people and can have many causes.
- Paranoia in particular has an impact on the risk of aggression in prison.

Differential diagnosis

- Different diagnoses are more likely depending on a range of features, such as age and stage of incarceration.
- Consider illicit drugs if visual hallucinations are reported.
- Recently imprisoned people have a higher risk of substance-related psychosis and antipsychotic medications may be inappropriately stopped following prison admission or transfer, leading to relapse.
- There is a peak incidence of first-onset psychosis in the late teens/early twenties.

Investigations

- Exclude physical causes.
- Screen for substance misuse, noting that there are often limits of commonly used investigations to detect PSs.
- Refer to specialist services if you think neuroimaging of the brain may be warranted, for example, if there is a history of a severe head injury or neurological signs are present.

Management

- Antipsychotics should be discussed, if possible, between the patient and doctor together, considering the risks and benefits of each, including metabolic, extrapyramidal, cardiovascular, and hormonal side effects.
- Mood stabilizers or antidepressants may also be warranted in addition if affective symptoms are present.
- Medications should be appropriately monitored including relevant physical health parameters.[2]
- As a minimum, all adults with schizophrenia should have monitoring of their weight, waist circumference, pulse, BP, fasting blood glucose, HBA1c, and lipid levels.
- Consider prescribing not in-possession and using oro-dispersible or depot formulations if compliance or diversion are a concern.
- Clozapine should ordinarily be initiated in an external hospital, due to the need for close monitoring for potentially lethal side effects, such as myocarditis and agranulocytosis, unless the relevant facilities exist for the relevant monitoring requirements.
- Risk assessment tools, such as OxRec, can be used to calculate the risk of violent reoffending[3] and ensure that there is appropriate follow-up care on release from prison. Tools should be brief, simple, scalable, and be externally validated.

References

1. Fazel S, Seewald K. Severe mental illness in 33,588 prisoners worldwide: systematic review and meta-regression analysis. Br J Psychiatry. 2012;200(5):364–373.
2. National Institute for Health and Care Excellence. Psychosis and schizophrenia in adults: prevention and management. Clinical guideline [CG178]. 2014. https://www.nice.org.uk/guidance/cg178
3. Fazel S, Chang Z, Fanshawe T, et al. Prediction of violent reoffending on release from prison: derivation and external validation of a scalable tool. Lancet Psychiatry. 2016;3(6):535–543.

Personality disorders

Introduction

PDs are entrenched patterns of behaviour that deviate markedly from norms of generally accepted behaviour, causing chronic difficulties in interpersonal relationships and social functioning. Estimates of the prevalence of PD vary considerably in studies of prison populations depending on the criteria used for diagnosis. Studies using diagnostic instruments report rates of up to 65%; however, estimates from clinical samples are much lower, in the range of just 7–10%. This difference could be due to the overlap between diagnostic criteria for antisocial PD and the reasons for incarceration, such as disregarding social norms, low threshold for violence, and an inability to profit from experience.[1]

While antisocial PD may be the most common, a number of other PDs are also important in the prison context, including emotionally unstable (borderline), narcissistic, and paranoid PDs (which are also called 'cluster B' PDs). It is important to recognize that many of the aetiological risk factors for developing these disorders are also recognized as criminogenic, such as exposure to violence and abuse as a child. PDs may coexist with other diagnoses and may complicate the clinical picture, including substance misuse, mood disorders, and psychotic illnesses. Treatment of comorbid mental illness may leave residual personality-related pathology.

Clinical features

Clinical features are dependent on the type of PD. There should be functional impairment and onset in childhood or late adolescence, although a diagnosis of PD cannot be made until a person is at least 18 years old. Criteria and terminology differ between commonly used classifications, such as the American Psychiatric Association's *Diagnostic and Statistical Manual of Mental Disorders*, fifth edition (DSM-5) and the WHO's 11th revision of the WHO International Classification of Diseases, ICD-11, although core features are usually similar. A person with antisocial PD may present due to repeated rule violations within the prison system, resulting in administrative segregation and revocation of privileges. A person with emotionally unstable PD may come to the attention of healthcare staff, due to repeated self-harm.

Antisocial personality disorder

- A pervasive disregard for and violation of the rights of others, that is manifested in childhood or early adolescence.
- Conflict with others, low frustration tolerance, and rejection of authority.

Emotionally unstable personality disorder

- Characterized by an enduring pattern of unstable self-image, mood instability, volatile interpersonal relationships, and impulsivity.
- Repeated self-harming behaviour and aggressive outbursts may result from impulsivity.

Narcissistic personality disorder

- An enduring pattern of grandiose beliefs and arrogant behaviour.

- An overwhelming need for admiration and a lack of empathy for others, that may lead to exploitative behaviour.

Paranoid personality disorder
- Pervasive belief that the motives of others are malevolent, resulting in suspiciousness, hypersensitivity, and mistrust.
- Fragile self-esteem which lead to querulousness and disproportionate response to perceived slights.

Investigations

- There is a limited role for physical investigations, but these can be useful to exclude physical differential diagnoses or to monitor comorbidities.
- Gathering informant history and background information is important, especially to establish whether the individual's pattern of behaviour has been present since adolescence and is found in different settings (including outside prison).

Management

- NICE recommends that practitioners should facilitate problem-solving, emotion regulation and impulse control, managing interpersonal relationships, reducing self-harm, and promoting the safe use of medicines.[2,3]
- The evidence base for psychological treatments is limited for people with PDs in prison, and there is little evidence in higher-quality trials. Group treatments may offer some modest benefits.[1]
- Poor engagement can limit the usefulness of psychotherapies.
- Therapeutic communities have been adapted for use in the prison context, but are available in very few prisons and their potential role is complicated by selection biases (in that people who are referred and accepted to such prisons are likely to be older, more stable, psychologically minded, motivated, and with higher IQs).
- Pharmacotherapy has a limited role, but can be used cautiously to treat symptomatic manifestations of PD. These should be time-limited prescriptions and reviewed regularly.

References

1. Fazel S, Hayes AJ, Bartellas K, et al. Mental health of prisoners: prevalence, adverse outcomes, and interventions. Lancet Psychiatry. 2016;3(9):871–881.
2. National Institute for Health and Care Excellence. Mental health of adults in contact with the criminal justice system. NICE guideline [NG66]. March 2017. https://www.nice.org.uk/guidance/ng66
3. National Offender Management Service, NHS England. Working with offenders with personality disorder: a practitioners' guide, 2nd ed. 2015. https://www.england.nhs.uk/commissioning/wp-content/uploads/sites/12/2015/10/work-offndrs-persnlty-disorder-oct15.pdf

Attention deficit hyperactivity disorder

Introduction

ADHD is a neurodevelopmental disorder characterized by developmentally inappropriate inattention, impulsivity, and hyperactivity. There is considerable controversy around the prevalence and impact of the disorder in prison population. Several studies have shown increased prevalence in prisons compared to the community. The source of this heterogeneity may result from using screening tools developed for community use in prisons, non-representative prison samples, over-reliance on self-reports, limited access to collateral information such as school reports, and inappropriate pooling of results and statistical modelling in systematic reviews. These sources of error are likely to lead to an overestimation of prevalence in many studies. Recent high-quality studies report prevalence rates between 11% and 17%,[1] and a comprehensive meta-analysis estimated that it was 12% in boys and 19% in girls under 20 years old.[2]

Clinical features

- Core features are inattention, impulsivity, and hyperactivity.
- Symptoms of impulsivity, emotional dysregulation, and a lack of self-control are of particular importance to recognize in people in prison due to the increased risks or aggression, violence, self-harm, and suicide.
- There must be an onset in childhood, but symptoms can persist into adulthood.
- Features need to be present in more than one context for diagnosis, including both the social and academic or occupational spheres.
- At least six symptoms with onset prior to the age of 12 years persisting for more than 6 months are required by the DSM-5, which need to directly result in impaired functioning in more than one sphere.
- Diagnosis requires well-documented, continuous symptoms, with onset in early childhood.
- Collateral information is very important, including parental report and school report.

Investigations

- Physical investigations can help to exclude differential diagnoses, such as thyroid overactivity.
- Rating scales can support the clinical diagnosis although it is important to use diagnostic instruments that have been validated for use in a prison context.

Management

- Psychoeducation around the condition and the use of organizational strategies can support functional improvement.
- Psychoeducation about the nature of ADHD and the use of the treatments can lead to increased engagement with treatments.
- Medication should be offered to adolescents and adults if their ADHD symptoms are still causing a significant impairment in at least one domain, and other managements approaches have failed.

- Psychotherapy can be useful as an adjunct where symptoms remain despite medication and as an alternative when medication is declined or problematic.
- Careful thought needs to be given to the prescription of stimulant medications in the prison context, especially the possibilities for diversion.
- Long-acting formulations of amphetamine-based medications, such as methylphenidate, should be used if possible, with shorter-acting preparations avoided due to the possibility of abuse or addiction.
- Atomoxetine can be used when stimulant medication is not tolerated, ineffective, or contraindicated.[3]
- Environmental modifications, such as alterations to lighting, seating, or work patterns, may be difficult to achieve, due to the restrictive nature of the prison environment.
- Psychosocial interventions such as skills building can help prepare people for life outside prison.

References

1. Fazel S, Hayes AJ, Bartellas K, et al. Mental health of prisoners: prevalence, adverse outcomes, and interventions. Lancet Psychiatry. 2016;3(9):871–881.
2. Fazel S, Doll H, Langstrom N. Mental disorders among adolescents in juvenile detention and correctional facilities: a systematic review and metaregression analysis of 25 surveys. J Am Acad Child Adolesc Psychiatry. 2008;47(9):1010–1019.
3. National Institute for Health and Care Excellence. Attention deficit hyperactivity disorder: diagnosis and management. NICE guideline [NG87]. 2018. https://www.nice.org.uk/guidance/ng87

Post-traumatic stress disorder

Introduction

Post-traumatic stress disorder (PTSD) is an anxiety disorder which is caused by highly frightening, stressful, or distressing events. It is characterized by hyperarousal, avoidance, emotional numbness, and re-experiencing of the traumatic event (through flashbacks and nightmares). Traumatic events can be single, repeated, or multiple and can include serious accidents, assaults, sexual abuse, torture, and conflict. Onset of symptoms can be delayed, sometimes for months or years after the precipitating event.

People in prison are usually young, of low socioeconomic status, and many have been exposed to traumatic and violent events, including previous military service and child abuse. These are all risk factors for developing PTSD, which has been shown to have an increased prevalence in prison populations compared to the general population, with rates of around 6% in males and 21% in females in prison, compared to 1% and 3% in the general population, respectively. PTSD that is untreated can lead to reduced daily functioning, worse treatment adherence, and an increased risk of self-harm and suicide.[1]

Clinical features

- Re-experiencing of the traumatic event(s) through flashbacks or nightmares.
- Avoidance of situations that are related to past trauma.
- Hyperarousal, including hypervigilance, anger, and irritability.
- Negative alterations in mood and thinking.
- Emotional numbing or dysregulation.
- Dissociative experiences.
- Negative self-perception.
- Interpersonal difficulties.
- In prison, PTSD may manifest as self-isolation, poor sleep, and avoidance of certain situations, such as association.

Investigations

- There is a limited role for physical investigations in suspected PTSD, although this may help to rule out physical health problems.
- People with undiagnosed PTSD may repeatedly present with physical health complaints.

Management

- The availability of psychological therapies varies between prisons and waiting lists may be long.
- For people with less severe symptoms or shorter sentences, it may be more appropriate to focus on symptomatic relief, such as sleep hygiene and relaxation groups.
- Trauma-focused CBT can be considered for individuals who present more than 1 month after the traumatic event, although the trial evidence for the effectiveness of such treatments is very limited in prisons.[2]

- Eye movement desensitization and reprocessing can be considered for adults with a diagnosis of PTSD who present more than 3 months after a non-combat-related trauma.
- CBT targeted at specific symptoms, such as sleep disturbance or anger management, can be considered for individuals in whom trauma-focused therapy is either ineffective or poorly tolerated.
- Venlafaxine or selective serotonin reuptake inhibitors can be considered if symptoms significantly interfere with normal functioning and other approaches are not possible or have not helped.
- Antipsychotics, such as risperidone, can be used with disabling symptoms, such as severe hyperarousal, which do not respond adequately to psychological therapy.[3]

References

1. Baranyi G, Cassidy M, Fazel S, et al. Prevalence of posttraumatic stress disorder in prisoners. Epidemiol Rev. 2018;40(1):134–145.
2. Yoon IA, Slade K, Fazel S. Outcomes of psychological therapies for prisoners with mental health problems: a systematic review and meta-analysis. J Consult Clin Psychol. 2017;85(8):783–802.
3. National Institute for Health and Care Excellence. Post-traumatic stress disorder. NICE guideline [NG116]. December 2018. https://www.nice.org.uk/guidance/ng116

Management of people with a history of sexual convictions

Introduction

In 2018, individuals convicted of sexual offences comprised ~19% of the sentenced prison population,[1] of whom roughly two-thirds offended against children (either directly or via the internet). Some are located in one of the small number of prisons housing only those convicted of sexual offences, but the majority are spread throughout the prison system on both general location and in 'vulnerable prisoner units'. Only a minority take part in specialist treatment programmes. Lengthy sentences and an increasing number of convictions for historical offences mean it is an ageing population.

Clinicians should be aware of the importance of language when working with this group, shifting the focus to the individual rather than the offence—'people with sexual convictions' rather than 'sex offenders'—and encouraging others to do the same.

Assessment

- Reconviction risk is based on static risk factors such as offence history and victim characteristics using actuarial instruments.[2,3]
- Treatment needs and treatment targets relate to clinical 'domains' associated with sexual interests and drive, relationships, attitudes and beliefs, and self-management. Take time to consider what the particular drivers for the patient's offending may be[4] and what treatment/referral options are available. For example, depressive symptoms may be managed through primary care; psychosis will require onward referral to psychiatry services; and sexual preoccupation will require highly specialist input.
- Assessment of security level takes into account length of sentence, institutional behaviour, and escape risk. Although healthcare services are unlikely to be involved in decision-making around security assessments, this will be an important factor to consider when making external referrals and should be discussed with the prison team.

Treatment

- Primarily cognitive behavioural treatment can be accessed through some prisons. Arrangements can be made to transfer patients to such estates if required.
- Evaluation of 'core' and 'extended' treatment programmes published in 2017[5] showed no reduction in recidivism, leading to significant revision of programmes. Further examination of the success of such programmes is underway.
- Behavioural programmes are available through some prisons for people with a history of sexual convictions or violence. The Horizon programme targets medium-risk individuals, and the Kaizen programme high-risk individuals. Seek local guidance as to the availability of such programmes; referral and transfer to other estates to access may be possible.

- 'Adapted' programmes 'Becoming new me plus' and 'Living as new me' for people with an IQ between 70 and 80.
- Healthy sex programme designed for individuals with offence-related arousal patterns.
- Additional focus on a 'good lives' model that encourages individuals to lead 'better lives' by both identifying personal goals and encouragement of pro-social living.
- Treatment programmes are primarily focused on males (females account for <1% of sexual convictions).
- Counselling psychology services are available in some specialist sites to manage trauma issues.

Medical treatment

- High rates of medical and psychiatric morbidity in males convicted of sex offences.
- People with autistic spectrum disorder, gender dysphoria, and dementia may require additional medical input.
- There is a relatively high number of transgender people in prison for sexual offences, who may need referral to specialist gender clinics.
- See Psychiatry, Chapter 8, Mental Health Assessment.

Medication to Manage Sexual Arousal (MMSA)

- MMSA programme is available in a limited number of prisons in England. The programme intends to facilitate referral, assessment, and treatment of individuals who may benefit from medication and takes voluntary referrals only.
- It sits within the Offender Personality Disorder Pathway, but a diagnosis of PD is not necessary for inclusion.
- The MMSA programme is based on medical need rather than risk of harm or reoffending.
- Selective serotonin reuptake inhibitors are recommended where sexual preoccupation or rumination is prominent, or where behaviour is associated with impulsivity or low mood.
- Testosterone-lowering medication (cyproterone acetate) or a gonadotropin-releasing hormone agonist such as triptorelin is recommended where treatment for a high sex drive is indicated.
- Assessment, treatment, and investigation protocols are available through the MMSA programme.

What happens after prison

- Most individuals are released to 'Approved Premises' (hostels run by the National Probation Service, voluntary sector organizations, and private sector providers).
- High-risk offenders are subject to mandatory polygraph testing.
- Most people will be subject to sex offender registration and many will be subject to a range of licence conditions, such as limiting contact with victims or vulnerable groups or subject to exclusion zones. Some people may be subject to GPS monitoring.
- GP registration upon release from prison may be a challenge, especially for people with no fixed abode. Support patients in navigating the

services available to them in the locality they will be released to, in particular any services specific to homeless persons or those on licence.

References

1. Ministry of Justice. Offender Management Statistics Bulletin, England and Wales. 2018. https://assets.publishing.service.gov.uk/government/uploads/system/uploads/attachment_data/file/750698/omsq-bulletin-2018-q2.pdf
2. Helmus LM, Hanson RK, Babchishin KM, et al. Sex offender risk assessment with the Risk Matrix 2000: Validation and Guidelines for combining with the STABLE-2007. J Sex Aggress. 2015;21(2):136–157.
3. OASys Sexual Reoffending Predictor (OSP).
4. Mann RE, Hanson RK, Thornton D. Assessing risk for sexual recidivism: some proposals on the nature of psychologically meaningful risk factors. Sex Abuse. 2010;22:191–217.
5. https://www.gov.uk/government/publications/impact-evaluation-of-the-prison-based-core-sex-offender-treatment-programme

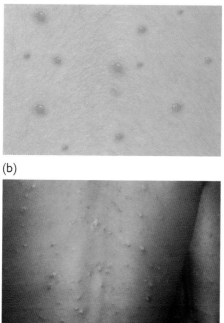

(a)

(b)

Fig. 7.1 Stage two chickenpox (blisters) presenting on (a) white skin and (b) dark brown skin.

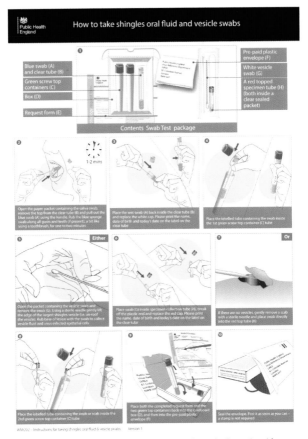

Fig. 7.2 How to take chickenpox oral fluid and vesicle swabs. Reproduced from Guidance on Infection Control for Chickenpox and Shingles in Prisons, Immigration Removal Centres and other Prescribed Places of Detention.

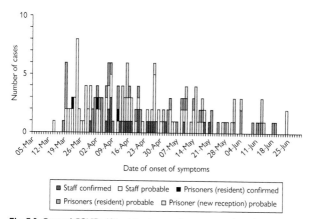

Fig. 7.3 Cases of COVID-19 by date of onset of symptoms or date of positive test result for asymptomatic people in prison and staff linked to a prison during an outbreak. Probable cases were individuals reporting one or more typical COVID-19 symptom (i.e. fever or temperature >37.8°C, new continuous cough, or anosmia). Confirmed cases were individuals with a positive SARS-CoV-2 test result. New reception is a resident in the reverse cohorting unit.

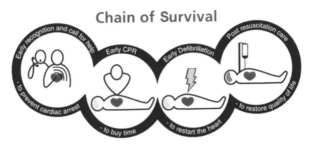

Fig. 15.4 Chain of Survival.

Safer custody

Prisons can be hostile environments. Bullying, physical assault, self-harm, and suicide present major challenges to the prison system which aspires to keep incarcerated people safe. Safety varies between prisons. This is influenced by many factors including how many people enter as new receptions and turnover (known as 'churn'), the prison regime, leadership, the culture in the prison, and the availability of illicit drugs.

The prison service in England is committed to reducing violent disorder in prisons. NHS England prioritizes reducing self-harm and self-inflicted deaths and the promotion of good health and well-being in custody.

Physical assault

Many but not all people in prison are serving sentences for committing violent crimes. Prisons represent a concentration of citizens who have experienced violence. Physical injury due to assault is common in prisons. Victims of violent crime in prisons often do not disclose the assault or injury to prison officers or healthcare staff for fear of retribution, reprisal, and being known as a 'grass', which can escalate further bullying and violence. Sexual violence and offending is also recognized as being a problem in prisons which is under-reported. There were 228 incidents reported in 2014.[1]

Homicide

In 2016, there were six murders in prisons compared with 571 homicides in total in England and Wales. The risk of being murdered in prison is approximately seven times that in the community.[2]

Self-harm

In 2018, 49,565 incidents of self-harm were reported in prisons, a rate of 585 per 1000 incarcerated people. Females in prison are at a higher risk of self-harm than males in prison.[3] Common self-harm practices include cutting, ligaturing, ingesting foreign bodies, inserting objects, and overdose.

People in prison who self-harm require careful assessment which should involve experienced healthcare staff. Self-harm is often a manifestation of emotional distress and difficulty coping and can indicate suicidal intent in some but not the majority of cases. Self-harm can be used as a behaviour or response to being denied medication or a desired outcome. PDs, mental illness, and substance misuse are often relevant comorbidities in self-harming people in prison.

'Suicide watch' is the colloquial phrase for the process used to keep people safe who are at risk of self-harm or suicide. Previously formally known as a 2052SH (self-harm) and now known as ACCT (Assessment, Care, Custody and Teamwork) this is a process supported by official documentation designed to keep at-risk people in prison safe.

Suicide

The safety and welfare of those detained is the responsibility of the state.

Self-inflicted death in custody mandates a coroner's inquest, as does any death of someone imprisoned. The Prisons and Probation Ombudsman will also independently investigate deaths in prisons. All prison suicides should be regarded as being preventable. A zero-tolerance approach to prison suicide is required. When someone kills themselves in prison, the statutory responsibility to keep that person safe has failed. Continuous improvement in prison systems and culture is required.

The highest rate recorded for prison suicide was 120 deaths in 2016, falling to 98 in 2018. The suicide rate in prison is ~15 times that of the whole population. While more men commit suicide in and out of prison than women, the risk for women is higher in prison.

NHS England health and justice regional commissioning teams and HMPPS actively seek to develop policy which makes prisons safer and reduces self-inflicted deaths. From an international perspective, the UK is mid-ranking in terms of its suicide rates in prisons. Hanging remains the most common method of prison suicide.

References

1. Sondhi J, Hinks S, Smith H. Sexual assaults reported in prisons: exploratory findings from analysis of incident descriptions. Ministry of Justice; 2018. https://www.gov.uk/government/publications/sexual-assaults-reported-in-prisons-exploratory-findings
2. Ministry of Justice. Safety in Custody Statistics Bulletin, England and Wales, deaths in prison custody to December 2016, assaults and self-harm to September 2016. 2017. https://www.gov.uk/government/statistics/safety-in-custody-quarterly-update-to-december-2016
3. Hawton K, Linsell L, Adeniji T, et al. Self-harm in prisons in England and Wales: an epidemiological study of prevalence, risk factors, clustering, and subsequent suicide. Lancet. 2014;383(9923):1147–1154.
4. Fazel S, Ramesh T, Hawton K. Suicide in prisons: an international study of prevalence and contributory factors. Lancet Psychiatry. 2017;4(12):946–952.

Segregation

Definition and rationale

Segregation, special accommodation, isolation, care and separation, removal from association, solitary, close supervision centres, cellular confinement, or 'the block' all refer to regimes where people are physically isolated and deprived of meaningful contact with others. Placement must be justified under a legal framework, most commonly 'Good Order or Discipline' or for a person's own protection. It is not intended to function as a form of punishment.[1] Segregation may also be orchestrated to transfer prison or escape debts or other aspects of life on ordinary location deemed to be intolerable.[2]

Duties

The regulation mandates a daily visit from a HCP, and only specifies a GP review every 3 days.[3] When safe, confidentiality should be facilitated by seeing the patient out of the hearing of officers. But confidentiality is not absolute; for instance, if someone states an intention to harm themselves, this information must be shared.[4]

HCPs may be drawn into procedures designed to meet the aims of the secure setting, such as discipline or judicial investigation. Despite these dual obligations, the HCP's primary obligation is to the health and well-being of patients.[4] Several international standards state that doctors should not be involved in 'fitting' someone for solitary confinement, which could be construed as collusion with discipline staff[5,6] and impair the doctor–patient relationship. UK legislation holds prison staff responsible for the decision to segregate.

Assessing mental health risk

However, HCPs have a vital role in advocating for the vulnerable, and escalating concerns about potential harm to the appropriate authority. There is unequivocal evidence of the detrimental impact isolation has on health and well-being.[7] Young offenders are particularly affected, and the BMA has called for an end to segregation in the youth estate.[8] The risk of suicide is raised threefold in segregation, with an average of ten deaths per year nationally. Half of these were on an ACCT procedure.[9] People at risk of self-harm or suicide (on ACCTs) should not be isolated other than in 'exceptional circumstances' such as 'violent or refractory behaviour',[1] and for the shortest possible time. Body belts are hazardous and should only be used by trained staff, and for the shortest possible time. Likewise, wearing tear-resistant clothing and being on constant observations via CCTV can feel dehumanizing and exacerbate distress.[1] Prisons and Probation Ombudsman reports have highlighted the inadequacy of cursory interactions between professionals and people in isolation, and an over-reliance on physical observations.[10] Active engagement with the person's concerns is key to re-integration. This plan is under CAREMAP in the ACCT documentation and updated at multidisciplinary review.[11] It might include increasing access to exercise, reading material, chaplaincy, or contact with family.

HCPs are required to perform a health screen within 2 hours of segregation. The current pro forma OTO14 highlights concerns such as drug withdrawal, psychosis, self-harm, and whether the person will 'cope' in isolation. Previous documentation and current presentation should be reviewed to consider:

- Has the person been in isolation before? Did their mental health or self-harming deteriorate?
- People with neurodevelopmental disorder are over-represented in isolation. Is there evidence of learning difficulties and disabilities? Has there been an MDT meeting to identify triggers and a care plan?
- How has the person's mental health and adherence to medication been recently? Do they need a formal mental health review?
- If there is an ACCT, are there any triggers or goals identified at a case review the HCP can help with?
- What alternatives have been considered, such as cellular confinement on the wing, constant observation cells, or the mental health unit?
- Does the person understand why they are isolated and what is needed to return to ordinary location?
- If kept in isolation, is it wise to set an early review after 24 hours?

Physical health

It is often difficult to gain access to examine patients. Work with officers to find the best time to visit, and request a handover, especially for those on ACCTs. Patients who are asleep at lunchtime may be manifesting a cause of their night-time insomnia, but care and separation units are often rowdy, so consider sleep packs as an alternative to hypnotics. Always seek verbal confirmation that there are no medical issues, and remember that all rounds may be recorded on CCTV. Not all problems can await return to ordinary location, which might be weeks away. Lack of access is not a medico-legal defence unless the HCP has done everything within their power to gain and document it. Particular risks include:

- suspected swallowed or secreted drugs: always consider transfer to hospital, which is standard care in the community
- fractures: do not delay stabilization and imaging if it would be indicated on ordinary location.

References

1. Ministry of Justice, HM Prison and Probation Service. PSO 1700. Segregation, special accommodation, body belts.
2. Prison Reform Trust. Deep Custody: segregation units and close supervision centres in England and Wales. 2015. http://www.prisonreformtrust.org.uk/deep-custody-segregation-units-and-close-supervision-centres-in-england-and-wales/
3. Ministry of Justice, HM Prison and Probation Service. PSI 17/2006. Segregation, special accommodation, body belts.
4. General Medical Council. The duties of a doctor registered with the General Medical Council. In: Good medical practice. 2013. https://www.gmc-uk.org/ethical-guidance/ethical-guidance-for-doctors/good-medical-practice/duties-of-a-doctor
5. United Nations Office of the High Commissioner for Human Rights. Principles of medical ethics relevant to the role of health personnel, particularly physicians, in the protection of prisoners and detainees against torture and other cruel, inhuman or degrading treatment or punishment. 1982. http://www.ohchr.org/EN/ProfessionalInterest/Pages/MedicalEthics.aspx
6. World Health Organization. Physical restraint. In: Health in prisons: a WHO guide to the essentials in prison health, p. 36. Geneva: World Health Organization.
7. Shalev S. The health effects of solitary confinement. In: A Sourcebook on Solitary Confinement, pp. 9–24. London: Mannheim Centre for Criminology, The London School of Economics; 2008.

8. British Medical Association. Solitary confinement and children and young people. 2021. https://www.bma.org.uk/collective-voice/policy-and-research/equality/the-medical-role-in-solitary-confinement
9. Freedom of information request to the Prisons and Probation Ombudsman, personal communication.
10. Prisons and Probation Ombudsman. Segregation. Learning Lessons Bulletin; June 2015. http://www.ppo.gov.uk/app/uploads/2015/06/Learning-Lessons-Bulletin-Segregation-final.pdf
11. HM Prison and Probation Service. PSI 64/2011. Management of prisoners at risk of harm to self, to others and from others (safer custody). 2011, revised July 2021. https://www.gov.uk/government/publications/managing-prisoner-safety-in-custody-psi-642011

Chapter 9

Substance misuse

Epidemiology

Alcohol and drug use are common in people prior to incarceration. The link between alcohol and drug use, including dependence, and criminal behaviour is well established. There is a positive correlation between substance misuse and rates of offending, and there are also strong links between alcohol use and violent crime.

The identification, assessment, and treatment when needed for drug and alcohol misuse and dependence is a priority for all prison healthcare systems.

Prevalence—use prior to incarceration

Alcohol

- Research on English prison populations[1] revealed that 87% of males and 75% of females had consumed alcohol in the 4 weeks prior to incarceration.
- Of these people, 63% met criteria for binge drinking (consuming a median amount of 12 units a day).

Of those who consumed alcohol in the month prior to incarceration, 32% stated that they drank daily, consuming a median amount of 20 units of alcohol a day.

Drugs

- In the prison population, 64% of people reported that they had used illicit drugs at some point in their life, much higher than the general population[1]:
  - Of those, 30% reported ever injecting and 27% reported having overdosed.
- Of people in prison, 55% of females and 39% of males reported ever using heroin:
  - Of these, ~80% reported using heroin 4 weeks or less prior to incarceration. Most used daily.
  - 56% reported smoking or chasing heroin and 53% injecting.
- 42% of males and 58% of females reported using crack cocaine.
- Over 70% of people in prison reported ever using cannabis with over half of those using it 4 weeks or less prior to incarceration. Many reported daily use.
- Synthetic cannabinoid use is uncommon outside of prisons, other than in certain subpopulations such as people who are homeless.

Reconviction

- People who reported drinking daily in the 4 weeks before incarceration were more likely to be reconvicted within a year, at 62% compared to 49%.[1]
- Of females in prison who binge drank alcohol, 75% were reconvicted within a year versus 37% who did not binge drink.
- Of those who used drugs in the 4 weeks prior to incarceration, 62% were reconvicted within the year versus 30% of those who had not.

Use of illicit drugs in prison

- The nature of illicit drug and alcohol use in prison varies by establishment and over time and can be difficult to estimate.
- In a prison sample of those who had ever used heroin, nearly 20% reported that their first use was in prison.
- Synthetic cannabinoids (PS) are a significant problem in many prisons and have been implicated in deaths in custody including suicides.
- Any drug given in-possession to a patient in prison has the potential to be diverted. Attempts may also be made to secrete drugs given in a supervised fashion.
- Illicitly brewed alcohol ('Hooch') remains a problem in certain prisons.

Numbers in treatment

- In the year 2017–2018, 55,413 adults accessed treatment in a secure environment[2]: 52% of the treatment population reported problematic use of opioids, with 70% of those with opioid problems also reporting problematic use of crack cocaine and 21% problematic benzodiazepine use. A further third of opioid users reported problems with alcohol.
- After opioid users the next most common primary substance that people sought treatment for was alcohol with 25,828 (47%) people in treatment.
- Of those in treatment for non-opioid drug use, 63% were in treatment for cannabis use, 49% for powder cocaine, 8% for amphetamine use, and 6% for benzodiazepine use.
- Nearly 9% of those in treatment stated that they had a problem with psychoactive substances (PSs).
- As reflected in the greater number of men incarcerated, 90% of those in treatment were male; however, problematic opioid use was only reported by 50% of the men in treatment, but 74% of the women in treatment.

Treatment interventions

- Of people in prison in treatment, 26% received pharmacological interventions for opioids, 9% for alcohol, and 4% for other drugs.
- Of those in treatment, 61% received a structured psychosocial intervention (PSI).
- The vast bulk of prescribing was for less than a year mainly due to relatively short periods of incarceration.

Young people

In 2017–2018 in England, a total of 1352 young people received substances treatment in secure settings with cannabis use interventions provided to 91% of those in treatment.[2] Interventions were provided to 47% for problematic alcohol use, 22% for nicotine use, and 16% for powder cocaine use.

References

1. Ministry of Justice. Gender differences in substance misuse and mental health amongst prisoners. 2013. https://assets.publishing.service.gov.uk/government/uploads/system/uploads/attachment_data/file/220060/gender-substance-misuse-mental-health-prisoners.pdf

2. Public Health England. Alcohol and drug treatment in secure settings: statistics summary 2017 to 2018. 2019. https://www.gov.uk/government/publications/substance-misuse-treatment-in-secure-settings-2017-to-2018/alcohol-and-drug-treatment-in-secure-settings-statistics-summary-2017-to-2018

3. HM Inspectorate of Prisons Changing patterns of substance misuse in adult prisons and service responses. 2015. https://www.justiceinspectorates.gov.uk/hmiprisons/wp-content/uploads/sites/4/2015/12/Substance-misuse-web-2015.pdf

4. Revolving Doors. Rebalancing act. 2017. https://revolving-doors.org.uk/publications/rebalancing-act/

Diagnosis

There are two main psychiatric classification systems used to diagnose issues with alcohol and drugs: the International Classification of Disease, 10th revision (ICD-10)[1] produced by the WHO and the DSM-5[2] produced by the American Psychiatric Association. For the purpose of this handbook the global ICD-10 will be used.

The two main diagnostic categories in ICD-10 are harmful use and dependence. *Important*: it is unlikely that a pharmacological intervention for alcohol or drugs would be needed without a diagnosis of dependence.

Each substance/class of substance is given a unique number code (where the dash represents the subcode) signified below for harmful use and dependence by the letter x:

• F10.– Alcohol.
• F11.– Opioids.
• F12.– Cannabinoids.
• F13.– Sedative hypnotics (benzodiazepines, Z drugs, etc.).
• F14.– Cocaine.
• F15.– Other stimulants (amphetamine, mephedrone, etc.).
• F16.– Hallucinogens.
• F17.– Tobacco.
• F18.– Volatile solvents.
• F19.– Multiple drug use and use of other PSs.

F1x.1 Harmful use

Diagnostic guidelines

The diagnosis requires that actual damage should have been caused to the mental or physical health of the user. Harmful use should not be diagnosed if dependence syndrome is present.

F1x.2 Dependence syndrome

Diagnostic guidelines

A definite diagnosis of dependence should usually be made only if three or more of the following have been present together at some time during the previous year:

• A strong desire or sense of compulsion to take the substance.
• Difficulties in controlling substance-taking behaviour in terms of its onset, termination, or levels of use.
• A physiological withdrawal state when substance use has ceased or been reduced, as evidenced by the characteristic withdrawal syndrome for the substance, or use of the same (or a closely related) substance with the intention of relieving or avoiding withdrawal symptoms.
• Evidence of tolerance, such that increased doses of the substances are required in order to achieve effects originally produced by lower doses.
• Progressive neglect of alternative pleasures or interests because of substance use, increased amount of time necessary to obtain or take the substance, or to recover from its effects.
• Persisting with substance use despite clear evidence of overtly harmful consequences; efforts should be made to determine that the user was actually, or could be expected to be, aware of the nature and extent of the harm.

References

1. World Health Organization. International statistical classification of diseases and related health problems 10th revision. 2016. https://icd.who.int/browse10/2016/en
2. American Psychiatric Association. Diagnostic and Statistical Manual of Mental Disorders, fifth edition. Arlington, VA: American Psychiatric Association; 2013.

Drug-specific harms and complications

Introduction

Drug use can be associated with many types of harm. These can include:
- intoxication, excessive consumption, and dependence
- harms associated with delivery route (e.g. BBVs such as hepatitis B and C)
- drug-specific harms.

Drug effects change depending on dose, the user's tolerance and experience, and the setting:
- Illicit drugs are used in prison, alongside the abuse of prescribed medications.
- Many illicit drugs within prisons may be mixed with adulterants or other drugs, which changes clinical presentation and response.

Commonly used drugs in prison

See Table 9.1.
- All people with prescribed medication need to have a risk assessment for issues of abuse and diversion (see Chapter 3).
- Overdosing on all drugs can result in fatalities and acute physical and psychological effects, including paranoia and hallucinations

For PSs, see Psychoactive substances, p. 228.

Table 9.1 Commonly used drugs in prisons

Illicit	
Opioids	
Cannabis	
Psychoactive substances	
Psychostimulants	Cocaine
	Amphetamines
	Methamphetamines
Prescribed	
Analgesics	Tramadol
	Codeine
	Gabapentinoids
Sedatives	Benzodiazepines
Antidepressants and antipsychotics	Mirtazapine
	Olanzapine

Alcohol

- Estimates of alcohol use disorder range from 16% to 51% in men and 10–30% in women in prison.[1]
- Alcohol is associated with many mental health problems: depression, anxiety, co-associated nicotine and other drug dependence, self-harm, and suicide.
- Alcohol can also be associated with domestic violence, parenting issues of neglect and abuse, impulsivity, financial problems, unemployment, and homelessness.
- Physical health problems are important, often dose related, and can present urgently or silently in prison. They include:
  - increase in cancer risk
  - alcohol-related liver disease
  - hypertension and cardiac problems
  - dependence with acute withdrawal
  - seizures
  - Wernicke–Korsakoff syndrome
  - related brain injury and related malnutrition.

Cocaine

- A stimulant drug from the leaves of the coca plant, more often used as powder or mixed with other drugs (e.g. synthetic opioids), or processed to make rock-crack.
- Short-term effects are usually of alertness, irritability, extreme energy, euphoria, paranoia or unpredictable behaviour, and physical effects of increased heart rate, dilated pupils, and hypertension.
- Seizures, strokes, rarely Parkinson's disease, extreme agitation, and chest pain (e.g. cardiac pain) are significant and severe effects.
- Method of use can result in problems, for example, snorting can cause chronic nose bleeds and anaemia, and injecting can lead to possible infection and virus transmission.

Amphetamines

- While these drugs have clinical use, especially in treatment of ADHD, their potential for abuse and dependence is high.
- They are psychostimulant drugs, causing excitement, increased attention, and concentration, though this is dose related.
- Side effects also include dry mouth, anxiety, grinding of teeth, sexual dysfunction, hypertension, and increased heart rate which can lead to cardiovascular events (e.g. strokes and seizures), and acute drug-induced psychotic symptoms.
- Chronic effects can be of dependence, tolerance, psychotic state presenting as paranoid behaviour and schizophrenia-like symptoms, and possible cognitive impairment.

Methamphetamine

- A stimulant drug, similar to amphetamine, used by smoking, orally ingesting, snorting, or injection.
- Effects are of wakefulness, rapid respiration and heart rate, and hypertension.

- Long-term effects are of cardiovascular events, possible cognitive impairment, seizures, Parkinson's disease, and paranoia.

Opioids

- Some people will misuse a range of opioids, including buprenorphine, codeine, heroin, morphine, dihydrocodeine, oxycontin, or other fentanyl analogues. Tramadol is used an analgesic with similar properties to opioids; dependence can develop.
- Use of prescription opioids is a risk factor for heroin use, nearly 80% of people in the US using heroin reported misusing prescription opioids first, though few people who use prescription opioids use heroin. However, prescription opioids and heroin have similar effects, though different risk factors.
- In the short term, opioids cause dose dependent effects of nausea, dry mouth, euphoria, and sedation.
- Long-term adverse effects including those related to route include venous damage, cardiac infections, lung complications, mortality related to overdose and reduced tolerance, dependence with withdrawal, and effects on liver, kidney, and menstrual dysfunction in females.
- Naloxone can treat an opioid overdose; this being given intramuscularly or intranasally. This should be available for urgent use in prisons.
- Great care is needed with prescription of opioids in prison to manage dependence, or in-possession because of the high risk of fatality to opioids either alone or in combination with other CNS depressant drugs.

Cannabis

- More often known as weed, dope, or grass, and is the most commonly used drug in the UK.
- The effects vary dependent on dose and person from relaxation, being more talkative, perceptual issues, sedation, to panic attacks, hallucinations, low mood, and anxiety.
- Longer-term effects can be of mental health problems, such as sleep difficulties, depression, irritability, increased risk of psychotic illness, and dependence in 10% of long-term users. Lung problems can occur, particularly in those who are tobacco smokers.

Benzodiazepines

- Sedative drugs, mainly taken orally, used clinically in the management of short-term anxiety and insomnia, and in treatment of alcohol withdrawal states, but can lead to dependence, with abuse of prescriptions and illicit supplies.
- The illicit supplies, frequently available from the internet, may resemble closely the pharmaceutical product but are often unreliable in terms of quality and purity.
- There are a wide variety of this group of drugs, mainly varying in length of action. The most well known are diazepam (Valium) and temazepam. Flunitrazepam is now illegal in some countries because of its association as a 'date rape' drug.

- While reducing anxiety and having anticonvulsant effects, which can be helpful during treatment, they can cause sedation and reduced respiration.
- Occasionally they can have paradoxical effects of increased unpredictable behaviour and aggression.
- Overdose can lead to confusion, decreased respirations, sedation, and particularly if combined with drugs such as opioids and alcohol can have fatal consequences, though death from use alone is rare.
- Dependence on illicit benzodiazepines is unusual, they are used more often in a binge pattern. The 'Drug misuse and dependence' guidelines[3] advise on management.

References

1. Fazel S, Yoon IA, Hayes AJ. Substance use disorders in prisoners: an updated systematic review and meta-regression analysis in recently incarcerated men and women. Addiction. 2017;112(10):1725–1739.
2. NHS Digital. Health survey for England 2017. 2018. https://digital.nhs.uk/data-and-information/publications/statistical/health-survey-for-england/2017
3. Clinical Guidelines on Drug Misuse and Dependence Update 2017 Independent Expert Working Group. Drug misuse and dependence: UK guidelines on clinical management [the Orange Book]. Department of Health and Social Care; 2017. https://www.gov.uk/government/publications/drug-misuse-and-dependence-uk-guidelines-on-clinical-management

Assessment

The substantive guidelines for the assessment and treatment for drug dependence including in prison are the 'Drug misuse and dependence: UK guidelines on clinical management [the Orange book]'[1] and for the treatment of alcohol dependence, the NICE (CG115) guideline 'Alcohol-use disorders: diagnosis, assessment and management of harmful drinking (high-risk drinking) and alcohol dependence'.[2]

Assessment

Assessment is an opportunity for a positive holistic healthcare interaction with a patient. Reception screening and subsequent clinical assessments should identify if there are any issues with substances. A comprehensive assessment should then take place at the earliest possible opportunity. The purpose is to identify problem substance use or dependence, psychological health issues, physical health issues, and any relevant social needs to inform a comprehensive care plan.

Screening tools may be of benefit in identifying needs for further substance use assessment and treatment.

- The Alcohol Use Disorders Identification Test (AUDIT) is a validated screening questionnaire for alcohol produced by the WHO.[3] It can be self-completed (Fig. 9.1).
- The Alcohol, Smoking and Substance Involvement Screening Test (ASSIST) is a validated screen questionnaire for drugs, alcohol, and tobacco produced by the WHO.[4]

The assessment should include the following:

History taking
- Alcohol and/or drug use: which substances are taken (including prescribed and over-the-counter medicines), quantity and frequency of use, pattern of use, routes of administration, withdrawal symptoms, and history of accidental overdose.
- Previous and ongoing treatment interventions for addictions, including medication prescribed.
- Physical consequences of alcohol and drug use; BBVs, hepatitis B/C, and HIV; liver disease; lung disease; deep vein thrombosis; abscess; and sexual health.
- Pregnancy in incarcerated females.
- Psychological health: history of abuse and trauma; self-harm and suicidality; and depression, anxiety, psychosis, and personality issues.
- Previous and current treatment interventions for physical and mental health including medication prescribed.
- Any relevant social issues liable to impact the person, including relationships, domestic violence, offending and the link to substance use, family issues, and financial.

Examination
- All patients should be examined physically, with special attention paid to issues raised in the history.
- Observations of pulse, BP, respiratory rate, and temperature should be taken.

Box 10

The Alcohol Use Disorders Identification Test: Self-Report Version

PATIENT: Because alcohol use can affect your health and can interfere with certain medications and treatments, it is important that we ask some questions about your use of alcohol. Your answers will remain confidential so please be honest.

Place an X in one box that best describes your answer to each question.

Questions	0	1	2	3	4	
1. How often do you have a drink containing alcohol?	Never	Monthly or less	2-4 times a month	2-3 times a week	4 or more times a week	
2. How many drinks containing alcohol do you have on a typical day when you are drinking?	1 or 2	3 or 4	5 or 6	7 to 9	10 or more	
3. How often do you have six or more drinks on one occasion?	Never	Less than monthly	Monthly	Weekly	Daily or almost daily	
4. How often during the last year have you found that you were not able to stop drinking once you had started?	Never	Less than monthly	Monthly	Weekly	Daily or almost daily	
5. How often during the last year have you failed to do what was normally expected of you because of drinking?	Never	Less than monthly	Monthly	Weekly	Daily or almost daily	
6. How often during the last year have you needed a first drink in the morning to get yourself going after a heavy drinking session?	Never	Less than monthly	Monthly	Weekly	Daily or almost daily	
7. How often during the last year have you had a feeling of guilt or remorse after drinking?	Never	Less than monthly	Monthly	Weekly	Daily or almost daily	
8. How often during the last year have you been unable to remember what happened the night before because of your drinking?	Never	Less than monthly	Monthly	Weekly	Daily or almost daily	
9. Have you or someone else been injured because of your drinking?	No		Yes, but not in the last year		Yes, during the last year	
10. Has a relative, friend, doctor, or other health care worker been concerned about your drinking or suggested you cut down?	No		Yes, but not in the last year		Yes, during the last year	
					Total	

Box 6

Risk Level	Intervention	AUDIT score*
Zone I	Alcohol Education	0-7
Zone II	Simple Advice	8-15
Zone III	Simple Advice plus Brief Counseling and Continued Monitoring	16-19
Zone IV	Referral to Specialist for Diagnostic Evaluation and Treatment	20-40

*The AUDIT cut-off score may vary slightly depending on the country's drinking patterns, the alcohol content of standard drinks, and the nature of the screening program. Clinical judgment should be exercised in cases where the patient's score is not consistent with other evidence, or if the patient has a prior history of alcohol dependence. It may also be instructive to review the patient's responses to individual questions dealing with dependence symptoms (Questions 4, 5 and 6) and alcohol-related problems (Questions 9 and 10). Provide the next highest level of intervention to patients who score 2 or more on Questions 4, 5 and 6, or 4 on Questions 9 or 10.

Fig. 9.1 (a) AUDIT. (b) Relevant interventions for the patient. Reproduced from Babor T et al. The Alcohol Use Disorders Identification Test: guidelines for use in primary care. Geneva: World Health Organization; 2001, with permission from the WHO.

- Given the high levels of comorbid mental illness in this population, a mental state examination should be carried out.
- If mental capacity concerns are identified, suitable examinations should be performed.
- If patients report injecting drug use, injecting sites should be examined and accurately documented.
- It should be noted if the patient is intoxicated or in withdrawal.

Completion of withdrawal scales

Withdrawal scales are of benefit in assessing withdrawal from alcohol and opioids and should be used. Their usefulness is both in the initial assessment and ensuring that ongoing treatment is effective in stopping withdrawals:

Assessment Protocol	Date							
CIWA-AR	Time							
Assess each morning prior to dispensing	Pulse							
	RR							
Chlordiazepoxide	BP							
Nausea/vomiting (0 - 7) 0 - none; 1 - mild nausea, no vomiting; 4 - intermittent nausea; 7 - constant nausea, frequent dry heaves & vomiting.								
Tremors (0 - 7) 0 - no tremor; 1 - not visible but can be felt; 4 - moderate w/ arms extended; 7 - severe, even w/ arms not extended.								
Anxiety (0 - 7) 0 - none, at ease; 1 - mildly anxious; 4 - moderately anxious or guarded; 7 - equivalent to acute panic state								
Agitation (0 - 7) 0 - normal activity; 1 - somewhat normal activity; 4 - moderately fidgety/restless; 7 - paces or constantly thrashes about								
Paroxysmal Sweats (0 - 7) 0 - no sweats; 1 - barely perceptible sweating, palms moist; 4 - beads of sweat obvious on forehead; 7 - drenching sweat								
Orientation (0 - 4) 0 - oriented; 1 - uncertain about date; 2 - disoriented to date by no more than 2 days; 3 - disoriented to date by ≥ 2 days; 4 - disoriented to place and/or person								
Tactile Disturbances (0 - 7) 0 - none; 1 - very mild itch, P&N, numbness; 2 - mild itch, P&N, burning, numbness; 3 - moderate itch, P&N, burning, numbness; 4 - moderate hallucinations; 5 - severe hallucinations; 6 - extremely severe hallucinations; 7 - continuous hallucinations								
Auditory Disturbances (0 - 7) 0 - no present; 1 - very mild harshness/ability to startle; 2 - mild harshness, ability to startle; 3 - moderate harshness, ability to startle; 4 - moderate hallucinations; 5 - severe hallucinations; 6 - extremely severe hallucinations; 7 - continuous hallucinations								
Visual Disturbances (0 - 7) 0 - no present; 1 - very mild sensitivity; 2 - mild sensitivity; 3 - moderate sensitivity; 4 - moderate hallucinations; 5 - severe hallucinations; 6 - extremely severe hallucinations; 7 - continuous hallucinations								
Headache (0 - 7) 0 - no present; 1 - very mild; 2 - mild; 3 - moderate; 4 - moderately severe; 5 - severe; 6 - very severe; 7 - extremely severe								
Total CIWA-Ar score:								

Fig. 9.2 CIWA-Ar. Reproduced from Sullivan JT et al. Assessment of alcohol withdrawal: the revised Clinical Institute Withdrawal Assessment for Alcohol scale (CIWA-Ar). British Journal of Addiction. 1989;84:1353–1357, with permission from Wiley.

Clinical Opiate Withdrawal Scale

For each item, circle the number that best describes the patient's signs or symptom. Rate on just the apparent relationship to opiate withdrawal. For example, if heart rate is increased because the patient was jogging just prior to assessment, the increase pulse rate would not add to the score.

Patient's Name: _____	Date and Time ___ / ___ / ___ : _____

Reason for this assessment: _____

Resting Pulse Rate: _____ beats/minute	GI Upset: over last 1/2 hour
Measured after patient is sitting or lying for one minute	0 no GI symptoms
0 pulse rate 80 or below	1 stomach cramps
1 pulse rate 81-100	2 nausea or loose stool
2 pulse rate 101-120	3 vomiting or diarrhea
4 pulse rate greater than 120	5 multiple episodes of diarrhea or vomiting
Sweating: *over last 1/2 hour not accounted for by room temperature or patient activity.*	**Tremor** *observation of out stretched hands*
	0 no tremor
0 no report of chills or flushing	1 tremor can be felt, but not observed
1 subjective report of chills or flushing	2 slight tremor observable
2 flushed or observable moistness on face	4 gross tremor or muscle twitching
3 beads of sweat on brow or face	
4 sweat streaming off face	
Restlessness *Observation during assessment*	**Yawning** *Observation during assessment*
0 no tremor	0 no yawning
1 tremor can be felt, but not observed	1 yawning once or twice during assessment
3 slight tremor observable	2 yawning three or more times during assessment
5 gross tremor or muscle twitching	4 yawning several times/minute
Pupil size	**Anxiety or Irritability**
0 pupils pinned or normal size for room light	0 none
1 pupils possibly larger than normal for room light	1 patient reports increasing irritability or anxiousness
2 pupils moderately dilated	2 patient obviously irritable or anxious
5 pupils so dilated that only the rim of the iris is visible	4 patient so irritable or anxious that participation in the assessment is difficult
Bone or Joint aches *If patient was having pain previously, only the additional component attributed to opiates withdrawal is scored*	**Gooseflesh skin**
	0 skin is smooth
0 not present	3 piloerrection of skin can be felt or hairs standing up on arms
1 mild diffuse discomfort	5 prominent piloerrection
2 patient reports severe diffuse aching of joints/muscles	
4 patient is rubbing joints or muscles and is unable to sit still because of discomfort	
Runny nose or tearing *Not accounted for by cold symptoms or allergies*	
0 not present	Total Score _____
1 nasal stuffiness or unusually moist eyes	The total score is the sum of all 11 items
2 nose running or tearing	
4 nose constantly running or tears streaming down cheeks	Initials of person completing assessment: _____

Score: 5-12 = mild; 13-24 = moderate; 25-36 = moderately severe; more than 36 = severe withdrawal
This version may be copied and used clinically.

Fig. 9.3 COWS. Reproduced from Wesson DR, Ling W. The Clinical Opiate Withdrawal Scale (COWS). Journal of Psychoactive Drugs. 2003;35(2):253–259, with permission.

- Alcohol: the Clinical Institute Withdrawal Assessment—Alcohol, revised (CIWA-Ar) scale[5] (Fig. 9.2).
- Opioids: the Clinical Opioid Withdrawal Scale (COWS[6]; Fig 9.3) or the Short Opioid Withdrawal Scale (SOWS).

Testing for drugs and alcohol

Drug testing can commonly be carried out on urine, oral fluids, and sweat. It can be used to confirm use and should be performed on all patients reporting substance use; however:

- a positive test does not confirm dependence

- a positive test for morphine/opiates does not confirm heroin use—codeine will give a positive result; only laboratory testing with liquid chromatography/gas chromatography–mass spectrometry can confirm heroin use
- drug testing is often limited in scope and will not usually identify many drugs such as pregabalin, tramadol, synthetic cannabinoids, and pethidine; it is important to clarify which drugs are tested for.
- the window after use for a positive test post shows considerable inter-substance and inter-individual variation
- unsupervised samples may be at risk of being adulterated.

Assessment of risks

Mental health
Patients with a history of drug and alcohol use are at heightened risk of self-harm and suicide in prison. This may relate to underlying psychiatric illness, social issues outside prison, or incarceration itself, but also untreated drug and alcohol withdrawals.

Physical health
The physical health of people in prison with addiction issues may be poor and any acute risks such as infected abscesses or severe liver disease should be identified and addressed.

Safeguarding
Any safeguarding issues regarding either the patient or someone in their care in the community (child or vulnerable adult) should be identified and addressed.

Polysubstance use
The use of multiple substances is common among alcohol and drug users. Symptoms of withdrawal from one substance can both mask and mimic those of another. Patients in withdrawal from multiple substances are at risk potentially of both over- and undertreatment. Such patients may need higher levels of assessment and observation.

Veracity of history
For a multiplicity of reasons the history given may be embellished. It is important to be aware of this risk and not start pharmacological treatment without a comprehensive assessment and convincing evidence of dependence.

Communication with outside agencies

This should be done at the earliest opportunity to confirm previous treatment in the community, especially regarding what medication was prescribed, was it supervised, and if it was collected. This often involves liaison with the community treatment provider, GP, and community pharmacy.

Any medication given in police or holding cells should be identified.

Treatment intervention and care plan

Based on the above assessments, a suitable care plan for treatment can be developed as set out in subsequent sections.

References

1. Clinical Guidelines on Drug Misuse and Dependence Update 2017 Independent Expert Working Group. Drug misuse and dependence: UK guidelines on clinical management [the Orange Book]. Department of Health and Social Care; 2017. https://www.gov.uk/government/publications/drug-misuse-and-dependence-uk-guidelines-on-clinical-management

2. National Institute for Health and Care Excellence. Alcohol-use disorders: diagnosis, assessment and management of harmful drinking (high-risk drinking) and alcohol dependence. Clinical guideline [CG115]. February 2011. https://www.nice.org.uk/guidance/cg115

3. World Health Organization. AUDIT: the Alcohol Use Disorders Identification Test, 2nd ed. 2001. https://apps.who.int/iris/bitstream/handle/10665/67205/WHO_MSD_MSB_01.6a.pdf;jsessionid=7E0846F347B121DE88D73C0F9B12411F?sequence=1

4. World Health Organization. The Alcohol, Smoking and Substance Involvement Screening Test (ASSIST). 2010. https://apps.who.int/iris/bitstream/handle/10665/44320/9789241599382_eng.pdf;jsessionid=DDAE0B370959D25FC46769FA60F6C930?sequence=1

5. Sullivan, JT, Sykora K, Schneiderman J, et al. Assessment of alcohol withdrawal: the revised Clinical Institute Withdrawal Assessment for Alcohol scale (CIWA-Ar). Br J Addiction. 1989;84:1353–1357.

6. Wesson DR, Ling W. The Clinical Opiate Withdrawal Scale (COWS). J Psychoactive Drugs. 2003;35(2):253–259. [Scale available at: https://www.drugabuse.gov/sites/default/files/files/ClinicalOpiateWithdrawalScale.pdf].

Alcohol withdrawal and management

Detoxification

Detoxification refers to the planned management of alcohol withdrawal. It requires careful assessment to determine the presence of dependence and associated comorbidities.

- Staff working in prisons should be competent to identify dependence, to assess if a person needs an acute intervention, manage withdrawal and any consequences, and assess risk from mental and physical comorbidities. Because of the high risk associated with alcohol withdrawal, management should start on arrival at prison reception.
- Those coming into prison may, because of court time and travel to prison, be in active withdrawal on arrival. This may be further complicated by concurrent use of illicit drugs, or suicidal thoughts or intent. A third of all suicides occur in the first week of prison and is significantly associated with both drug and alcohol withdrawal.
- Detoxification in the prison setting can be complicated by significantly reduced observations, by little knowledge of the person and lack of medical records on first night, and multiple comorbidities. It is crucial that there is adequate assessment and early management of withdrawal with adequate doses to prevent development of complications. Careful and comprehensive recording of symptomatology and response to medications regimen is important.

Assessment of alcohol withdrawal

Components of this are:
- consumption, both current and historical patterns of use
- diagnosis of dependence
- associated risks
- other illicit and prescribed drug use
- physical health problems
- mental health issues, both current and historical.

The AUDIT questionnaire (see Fig. 9.1, p. 215) is very useful as a screening tool and can support the diagnosis of dependence. A timeline from the last use of alcohol or treatment (which might have been initiated in police custody) is useful to determine the severity of withdrawals and aid diagnosis.

Symptoms of acute withdrawal
- Agitation, increasing over time.
- Anxiety.
- Nausea and vomiting.
- Paroxysmal sweats.
- Perceptual disturbances.
- Tremors.

Particular concerns should be noted
- History of epilepsy.
- Experience of withdrawal seizures.
- The need for concurrent withdrawal from other drugs such as benzodiazepines.
- Physical health problems.

A formal measure of withdrawal symptoms, the CIWA-Ar (see Fig. 9.2, p. 216), can be an adjunct to clinical decision-making and aid observation and dose.

Treatment

- While NICE[1] considers a symptom-triggered regimen as the preferred option, this requires much observation and skilled nursing, and is not suitable for prison settings.
- Most prisons that receive individuals on first night have protocols and procedures to initiate and continue treatment for alcohol withdrawal. Prescribing and administering of medication is completed within a standard clinical protocol that has been agreed and is reviewed by the prison clinical team.
- Benzodiazepines can be used, either diazepam or chlordiazepoxide, though chlordiazepoxide remains the more usual drug prescribed in prison. Fixed dose suggestions are given by NICE.[2]
- In a fixed dose regimen, the initial dose is usually titrated to the severity of the dependence and the severity of withdrawal symptoms. For those with severe withdrawal symptoms, there may need to be further dosing dispensed to manage the withdrawals.
- In prison, the dose should be supervised by a registered professional.
- Those who give a history of dependence in the past and note high levels of consumption should have the regimen initiated as early as possible. It is important to be assured that the person is dependent.
- Monitoring of the regimen, particularly in the first 48 hours, is essential as complications can occur as well as an increased risk of suicide.
- Continued withdrawal symptoms would generally suggest that the dose is insufficient and will require an increase.
- If the person is sedated, the dose should be withheld and the person observed and checked for any problems (e.g. other concurrent illicit drug use, infection).
- Some patients require adjunctive medication for support (e.g. for nausea or headache).
- Ensure adequate hydration and supportive care.[1]

Complications

- *Wernicke's encephalopathy*: for those at risk of developing Wernicke's who are undergoing a detoxification or are malnourished, oral thiamine should be given in doses towards the high end of the BHF formulary and continued for at least a month. If the person presents with suspected Wernicke's (a diagnosis of ophthalmoplegia, ataxia, nystagmus, confusion, and sometimes neuropathy), parental thiamine must be given for at least 5 days and then followed by oral thiamine. Acute referral to hospital is necessary.
- *Seizures*: there is no requirement for prophylactic antiepileptic treatment for those with alcohol withdrawal unless the person has epilepsy, in which case treatment continues. Adequate doses of benzodiazepines must be given during withdrawal regimen to avoid seizures.

- *Delirium tremens*: this is a serious complication from alcohol withdrawal and has a significant mortality—up to 2% even if treated. Adequate prevention comprises chlordiazepoxide to ensure the person has no withdrawal symptoms and supportive care. If concerns of delirium tremens, the dose regimen of chlordiazepoxide must be urgently reviewed and increased and/or with use of lorazepam. Antipsychotic medication may also be required for sedation. Hospital care should be sought urgently.

Relapse prevention

- After successful withdrawal for those with moderate and severe dependence, acamprosate or naltrexone should be offered for up to 6 months,[2] in combination with psychological therapies.
- Side effects and adherence to the medication should be discussed with the patient and an assessment of liver function conducted.
- Disulfiram is a second-line drug useful in supervision for some with alcohol dependence.
- The advice to prescribe will depend on the individual, the alcohol history and its consequences, and the length of sentence. Continuity of care is an important issue: the prison setting supports the attainment and continuation of abstinence; alcohol is more readily available in the community. All relapse prevention drugs should be considered prior to discharge, if not prescribed after detoxification, and the community GP informed.

References

1. National Institute for Health and Care Excellence. Alcohol use disorders: diagnoses and management of physical complications. Clinical guideline [CG100]. 2010 (updated April 2017). https://www.nice.org.uk/guidance/cg100
2. National Institute for Health and Care Excellence. Alcohol use disorder: diagnosis, assessment and management of harmful drinking (high-risk drinking) and alcohol dependence. Clinical guideline [CG115]. February 2011. https://www.nice.org.uk/guidance/cg115

Opioid detoxification

Opioid detoxification

- There is strong evidence that ongoing opioid substitution therapy (OST) is protective against overdose mortality and reduces reoffending. For some, imprisonment will be an opportunity to detoxify from opioids and establish a drug-free lifestyle.
- Careful and comprehensive clinical assessment and review is needed to establish whether ongoing OST or detoxification is most appropriate for each patient.
- Patients with opioid dependency are provided with a full range of information regarding either ongoing OST or detoxification and the risks associated with each. They should be warned of the risk of fatal overdose.
- Patients should be enabled to make an informed choice about what they perceive to be in their best interests.

There is no clinical evidence that people in prison serving longer duration sentences benefit from enforced detoxification; indeed, there is clear evidence that coerced detoxification is likely to lead to relapse and increased harm.

There are four important factors which influence detoxification:

- The patient's wishes and needs.
- Severity of dependence.
- The opinion of the treating team in prison and, if possible, the community.
- The length of sentence.

Any detoxification regimen should be in line with the 'Orange Book'[1] and NICE[2] guidelines on detoxification:

- Sufficiently slow to minimize withdrawal symptoms.
- Regular assessment of progress by clinical staff.
- Completed in 12 weeks or less, but with flexibility to extend or shorten.
- If the patient changes their plan or destabilizes (e.g. significant withdrawal), or there is emergence of psychological distress or illicit drug use, the planned detoxification may need to stop and OST be optimized.
- A programme of psychosocial support should be in place during and after detoxification. This should carry on into the community.
- Patients should be made clear of the routes back into OST in the community after release should they relapse.
- They should be provided with naloxone on release.

Detoxification regimens

- Patients should first be stabilized on OST for 5 days. Once stabilized, withdrawal should commence with a gradual reduction of the medication that was used in stabilization—methadone or buprenorphine.
- In line with NICE guidance,[2] patients usually are not swapped between methadone and buprenorphine during detoxification; however, buprenorphine has pharmacological advantages in detoxification.

- Some patients choose reduction regimens quicker than those set out below; others slower. Many patients prefer quicker rates of reducing early in the detoxification process, seeking a more gradual reduction when they reach lower doses.

Methadone

Usually methadone will be reduced at a rate that reaches zero over 12 weeks, most often involving a reduction of 5 mg every 1–2 weeks.

Buprenorphine

Buprenorphine can be reduced by 2 mg every 1–2 weeks to 2 mg. Usually from this point reductions are made in 400-microgram steps.

Lofexidine

Lofexidine, an alpha-adrenergic agonist and not a controlled drug, may be used to detoxify those on small amounts of opioids. It should only be used in those who have uncertain tolerance or have declined methadone or buprenorphine. A starting dose is 800 micrograms raising to a maximum of 2.4 mg in divided doses. It is then gradually reduced over the subsequent 7–10 days. The patient needs close monitoring for hypotension and brady-cardia. They often need further symptomatic relief from opioid withdrawal.

Symptomatic relief

Symptomatic relief is usually not needed in well-structured detoxification regimens with methadone or buprenorphine. The following may be pre-scribed if needed, appropriately supervised:
- Diarrhoea: loperamide 4 mg initially followed by 2 mg after each loose stool. To a maximum of 16 mg daily.
- Nausea and vomiting: metoclopramide 10 mg three times daily or prochlorperazine 5 mg three times daily for a maximum of 5 days.
- Stomach cramps: mebeverine 135 mg three times daily.
- Agitation, anxiety, and insomnia: consider stopping reduction regimen and increasing dose of opioid if on methadone/buprenorphine reduction. Consider opioid stabilization if on lofexidine reduction. Consider psychiatric assessment.
- Muscular pains and headache: paracetamol, aspirin, or other NSAID.

Medication for relapse prevention

Naltrexone, an opioid antagonist, may be used to support abstinence as part of a wider psychosocial package of care. It needs to be adequately supervised. Prior to prescribing, note the following:
- Due to potential hepatotoxicity, LFTs should be taken before and during treatment.
- It should only be prescribed once opioid-free status is confirmed, usually 7–10 days post methadone or 3–4 days post buprenorphine. This should be confirmed with a negative urine test. If uncertain, a naloxone challenge may be carried out. Patients should be warned of the risk of significant and prolonged withdrawal if opioid use was more recent.
- Patients should be informed that opioid pain relief will not work once treatment has commenced.

- Patients should be warned of the risk of overdose if they stop naltrexone and use opioids.
- Patients should be advised of side effects such as light headedness and dizziness.

Dose of naltrexone

On day 1, 25 mg with a period of observation for withdrawals post dose of 1 hour. If no withdrawal or significant side effects, increase dose to 50 mg daily from day 3.

Psychosocial interventions

Detoxification and the maintenance of abstinence should take place in a wider package of care such as:

- mutual aid—'12 steps' or SMART Recovery
- meaningful daily activity such as work or education
- cognitive-based relapse prevention.

References

1. Clinical Guidelines on Drug Misuse and Dependence Update 2017 Independent Expert Working Group. Drug misuse and dependence: UK guidelines on clinical management [the Orange Book]. Department of Health and Social Care; 2017. https://www.gov.uk/government/publications/drug-misuse-and-dependence-uk-guidelines-on-clinical-management
2. National Institute for Health and Care Excellence. Drug misuse in over 16s: opioid detoxification. Clinical guideline [CG52]. July 2007. https://www.nice.org.uk/Guidance/CG52

Psychoactive substances

Synthetic cannabinoids

Use of synthetic cannabinoids such as 'spice' is uncommon in the community outside of certain populations such as people who are homeless. Use is higher in prison due in part to difficulties in detection of use by drug testing and the high potency of small volumes. The class of synthetic cannabinoids contains a multiplicity of different substances that exert effects on the endocannabinoid system; this leads to a wide variety of desired effects, side effects, and withdrawal symptoms.

Consequences of synthetic cannabinoid use

Dependence

Daily regular use may lead to tolerance and a withdrawal syndrome similar to cannabis withdrawal including:
- low mood and anxiety
- irritability and aggression
- insomnia
- gastrointestinal disturbance.

Intoxication

Intoxication may cause several different toxic effects including:
- cardiovascular: arrhythmia, hypertension and tachycardia, bradycardia, chest pain, and myocardial infarction
- psychiatric: psychosis including paranoia and hallucinations, anxiety, agitation, depressed mood, and suicidality
- neurological: delirium, excited delirium, seizures, and cerebrovascular accident
- hyperpyrexia.

Treatment of dependence
- Detoxification.
- There are no standard regimens for the treatment of synthetic cannabinoid withdrawal. Treatment should be symptomatic. Brief courses of benzodiazepines or second-generation antipsychotics may be useful in the treatment of agitation, anxiety, and insomnia. The patient should be closely monitored. PSIs should be offered in line with those offered for other substances.

Treatment of effects of intoxication

Treatment should be in line with the principle of 'treat what you see'. In the prison context, synthetic cannabinoids have been implicated in several suicides. Patients should not be excluded from appropriate psychiatric treatment and observation due to the use of drugs. For many, the psychiatric effects remit within 6–12 hours; however, suicidality, mood changes, and psychosis may persist for longer periods and need the ongoing involvement of psychiatric services.

A further concern should be the potential for excited delirium, leading to restraint. In such situations, patients should be especially closely physically monitored due to additional cardiovascular risks.

Cardiovascular instability should lead to consideration of emergency hospital admission.

Other PS drugs—psychostimulants

Other illicit drug use including psychostimulant use is less common. There are generally no specific detoxification regimens and treatment is symptomatic.

Further information on individual substances can be found on TOXBASE (https://www.toxbase.org/) and on the treatment of PS in Project NEPTUNE (http://neptune-clinical-guidance.co.uk/).

Gabapentinoids

Pregabalin and gabapentin have the potential to produce a positive psychoactive effect, to cause dependence, and are implicated in fatal overdose, especially associated with opioids.

If a decision is made to stop a patient's prescribed pregabalin or gabapentin due to the lack of a medical reason to prescribe it, it should not be stopped abruptly and should be tapered over at least a week. Although evidence is weak, it has been suggested that pregabalin should be reduced at most by 50–100 mg a week and gabapentin 300 mg every 4 days. There is no evidence for substitution with other medications. Patients should be observed for the emergence of withdrawal symptoms. In most prison settings, as pregabalin and gabapentin are controlled drugs, they should not be given in-possession.

Further reading

Public Health England. Advice for prescribers on the risk of the misuse of pregabalin and gabapentin. December 2019. https://assets.publishing.service.gov.uk/government/uploads/system/uploads/attachment_data/file/385791/PHE-NHS_England_pregabalin_and_gabapentin_advice_Dec_2014.pdf

Psychosocial interventions

- PSIs are endorsed internationally for recovery and harm reduction in all illicit/licit substance misuse.
- Prison PSI access/quality must be (at least) equivalent to community services.
- PSIs range from social support to structured, psychologist-led sessions.
- Used with any other treatment modality but are the mainstay for PSs/cannabis, depressants, stimulants, dissociatives, and hallucinogens.
- Effective at any stage of change or detention.
- Prison-specific challenges: remand, self-harm/suicide, release planning, and post-release overdose.

Core elements

- *Governance*: organizational commitment to staff competencies (e.g. https://www.skillsforhealth.org.uk/) through training/skilled clinical supervision is vital. Must audit PSI effectiveness/outcomes.
- *Access*: prison PSI provision must be comparable to the community and account for regimen challenges. Continuity between prison(s)/court/community is crucial. Drop-out rate reduced by addressing other health issues or stigma and integrating care models/databases.
- *Therapeutic alliance*: non-specific, non-technical positive therapist characteristics (e.g. positive, caring, non-judgemental, flexible) used to form unique, collaborative relationship.
- *Evidence base*: relative dearth of high-quality PSI prison research in the UK. Contingency management and behavioural couples therapy have a strong evidence base (NICE endorsed) but systematic reviews/meta-analyses suggest equivalent, moderate effect sizes across many PSI types. Outcomes: cannabis (best) > cocaine > opioids > polydrug use (worst). Groups allow greater coverage/mutual aid but need significant supervision and can have high drop-out rates.
- *Social networks*: avoiding drug-using groups and promoting peer mentors to allow positive change. All patients should be asked if they want family/partners involved in their care.
- *Monitoring and evaluation*: self-reports, family/carer opinions, and strategic care plan reviews should be routinely used to monitor abstinence duration, quality of relationships, and so on.

Categories

Select according to patient choice, evidence base, and trained staff availability.

- *Brief interventions*: often in screening/primary care. Information/advice to increase understanding and motivation for change. Often used for milder dependence (e.g. cannabis).
- *Motivational interviewing/enhancement techniques*: empathic and reflective exploration ('rolling with resistance'), rather than forceful/direct persuasion, of differences between current behaviour and goals. Motivational enhancement technique (see Project MATCH) analyses feedback.
- *Contingency management*: patient-agreed reinforcement (e.g. extra visits) of positive behaviour (e.g. regular engagement). Incentives must be given promptly and consistently.

- *Family and couple interventions*: communication skills/problem solving to improve relationships and stress (e.g. Storybook Mums/Dads). Supplemented by 'node link mapping'. Family/carers need to be offered information, assessment and support (e.g. Al-Anon).
- *CBT*: identifies thoughts/behaviours/emotions/physical feelings in high-risk situations. Can be regular, structured one-to-one or group sessions (e.g. Enhanced Thinking Skills), informal CBT-informed interventions (those on remand), in-cell computer-based CBT (e.g. http://www.breakingfreeonline.com), or trauma focused.
- *Psychodynamic psychotherapy*: regular outcome monitoring is recommended.
- *Therapeutic communities*: peers/education promote personal responsibility and social norms. Invariably involve reducing/stopping OST. Patients making an informed decision to abstain post release should be considered for community residential treatment.
- *Mutual aid*: largely cost-free but need adequate staffing (http://www.clinks.org):
  - 12-step programmes such as Alcoholics Anonymous (AA) and Narcotics Anonymous (NA); addiction seen as a spiritual/mental/physical disease; medication sometimes discouraged.
  - SMART Recovery: more common alternative to 12 steps; addiction seen as a choice; secular; CBT/motivation interviewing based; medication accepted. Mutual aid also useful for gambling disorder (https://www.gamcare.org.uk/).

Psychosocial interventions and recovery

Person-centred recovery needs PSI stratification as seen in the 'phases and layers' model (Table 9.2). Patient reviews determine what phase/layer is appropriate ('stepped care').

Table 9.2 Phases and layers model in psychosocial interventions

Layers	Phases			
	Assessment	Engagement	Behavioural change	Early recovery
Standard	Harm reduction advice	Brief interventions, motivational interviewing, monitoring attendance	Set goals, build confidence and coping skills	Mutual aid, relapse prevention
Enhanced	Identify comorbidity	Formal motivational interviewing, contingency management	CBT, trauma-therapy, vocational training, accommodation	Day programmes, therapeutic communities, relapse medication

Source: data from Clinical Guidelines on Drug Misuse and Dependence Update 2017 Independent Expert Working Group. Drug misuse and dependence: UK guidelines on clinical management. London: Department of Health; 2017.

Phases
Different balances of PSI (Table 9.2); time taken and progression is highly individual but usually progress from identifying risks to characterizing strengths/recovery capital and useful deficits.
- *Assessment*: balances patient engagement against information collation; however, must clarify patient goals, reason for drug use, motivation for change, and risks at initial contact.
- *Engagement*: need low thresholds to engage/re-engage those with severe/complex comorbidity (e.g. ADHD or cognitive impairment).
- *Behavioural change*: 'SMART'—specific, measurable, agreed-upon, realistic, time-limited—and prioritized goals, formal psychological sessions, social skills, vocational training, and housing support.
- *Early recovery*: integrate skills/positive changes into social networks (e.g. Inside-Out prison exchange programme), 'active linkage' (i.e. introducing) to current members of mutual aid (e.g. sports groups), appropriately trained peer mentors, intensified PSI, or relapse prevention medication (nicotine, alcohol and opiates).

Layers
Balance the best chance of success against over-burdening patients:
- *Enhanced care*: formal PSI and care coordination/case management by staff with formal qualifications/training—usually clinical substance misuse or mental health teams.
- *'Recovery check-ups'* and rapid re-engagement, especially if previously on OST, must remain an option for all.

Further reading

Day E, Micheson L. Psychosocial interventions in opiate substitution treatment services: does the evidence provide a case for optimism or nihilism? Addiction. 2017;112(8):1329–1336.
Dutra L, Stathopoulou G, Basden SL, et al. A meta-analytic review of psychosocial interventions for substance use disorders. Am J Psychiatry. 2008;165:179–187.

Opioid substitution therapy

Few treatments in mental health, certainly substance misuse, have had a greater impact than OST. Methadone/buprenorphine are both WHO essential medicines. Of ~55,000 people in English prisons/year in substance misuse treatment, around 25% are on OST.

Evidence of OST benefits

- Over 60 years of randomized controlled trials/systematic reviews/ meta-analyses (mostly methadone/generic buprenorphine) demonstrate cost-effective benefits of OST including decreased opioid use/injecting/crime/mortality, and increased treatment retention.
- OST's cost-effective benefits translate to prison where the standardized mortality rate is ~50% higher than the general population. Peak death rate: first 4 weeks post release, some cohorts 70× risk of death versus age/sex-matched community peers. Substance misuse main cause. OST at release saves lives: 20 mg or more of methadone/day decreases deaths by at least 75% in first month by increasing opioid tolerance.
- OST half-life ($t_{1/2}$) of 24 hours or greater (both methadone/ buprenorphine): allows decreased intoxication/withdrawal. Positive, reinforcing psychoactive effects but also decreases respiratory rate— OST's inherent risk balance. Like natural endorphins and illicit opioids, OST acts at mu-opioid receptors to decrease cAMP/noradrenaline neuronal firing.

Pharmacological options for OST

- Methadone (liquid). Full mu-opioid receptor agonist. Peak plasma concentration ~4 hours after oral dose; $t_{1/2}$ ~24 hours, steady state ~5 days. Usual therapeutic dose 60–120 mg daily, no upper dose limit. ECG for increased QTc/risk of arrhythmia when greater than 100 mg daily. Concentrated form (10 mg/1 mL) if larger volumes not tolerated. Evidence suggests methadone keeps patients in treatment for longer than buprenorphine. Commonest prison OST.
- Buprenorphine sublingual tablets (generic). High-affinity partial mu-opioid receptor agonist—better safety profile, can block opioids used 'on top' but precipitate withdrawals if displacing other opioids. Peak plasma concentration ~2 hours after oral dose; $t_{1/2}$ greater than 24 hours, steady state ~5 days. Usual therapeutic dose 12–16 mg daily, 32 mg maximum. Increased $t_{1/2}$ allows less than daily dosing. Diversion risk due to slow dissolution, crushing (off-licence) recommended. Rarely used.
- Buprenorphine wafer. Compared to generic: maximum dose 18 mg daily, increased bioavailability (30%), quick dissolution potentially decreases administration times/diversion. As with tablets and depot, baseline/regular LFTs recommended. Increasingly used in UK prisons.
- Buprenorphine depot. Weekly/monthly subcutaneous injection. Oral test dose if no prior buprenorphine or recent use of other opioids; if swapping from oral start 1 day after last dose. Recommended weekly start dose 16 mg, then up to two additional 8 mg daily administrations—to maximum 32 mg in first week. Second week dose

= combined first week total. Can then convert the weekly dose to a monthly preparation given every four weeks.

Maintenance OST

- Staff must support patient around whether to maintain OST or reduce/stop *if/when* stable—that is, no opioid withdrawals/intoxication/illicit opioid or possibly non-opioid misuse. Could be stable from day 5 review—soonest OST steady state—but usually takes weeks.
- Maintenance OST is often the first step to recovery—crucial platform for PSI. If prior relapse/overdose/severe dependence and on short sentence (<6 months), then maintenance OST is the most appropriate/evidence-based approach.
- Stopping/reducing OST should not be enforced, regardless of sentence length or challenging behaviour. Needs thorough clinical/risk assessment and patient/team/prescriber collaboration. Staff must offer support and discuss risks—specifically increased death rates in prison and at/after release as well as drug dependence's chronic relapsing course. Often stopped in 12 weeks (decrease by 5 mg/1–2 weeks). No evidence for linear or exponential approach.

Optimization

- A 13-week/strategic care plan reviews monitor effectiveness of OST.
- Instability often presents as opioid cravings/withdrawals/'on top' use requiring ↑ OST dose.
- Crucially, effective OST doses are determined by subjective cravings, not just objective withdrawals, and can be higher than 'the dose that helps a patient to "feel OK" '.[1]
- Need at least 3 days between any incremental increase in OST dose—5–10 mg methadone or 2–4 mg buprenorphine—and ongoing reviews.
- Seek advice from senior prison addiction specialist if cravings/withdrawals/'on top' use continue at high doses (e.g. methadone ≥120 mg daily).

Common regimen challenges

- *Intoxication*: needs skilled risk balance. Intoxication/sedation must result in OST/any CNS depressant medication being temporarily withheld. Closely monitor in a safe area. Any cardiorespiratory instability needs hospital admission. Otherwise needs medic review to restart OST as soon as possible—may need symptomatic treatment. Opioid withdrawal is not fatal but must take account of self-medicating/self-harm risks—no guaranteed 'drug-free' areas in prison. If medic review is not possible before next dose (e.g. weekend) can restart OST if not intoxicated/sedated. Try to clarify reason for intoxication. Not always due to suboptimal OST; however, in addition to withdrawals/cravings, OST optimization may be needed if subtherapeutic dose (i.e. <60 mg methadone daily or <12 mg buprenorphine (generic oral)); recently decreased OST dose; previously stable at higher OST doses. Repeated intoxicated needs MDT meeting/strategic care plan review. Patients secreting drugs/alcohol who are not intoxicated/sedated should

continue OST. Withholding OST can increase risks of self-medicating/harming. Advise/document risks and bolster support.
- *Diversion*: examine mouth before/after OST. Also drink ~200 mL water and talk afterwards. Security staff should try to decrease challenging behaviour to decrease diversion risks.
- *Administration*: OST must be given in a timely, safe, and integrated manner with security. Need protocols to administer OST when access restricted/equipment fails. Automated dispensing equipment/stock supply medication can improve efficiency/decrease errors.

Reference

1. Clinical Guidelines on Drug Misuse and Dependence Update 2017 Independent Expert Working Group. Drug misuse and dependence: UK guidelines on clinical management [the Orange Book]. Department of Health and Social Care; 2017. https://www.gov.uk/government/publications/drug-misuse-and-dependence-uk-guidelines-on-clinical-management

Further reading

Gisev N. A cost-effectiveness analysis of opioid substitution therapy upon prison release in reducing mortality among people with a history of opioid dependence. Addiction. 2015;110(8):1975–1984.

Marsden J, Stillwell G, Jones H, et al. Does exposure to opioid substitution treatment in prison reduce the risk of death after release? A national observational study in England. Addiction. 2017;112(8):1408–1418.

Discharge planning

- Transitions between police custody, prison, and community increase risks for substance misuse patients. Seamless, carefully documented, and person-centred care decrease risks.
- Vital from initial contact: skilled risk assessments; discussions of relapse/opioid-related overdose associated with reducing/stopping OST; proactive efforts to engage patients in pre-discharge plans; continuity of care by systematic communication between and within community/prison services. Person-centred care needs valid consent which entails: discussing risks/benefits of treatment and any alternatives, including no treatment, relevant to that patient as well as a reasonable person in their position ('Montgomery ruling'). As a minimum, valid consent must be sought at all 13-week/strategic care plan reviews and pre-release reviews (≥2 weeks before release).
- Staff supporting patients on OST/those who have stopped it must be competent in their knowledge of OST and broader community recovery support. This requires clear organizational commitment to effective, high-quality teaching and training.

Pharmacological relapse prevention (PReP)

NB: PrEP may also refer to pre-exposure prophylaxis for HIV. For HIV, see HIV care in prisons, p. 150.

Cost-effective and evidence based. Decreases relapse risk during/after prison. Caution in severe renal/hepatic impairment. Must consider PReP (and document this) if ongoing/historical opioid and/or alcohol misuse. Should be used alongside evidence-based PSIs. NICE recommended and is part of NHS England's minimum standards of prison substance misuse care.[1]

Opioid PReP

Naltrexone[2]—non-selective opioid receptor antagonist:
- Start if *opioid free for at least 7 days* (~4 days for buprenorphine) and clear opioid urine screens (e.g. days 0 and 7).
- 25 mg initial dose (monitor withdrawals for ≥1 hour), then 50 mg daily.
- Can give as doubled dose on alternate days (plasma terminal $t_{1/2}$ ~96 hours) to increase concordance.
- Side effects include gastrointestinal upset/headache (>1%); rarely, fatal overdose if try to overcome opioid blockade.
- Can preclude opioid analgesia—offer medical alert card.
- Baseline/regular reviews (weekly initially)/LFTs.
- Continue if beneficial/abstinent.
- Depot unlicensed in UK for opioids/alcohol misuse.

Alcohol PReP

- Patient goal: abstinence.
- I effect 'not in-possession'.
- Baseline: U&E/LFTs with gamma-glutamyltransferase.

- Avoid in severe hepatic/renal impairment or pregnancy/breastfeeding.
- Acamprosate: for moderate/severe dependence (SADQ >15), also mild dependence/harmful drinking if PSI alone fails/patient requests medication, can decrease cravings. Glutamate NMDA receptor antagonist. Optimum effect: start when abstinent, possible neuroprotective role. 1998 mg PO daily, or 1332 mg if patient weighs less than 60 kg. Benefits at 1 week but can improve for months. Side effects: headache/gastrointestinal upset/decreased sexual drive (>1%); rarely: anaphylaxis. No significant interactions. Review monthly for 6 months, then less. Continue as long as reported benefits; if still drinking continue for up to 6 weeks.
- Naltrexone: indication/review/continuation as in acamprosate. Can decrease cravings. Optimum effect: when alcohol-free *but must also be opioid free for at least 7 days* with clear urine screens (days 0 and 7). If still drinking, continue for up to 6 weeks. Otherwise as for opioid PReP.
- Disulfiram: for moderate/severe dependence if acamprosate/naltrexone fail or specifically requested. Action: decreases aldehyde dehydrogenase, increases acetaldehyde if alcohol consumed, causes flushes/arrhythmia/collapse. Optimum effect: start when abstinent *but must be alcohol-free for at least 24 hours*. 200 mg PO daily, increase to 500 mg daily if needed. Side effects: include halitosis (possible monitoring tool)/fatigue/gastrointestinal upset (>1%); rarely, hepatotoxicity, dermatitis. Contraindications: include psychosis, severe PD, high suicide risk, heart disease, stroke. Must warn of alcoholic food/toiletries/medication. Review fortnightly for 2 months, then monthly for 4 months, then 6-monthly. Continue as long as reported benefit.

Restarting/increasing OST

- Must consider restarting OST before release if stopped in prison and prior opioid relapse/overdose or disengagement after release, long dependence history, injecting pre-detention, polydrug use; also if patient feels they cannot abstain post release. Need thorough discussion with patient and substance misuse community/prison team but not ongoing opioid withdrawal/use. Careful induction required (e.g. methadone 5–10 mg or buprenorphine 2–4 mg increases every ≥3 days); if sedated, withhold next dose/other sedatives until medically reassessed. Restarting buprenorphine: must be heroin-free for at least 12 hours/methadone-free for at least 24 hours; need LFTs. Must consider increasing OST dose pre-release if decreased in prison/community stability at increased dose. Risks/benefits as in restarting OST. Increasing/restarting OST need close clinical monitoring.
- Target OST dose: that at which patient is stable historically; evidence-based therapeutic doses for methadone (60–120 mg daily) or generic buprenorphine (12–16 mg daily) should also be noted; guided primarily by ongoing assessment/review. Aim to stabilize prior to release.
- If decline restart/increase in OST: must discuss/document decreased opioid tolerance and risk of fatal overdose. Also need to inform community team and organize day-of-release review.

Proactive contact with community services

- Need a prearranged community substance misuse services appointment if on OST at release.
- Contingency plans should be made for release outside of community service opening hours (i.e. bridging scripts), taking care to avoid double-scripting/dosing.
- Prison services must inform community substance misuse teams about temporary releases and expected/actual release dates, current OST dose/recent changes, other prescribed sedating medication (e.g. benzodiazepines, gabapentinoids), if OST restarted/stopped, or PReP prescribed (also inform community GP).
- Communications must be documented.
- Offer family/carer involvement in care plans if on OST or OST stopped.
- Prison staff should attend community MDT meetings and vice versa, especially if polypharmacy, pregnant, or on Criminal Behaviour Orders.

Additional overdose prevention

- Always:
    - give patient OST before release/attending court
    - offer naloxone, and document this
    - consider OST pre-release if an opioid misuse risk
    - try to integrate substance misuse care plans with 'through the gate' services/ community rehabilitation companies
    - write clear OST protocols for unplanned releases
    - use integrated data systems to reconcile medicines and share clinical data within/between police custody/prison/community (e.g. region-wide single point of contact (SPoC) and SystmOne).

References

1. NHS England. Service specification: Integrated Substance Misuse Treatment Service in Prisons in England. 2018. https://www.england.nhs.uk/publication/service-specification-integrated-substance-misuse-treatment-service-prisons-in-england/
2. Clinical Guidelines on Drug Misuse and Dependence Update 2017 Independent Expert Working Group. Drug misuse and dependence: UK guidelines on clinical management [the Orange Book]. Department of Health and Social Care; 2017. https://www.gov.uk/government/publications/drug-misuse-and-dependence-uk-guidelines-on-clinical-management

Women's health in prison

Health needs of women in prison

Introduction

- Women make up a small proportion of prison populations—about 5% of the 85,000 people in prison in England and Wales. However, this number has doubled over the last 25 years, from 1562 in 1992 to 3975 in 2017.
- Women commit more acquisitive crime and are less likely to have committed a violent offence than men. In 2018, 82% of women's prison sentences were for non-violent offences.
- Prison is often experienced by women as harsher because prisons and the practices within them have largely been designed by and for men.
- When women are imprisoned, there are likely to be profound consequences for their families; unlike imprisoned men, women are often the primary caregivers for dependent children.
- Imprisoned women often come from the most socially and economically disadvantaged sectors of society; almost one-third of female offenders spent time in care as a child.
- The majority of imprisoned women will have experienced some form of trauma and abuse as a child or adult.
- Although a small proportion of the prison population, imprisoned women have specific and complex health and social care needs that are distinct from the needs of imprisoned men.

Health needs

- The health of imprisoned women is worse than that of their female peers in the community and is also worse than that of imprisoned men.
- They have higher rates of mental health disorders and higher rates of both self-harm and self-inflicted deaths than women in the community and imprisoned men. Self-harm rates are more than ten times higher in imprisoned women than men.[1]
- Women in prison also have high rates of drug dependence; imprisoned women have a two- to fourfold excess of alcohol dependence and at least a 13-fold increase in drug dependence compared to women in the community.[2]
- Imprisoned women also have poor physical health; they are at high risk of communicable[3,4] and non-communicable diseases.[4,5]
- Pregnant women in prison are a high-risk obstetric group with a range of poor outcomes when compared to the community. High-quality perinatal care can improve both short- and long-term outcomes.[6]
- Although disempowered by the prison system, many women are interested in their health and have a clear and accurate view of the key health issues they face and the potential ways that this could be achieved within the confines of prison.[7]

Gender-specific standards

- International standards for women of particular note include the WHO's Kyiv Declaration on Women's Health in Prison (2009) and the UN's Bangkok Rules (2010) (see also Women in prison, p. 26) There is international recognition that imprisonment should be seen as a last resort for women and alternatives to imprisonment must be considered.

- In the UK, the 'Prison safety and reform' White Paper published in November 2016 highlighted the vulnerability of imprisoned women.[8]
- In 2018, PHE published 'Gender specific standards to improve health and wellbeing for women in prison in England'. This set out six overarching principles and 122 standards, across ten key areas, to guide providers and commissioners of health, social care, and prison services for women.

References

1. Hawton K, Linsell L, Adeniji T, et al. Self-harm in prisons in England and Wales: an epidemiological study of prevalence, risk factors, clustering, and subsequent suicide. Lancet. 2014;383(9923):1147–1154.

2. Fazel S, Yoon IA, Hayes AJ. Substance use disorders in prisoners: an updated systematic review and meta-regression analysis in recently incarcerated men and women. Addiction. 2017;112(10):1725–1739.

3. Dolan K, Wirtz AL, Moazen B, et al. Global burden of HIV, viral hepatitis, and tuberculosis in prisoners and detainees. Lancet. 2016;388(10049):1089–1102.

4. Escobar N, Plugge E. Prevalence of human papillomavirus infection, cervical intraepithelial neoplasia and cervical cancer in imprisoned women worldwide: a systematic review and meta-analysis. J Epidemiol Community Health. 2020;74(1):95–102.

5. Herbert K, Plugge E, Foster C, et al. A systematic review of the prevalence of risk factors for non-communicable diseases in worldwide prison populations. Lancet. 2012;379(9830):1975–1982.

6. Bard E, Knight M, Plugge E. The outcomes of pregnancy among imprisoned women and the effect of perinatal health care service on these outcomes: a systematic review. BMC Pregnancy Childbirth. 2016;16(1):285.

7. Plugge E, Douglas N, Fitzpatrick R. Imprisoned women's concepts of health and illness: the implications for policy on patient and public involvement in healthcare. J Public Health Policy. 2008;29(4):424–440.

8. Ministry of Justice, National Offender Management Service. Prison safety and reform. 2016. https://assets.publishing.service.gov.uk/government/uploads/system/uploads/attachment_data/file/565014/cm-9350-prison-safety-and-reform-_web_.pdf

9. Public Health England. Gender specific standards to improve health and wellbeing for women in prison in England. 2018. https://www.gov.uk/government/publications/women-in-prison-standards-to-improve-health-and-wellbeing

Contraception

Introduction

- Imprisoned women need easily accessible, comprehensive contraception services. Unpredictable lengths of stay, prison transfers, and unexpected release from court all highlight the need for rapid access to reliable contraception.
- Because of the chaotic lifestyles prior to imprisonment, few women access long-acting reversible contraception (LARC) in the community; the relative stability of the prison environment is an opportunity to encourage women to address their contraceptive needs.
- Contraceptive methods with minimal user failure are important for many women with chaotic lifestyles and/or substance use problems.

Contraceptive choices: LARC

Many women have repeat custodial sentences and so it is sensible to set up scheduled reminders through SystmOne for contraception renewal when fitting LARCs. Common comorbidities/contraindications and interactions seen in imprisoned women are shown in the Table 10.1.

Contraceptive choices: non-LARC

These types of contraception have higher user failure rates than LARC. Common comorbidities/contraindications and interactions seen in imprisoned women are shown in Table 10.2.

Barrier contraception should be offered to all people at the time of release from prison.

Quick start contraception

The scenario in remand prisons of a female wanting contraception, at high risk of unwanted pregnancy with imminent possible release, is common. If pregnancy cannot confidently be excluded, then guidance is to give contraception anyway as either combined hormonal contraception (ethinylestradiol-ethinyloestradiol, cyproterone), the progesterone-only pill, or an implant as first-line choices. Depot medroxyprogesterone acetate (DMPA) may also be given but it must be advised that there is lack of evidence for use in early pregnancy. See Faculty of Sexual and Reproductive Healthcare guidance.[1]

Emergency contraception

Guidance is to offer the copper IUD first line in emergency contraception but in practical experience this is not often taken up by women. There is a decision-making table in the Faculty of Sexual and Reproductive Healthcare emergency contraception guideline[2]:

- *Copper IUD*: can be fitted up to 120 hours after unprotected sexual intercourse or 5 days after expected ovulation, whichever is longer. If high risk of STI, the IUD can still be fitted but swab at the time and consider antibiotic cover.
- *Ulipristal*: can be given up to 120 hours after unprotected sexual intercourse. Efficacy may be reduced if on concurrent enzyme inducers. The patient should avoid progesterones in the 5 days after taking it as this may reduce its effectiveness.

Table 10.1 Common comorbidities and contraindications for types of LARC

	Implant	DMPA 12-weekly intramuscular injection. Consider setting up PGD for nurse delivery of this in prison	IUS/IUD screen for STIs prior to fit or prophylactic treatment given at time of fit if screening not possible
Viral hepatitis	UKMEC 1 but UKMEC 3 if severe decompensated cirrhosis	UKMEC 1 but UKMEC 3 if severe decompensated cirrhosis	UKMEC 1 but IUS—UKMEC 3 if severe decompensated cirrhosis
Venous thromboembolism	UKMEC 2 for current or historic	UKMEC 2 for current or historic	IUD—UKMEC 1 for current or historic IUS—UKMEC 2 for current or historic
HIV (if on antiretrovirals check https:// www.hiv-druginteractions.org/)	UKMEC 1	UKMEC 1	UKMEC 2 but UKMEC 3 if CD4 <200 cells/mm^3
Enzyme inducers	UKMEC 4	UKMEC 1	UKMEC 2
History of subacute bacterial endocarditis	UKMEC 1	UKMEC 1	UKMEC 2
Pelvic inflammatory disease	UKMEC 1	UKMEC 1	Current: UKMEC 4 for initiation UKMEC 2 for continuation Past (no current risk factor): UKMEC 1
Long QT syndrome	UKMEC 1	UKMEC 2	UKMEC 3 for initiation UKMEC 2 for continuation

DMPA, depot medroxyprogesterone acetate; IUD, intrauterine device; IUS, intrauterine system; UKMEC, UK Medical Eligibility Criteria for Contraceptive Use; category 1, use method; 2, generally use method but higher-level judgement and more careful follow-up required; 3, probably don't use (needs expert judgement/specialist referral); 4, do not use.

Table 10.2 Common comorbidities and contraindications for non-LARC contraceptive types

	Combined hormonal contraception	Progesterone-only pill (POP) (highest user failure rates of contraceptives listed here)
Viral hepatitis	Acute or flare: Initiation—UKMEC 3 Continuation—UKMEC 2 Chronic: UKMEC 1 but UKMEC 4 if severe decompensated cirrhosis	UKMEC 1 but UKMEC 3 if severe decompensated cirrhosis
Venous thromboembolism	UKMEC 4 for current or historic	UKMEC 2 for current or historic
HIV (if on antiretrovirals check https:// www.hiv-druginteractions.org/)	UKMEC 1	UKMEC 1
Enzyme inducers	UKMEC 4	UKMEC 4
History of subacute bacterial endocarditis	UKMEC 4	UKMEC 1
Pelvic inflammatory disease	UKMEC 1	UKMEC 1
Long QT syndrome	UKMEC 2	UKMEC 1

UKMEC, UK Medical Eligibility Criteria for Contraceptive Use; category 1, use method; 2, generally use method but higher-level judgement and more careful follow-up required; 3, probably don't use (needs expert judgement/specialist referral); 4, do not use.

- *Levonorgestrel:* can be given up to 72 hours after unprotected sexual intercourse. Give double dose if taking enzyme-inducing drugs. There is no restriction on using progesterone quick start contraception after giving Levonelle (Levonorgestrel).

Follow-on contraceptive care

- Inform community GP when contraceptives have been started and when the patient will need a review or replacement.
- Consider linking with the PAUSE project, a nationwide scheme for women who have had two or more children taken into care and are at risk of having further children taken into care. The project provides intensive treatment to give women the opportunity to pause and take control of their lives to break the destructive cycle that causes them and their children deep trauma (see http://www.pause.org.uk).

References

1. Faculty of Sexual and Reproductive Healthcare. FSRH guideline: quick starting contraception. April 2017. https://www.fsrh.org/standards-and-guidance/documents/fsrh-clinical-guidance-quick-starting-contraception-april-2017/
2. Faculty of Sexual and Reproductive Healthcare. FSRH Clinical Guideline: Emergency Contraception. March 2017 (amended December 2020). https://www.fsrh.org/standards-and-guidance/documents/ceu-clinical-guidance-emergency-contraception-march-2017/

Pregnancy care

Introduction

- Every year an estimated 600 pregnant women are held in prisons in England and Wales and some 100 babies are born to women in prison.
- All women who enter prison are offered a urine pregnancy test and a UDS test. Some women may enter prison in the advanced stages of pregnancy.
- Antenatal care is carried out where possible by visiting clinicians but attendance at local hospitals is essential for most patients for anomaly scans and more complex care needs.
- Delivery will be planned at a local maternity hospital. None of the female prisons in England have a birthing suite.
- Pregnant women in prison should receive equitable care to women in the community.

Antenatal care

- Antenatal visits may include up to ten appointments throughout pregnancy.
- A midwife will visit the patients in the prison for antenatal appointments. Where there is a complex need, such as substance misuse, a visit to a consultant obstetrician will be required.
- An ultrasound 8–14-week dating scan can include a nuchal translucency scan if screening is chosen.
- An ultrasound 18–21-week anomaly scan can check for structural abnormalities.
- Other scans may be done if there is concern about growth.
- Some prisons will do the scanning within the prison to avoid escorting patients to an outside hospital.
- If the child is to remain in custody of the mother, an application should be made for a place on the mother and baby unit (MBU); this should occur not less than 3 months before the expected delivery date.

Common problems seen in pregnancy in prison

- Many imprisoned pregnant women will need support with the management of their substance misuse throughout their pregnancy.
- Imprisoned women are more likely than the general population to have mental and physical health problems and these may affect the pregnancy.
- Women should be offered support if they wish to terminate their pregnancy. They should be offered abortion counselling before and after the procedure and scans should occur in a timely manner to allow them to make their decision. Many female prisons work with local charities that come in to offer counselling for such women.

Substance misuse

- The management of opioid substitution treatment and detoxification of other drugs such as benzodiazepines needs to be under the guidance of a specialist midwife and a consultant with an interest in substance misuse following local or national guidance. They will then work with the healthcare prescribers on site.

- Social services should be involved and information from them regarding any child protection issues should be sought early on.

Nutrition and diet
- Folic acid and vitamin D supplementation is recommended for all imprisoned women who are pregnant and should be made available.
- In early pregnancy nausea may be a problem and facilitating small and frequent snacks should be considered.
- Women should receive the same advice on diet and nutrition as pregnant women in the community.

Labour and delivery
- Women should not be transported in cellular vans when heavily pregnant in labour or returning with their baby.
- Women should have the opportunity to have a birth supporter with her who may be a family or friend.
- Prison officers escorting women in labour should receive clear guidance on how to manage this; they should be respectful and allow privacy when breastfeeding or during intimate medical examinations.
- When in full labour the prison officers should only be in the room if the woman wishes them to be.

Postnatal care
Some babies will return with their mother to the MBU where a supportive and nurturing environment should be provided. Some mothers return to prison without their baby and there are a number of reasons why this might be temporary for some, and permanent for others:
- Temporary separation might be because the baby needs additional care or because a place in the MBU is not available. In these cases, the mother should be supported in expressing breast milk with the hope that when she is reunited with her baby, breastfeeding can be re-established. It can also help to alleviate some distress from the mother by feeling that she is doing something for her baby.
- It is not unusual for mothers to be permanently separated from their baby at birth because of child protection orders or the length of time a mother is to serve in her sentence. The mother's physical and mental health well-being should be monitored and support offered.

Further reading
Birth Companions. Birth charter for women in prisons in England and Wales. March 2016. https://www.birthcompanions.org.uk/resources/5-birth-charter-for-women-in-prison-in-engl and-and-wales

Gov.uk. Prison life: pregnancy and childcare in prison. n.d. https://www.gov.uk/life-in-prison/pregna ncy-and-childcare-in-prison

HM Prison and Probation Service, Ministry of Justice. Managing prisoners who pose an escape risk: PSI 10/2015. March 2015. https://www.gov.uk/government/publications/managing-prison ers-who-pose-an-escape-risk-psi-102015

National Institute for Health and Care Excellence. Antenatal care. NICE guideline [NG201]. August 2021. https://www.nice.org.uk/guidance/ng201

National Institute for Health and Care Excellence. Pregnancy and complex social factors: a model for service provision for pregnant women with complex social factors. NICE guideline [CG110]. September 2010. https://www.nice.org.uk/guidance/cg110

Common gynaecological problems

A high proportion of general practice consultations in women's prisons are for gynaecological issues. Gynaecological problems cause particular anxiety because many women in prison have histories of sexual abuse, sexual assault, and commercial sex work.

Some of the commonest presenting gynaecological problems seen in the female estate are outlined below:

Secondary amenorrhoea

- Hypothalamic amenorrhoea is common in female opioid-dependent individuals due to:
  - low BMI
  - chronic opiate use
  - stressful lifestyle associated with drug use.
- Often entry into prison with regular meals, resulting in an increase in BMI, and stabilization onto opiate substitution therapy are enough for menstruation to return. If there are no other concerning features in the history and amenorrhoea coincides with opiate misuse history, it is reasonable to wait 3–6 months to see if menstruation returns naturally.
- NICE gives clear guidance on investigating possible other causes of amenorrhoea.[1]
- It is important to advise amenorrhoeic women that they still require contraception if they do not wish to become pregnant as this is a common misconception.
- Consider if osteoporosis prophylaxis is required in those with amenorrhoea lasting longer than 12 months.

Menorrhagia

NICE guidance has excellent charts for diagnosing and managing menorrhagia.[2]

Specific considerations for prison population include the following:

Patients on anticoagulation therapy with menorrhagia

- Caution should be used if considering tranexamic acid due to increased risk of coagulopathy.
- Mefenamic acid should be used with caution due to increased risk of gastric bleeding and with proton pump inhibitor cover.

Drug management with history of venous thromboembolism

- Tranexamic acid should be avoided if history of venous thromboembolism.
- Do not prescribe norethisterone to those with a history of venous thromboembolism.

Vaginal discharge

Many women in prison are at higher risk of STIs. It is important to take a good history, including sexual history, and whether or not the woman practises vaginal douching as this can lead to bacterial vaginosis. Examination should be performed including:

- speculum examination—to visualize discharge and cervix and to take relevant swabs

- bimanual examination if associated with pain—to check for cervical excitation and adnexal tenderness.

Commonest causes of non-STI discharge in females in prison

Good guidance is available on the British Association of Sexual Health and HIV website (http://www.bashhguidelines.org/current-guidelines/vaginal-discharge). See Table 10.3.

Table 10.3 Common causes of non-STI discharge

	Bacterial vaginosis	Candida/thrush
Symptoms	Offensive fishy smelling vaginal discharge	Thick white vaginal discharge, with vulval itch and soreness. External dysuria and superficial dyspareunia
Swabs to take	MCS vaginal swab	MCS vaginal swab
Treatment	Only treat if symptomatic or a/w surgery First line: metronidazole—2 g stat or 400 mg twice daily for 5–7 days. Intravaginal gels and creams are also options if the women prefers[a] Second line: metronidazole 400 mg twice daily for 5–7 days	Only treat if symptomatic Multiple treatment options depending on patient preference and availability[a] First-line options: Fluconazole capsule orally 150 mg stat Clotrimazole 500 mg pessary stat
Relapse prevention advice	Avoid vaginal douching, use of shower gel, and use of antiseptic agents or shampoo in the bath	Use vulval moisturizers as soap substitute Avoid tight-fitting synthetic clothing Avoid irritants, e.g. perfumes/soaps
Recurrent episodes	3 or more proven episodes in 6-month period 50% reduction achieved from metronidazole 2 g orally once monthly. Alternative—twice-weekly metronidazole vaginal gel	4 or more symptomatic episodes a year with *Candida* shown on swab in at least 50% Treat initial episode with longer treatment course such as fluconazole: Oral 150 mg, 3 courses in 7 days Oral 50 mg once daily for 7–14 days Follow this with fluconazole 150 mg weekly or clotrimazole 500 mg weekly for 6 months

[a] See British Association of Sexual Health and HIV guidelines: http://www.bashhguidelines.org/current-guidelines/vaginal-discharge

For specific guidance on diagnosis and management of STIs, see Sexually transmitted infections, p. 64.

Pelvic pain

A high proportion of women within the prison estate have a history of sexual abuse, sexual assault, and domestic violence. This needs to be considered in women presenting with pelvic pain together with other common causes including:

- endometriosis
- dysmenorrhoea
- pelvic inflammatory disease
- ectopic pregnancy.

Cervical cancer screening

- Imprisoned women are less likely to be up to date with cervical screening yet more likely to be HPV positive or have had an abnormal result than women in the community.
- Past experience of sexual abuse and/or assault may mean some women are reluctant to participate in screening.
- A robust smear programme identifying women due for screening, with easy-to-access, clear information on smear taking and how abnormal results are treated can help to increase screening numbers.
- Consider developing a special arrangement with the local processing laboratory to ensure samples sent out of the normal screening times are not rejected.
- Colposcopy—if referred, make women aware of the prison policy for officers escorting women during intimate examinations. Women are more likely to attend if they know their privacy will be respected.

References

1. National Institute for Health and Care Excellence. Amenorrhoea. February 2022. https://cks.nice.org.uk/topics/amenorrhoea/
2. National Institute for Health and Care Excellence. Tools and resources. In: Heavy menstrual bleeding: assessment and management. NICE guideline [NG88]. 2018 (updated May 2021). https://www.nice.org.uk/guidance/ng88/resources

Mother and baby units

Introduction

There are six prisons that have a MBU in England and Wales (and two regional MBUs in Scotland). These are HMP Bronzefield, HMP Eastwood Park, HMP Styal, HMP New Hall, HMP Peterborough, and HMP Askham Grange. There are 64 places available between them and an application needs to be submitted and an admission process has to be followed. Babies can stay with their mothers up to 18 months of age, beyond this it is felt that the benefits to the child are no longer outweighed by the restrictions of the environment.

It is recognized that the quality and sensitivity of mother and child interaction at 6–15 weeks correlates directly with the attachment relationship at 18 months. This is why for women who are serving a short sentence and retaining custody of their children it is so important to facilitate their time together in a nurturing environment.

Application

- The mother should be referred to the nominated mother and baby liaison officer.
- The mother makes an application. A dossier should be put together with support from the mother and baby liaison officer with input from:
  - local authority children's services report
  - adult social service report, where appropriate
  - security report
  - relevant medical reports
  - personal officer report
  - report from community offender manager.
- A recommendation is then made to the prison governor by a multiagency admission board chaired by an independent chair.
- The recommendation needs to be endorsed by the governor. They need to consider the health and safety of the other mothers and babies on the unit and ensure that good order and discipline is maintained on the MBU.

Assessment

- The decisions made need to be in the child's best interest at all times.
- Information will be sought from the previously listed multiagency teams. Previous children being removed from the mother's care would not preclude admission but would need to be reviewed and considered.
- Sentence length is considered.

Life on the mother and baby unit

- The MBU is a designated separate area within the prison walls but away from normal location; each room has a cot and en suite bathroom.
- There is an outside space with play equipment.
- There is an inside nursery area and a nursery nurse available to monitor development of the children and care for them while the mother engages with aspects of the prison regime. The unit is very much child focused.

- Mothers are supported by a visiting health visitor to help with feeding, establishing routines, bonding, and weaning, similar to that in the community.
- Some units will have kitchen staff who will teach the mothers how to cook healthy and nutritious food on a budget.
- Staff take the babies out to supermarkets, libraries, and garden centres to broaden their range of experiences, sights, and sounds.
- The mothers will be with their babies 24/7 for the first 8 weeks and not go to work but beyond that they may leave their baby in the nursery while they attend work, education, and so on as it is important that the mothers participate in the prison regime and rehabilitation.
- Visits may be provided on the MBUs, and where possible visits from siblings are encouraged.
- Where possible, release on temporary licence may be facilitated to enable family bonding.

Separation

There may come a time when the mother and baby may need to be separated. This may be because the mother's sentence extends beyond 18 months, because of child protection concerns, or if the mother has lost her place on the unit due to her behaviour. A separation plan is decided as part of the admission process on to the MBU and must be a MDT decision. It can be reviewed and is flexible to ensure the minimum distress. Separation plans are considered at the time of admission; for example, if the sentence is 5 years, separation may be better to do at 6 or 9 months rather than 18 months.

- The mother should nominate two appropriate and responsible adults.
- The local authority will assess the suitability of the chosen carer and submit a written report to the prison.
- If there is a failure to find a suitable adult, the child will be placed in the care of the local authority.
- Release on temporary licence where possible should be arranged to help with the transition to the new carer.
- Pre- and post-separation counselling must be made available for the mother.

Further reading

Birth Companions. Birth charter for women in prisons in England and Wales. March 2016. https://www.birthcompanions.org.uk/resources/5-birth-charter-for-women-in-prison-in-engl and-and-wales

Gov.uk. Prison life: pregnancy and childcare in prison. n.d. https://www.gov.uk/life-in-prison/pregna ncy-and-childcare-in-prison

Ministry of Justice, HM Prison and Probation Service. Pregnancy, MBUs and maternal separation in women's prisons policy framework. September 2021. https://www.gov.uk/government/publi cations/pregnancy-mbus-and-maternal-separation-in-womens-prisons-policy-framework

Ministry of Justice, HM Prison and Probation Service. Women's policy framework. June 2021. https://www.gov.uk/government/publications/womens-policy-framework

National Institute for Health and Care Excellence. Pregnancy and complex social factors: a model for service provision for pregnant women with complex social factors. NICE guideline [CG110]. September 2010. https://www.nice.org.uk/guidance/cg110

Sexual violence

Sexual violence is defined as 'any sexual act, attempt to obtain a sexual act, unwanted sexual comments or advances, or acts to traffic, or otherwise directed, against a person's sexuality using coercion, by any person regardless of their relationship to the victim, in any setting, including but not limited to home and work'.[1]

- Experience of sexual violence is relatively common in the prison population and can be hard for victims to disclose.
- Sexual violence can cause severe and long-lasting physical and psychological harm.
- Most sexual violence is perpetrated by someone known to the victim. It can happen prior to imprisonment and may be linked to domestic violence or can be used as a tool of victimization in prison.

Consider sexual violence as a possible cause of a patient presenting with relevant physical or psychological symptoms. Sexual assault strips an individual of control. The HCP's response can play an important part in the survivor beginning to regain that control. The role includes:

- listening and recording
- assessing what a person might need—including medical, psychological, and forensic needs
- explaining this to them sensitively
- offering them informed choices
- following up.

Management

Key issues to consider include the following:

- Are they safe from the perpetrator/others? Are any safeguarding measures required?
- Assess and manage any injuries.
- Are they at risk of self-harm? Should an ACCT be opened? What psychological support is available?

Recent abuse

- If sexual assault has happened within the last 7 days there may be forensic evidence that can be gathered.
- If the individual consents to referral, this should be conducted at a sexual assault referral centre (SARC).
- This should be arranged as soon as possible and they should be advised not to wash and to bring any clothing/items from when the assault took place.
- Do not attempt forensic examination if you have not been appropriately trained.

SARCs offer medical, practical, and emotional support and are open 24/7. The individual *does not* have to report the crime to the police to receive support from a SARC. If they are not sure if they would like to report it, forensic medical evidence can be collected at the SARC and stored while they have more time to think about whether they want to make a report.

The following issues should be managed by the SARC if the individual consents to go there. If the victim makes an informed decision not to go to a SARC, and they have capacity to refuse, these needs should be managed as best as possible in the prison:

- Is emergency contraception required? Is a pregnancy test required?
- Is post-exposure prophylaxis after sexual exposure required? See British Association for Sexual Health and HIV guidance.[2]
- STI screening and sample storage. Follow-up testing may be required after exposure:
  - 2 weeks for chlamydia and gonorrhoea.
  - 1 month for HIV.
  - 3 months for syphilis and hepatitis.

Non-recent sexual abuse

- Imprisonment can be a time where traumatic memories can resurface.
- If someone has been a victim of sexual assault in the past, including childhood sexual abuse, they should be able to access support for this. This may include understanding the legal process if they are considering reporting the assault to the police but should not be limited to this.
- If the patient would like to be referred for at least telephone support from a local service (see Further reading), they should be supported to do so.
- If they decline referral for support, it is still important to listen to their experience if they would like to talk about it or provide an opportunity for them to do so in the future.

Documentation

It is important to make comprehensive contemporaneous notes and a body map for injuries. The notes may be used as evidence in court months or even years later.

Self-care and clinician support

Consider involving a senior clinician for advice and support. These cases can be distressing to hear and manage—ensure there is appropriate support and space to process this.

References

1. Jewkes R, Sen P, Garcia-Moreno C. Sexual violence. In: Krug EG, Dahlberg LL, Mercy JA, et al. (eds), World Report on Violence and Health (pp. 147–182). Geneva: World Health Organization; 2002. https://apps.who.int/iris/bitstream/handle/10665/42495/9241545615_eng.pdf
2. British Association of Sexual Health and HIV. UK guideline for the use of HIV post-exposure prophylaxis 2021. 2021. https://www.bashhguidelines.org/current-guidelines/hiv/post-exposure-prophylaxis-following-sexual-exposure/

Further reading

Details of local SARCs: https://www.nhs.uk/Service-Search/Rape-and-sexual-assault-referral-centres/LocationSearch/364

Details of local support agencies for survivors of sexual assault: http://thesurvivorstrust.org/find-support/

Domestic violence

Is domestic violence a prison issue?

- The majority of women in prison have experienced domestic violence as adults. There are strong links between women's experience of domestic and sexual abuse, coercive relationships, and criminal offending.
- Men can also experience domestic violence but it is less common and less is known about this.
- Domestic violence is defined as 'Any incident or pattern of incidents of controlling, coercive, threatening behaviour, violence or abuse between those aged 16 or over who are or have been intimate partners or family members regardless of gender or sexuality'.[1]
- A victim of domestic violence may experience a profoundly damaging abuse pattern, without a single episode of physical violence—emotional abuse can be just as harmful as physical violence.
- Domestic violence is about *power* and *control*. Controlling or coercive behaviour is often part of this pattern, and these are defined as follows:
  - *Controlling behaviour* is a range of acts designed to make a person subordinate and/or dependent by isolating them from sources of support, exploiting their resources and capacities for personal gain, depriving them of the means needed for independence, resistance, and escape, and regulating their everyday behaviour.
  - *Coercive behaviour* is an act or a pattern of acts of assault, threats, humiliation, and intimidation or other abuse that is used to harm, punish, or frighten the victim.

Controlling and coercive behaviour in an intimate or family relationship is now an offence under the Serious Crime Act 2015.

- Domestic violence is a gendered crime. While both men and women may experience incidents of domestic violence, women are considerably more likely to experience repeated, sustained, and severe forms of abuse, and are more likely to be injured, hospitalized, or killed than men.
- Domestic violence is associated with a range of physical and mental health conditions, as outlined in Box 10.1. Women experiencing domestic violence seek health services more than the general population.

Healthcare professionals can play a crucial role in identifying domestic violence, and referral to specialist support.

How to ask about domestic violence

Survivors say their doctor is one of the few people they can disclose violence to and want them to respond appropriately. They often don't bring it up and therefore HCPs need to ask about this (Box 10.2).

How to respond to a disclosure

The immediate response is important
- It might have taken months or years to disclose domestic violence to someone; the victim may have been told by the perpetrator that

> **Box 10.1 Examples of clinical conditions associated with intimate partner violence**
> - Symptoms of depression, anxiety, PTSD, sleep disorders.
> - Suicidal ideation, behaviours, or self-harm.
> - Alcohol or other substance misuse.
> - Unexplained chronic pain or gastrointestinal, neurological, or genitourinary symptoms.
> - Adverse reproductive outcomes, including multiple unintended pregnancies.
> - Repeated vaginal bleeding or STIs.
> - Traumatic injury.
> - Repeated health consultations with no clear diagnosis.

> **Box 10.2 Suggested ways to ask about domestic violence**
> - 'Sometimes people who have these symptoms/injuries have been frightened or hurt by someone at home. Has anyone's behaviour upset you?'
> - 'Are there things that have happened at home that scare you? Are you afraid of anyone at home?
>   - This could be from other members of the household—this is still domestic violence.
>
> It can be useful to look at a power and control wheel[2] with the patient if the HCP is not sure whether this is domestic violence or not.

they will not be believed, it is their fault, and that no one is going to help them.
- It is important to counter this with phrases such as 'Thank you for telling me', 'I believe you', 'This is not your fault and it's not ok for someone to do this to you'.

Ongoing response
- Discuss and offer a referral to a local domestic violence service—this can be arranged as a phone call as a starting point. This connection enables people to understand more about domestic violence, be heard, be risk assessed, and be informed of what options and support are available.
- Some survivors may make an informed decision to decline referral for support at this time; even if all they are ready for now is to be listened to, that is still therapeutic.
- It may be appropriate to liaise with the prison release team to plan for a space in a safe house/refuge on release.
- It is important to empower the survivor to feel *in control* of her options as much as is possible. There are situations where safeguarding concerns may override this, but this is rare.

References

1. Home Office. UK cross government definition of domestic violence. September 2012. https://www.gov.uk/government/news/new-definition-of-domestic-violence
2. Domestic Abuse Intervention Programs. Power and control wheels. n.d. [Can be helpful to look at with a patient to see if they have experienced these behaviours; translated versions available.] https://www.theduluthmodel.org/wheel-gallery/

Further reading

Identification and Referral to Improve Safety (IRIS) [a general practice-based domestic violence and abuse training and referral programme]. http://irisi.org/

Men's Advice Line [a confidential helpline for any man experiencing domestic violence and abuse from a partner (or ex-partner). Tel. 0808 801 0327]. http://www.mensadviceline.org.uk/

Ministry of Justice. Thinking differently about female offenders. Transforming rehabilitation. Guidance document. London: Ministry of Justice, National Offender Management Service; 2014.

National Domestic Violence Helpline [a 24-hour helpline for women experiencing domestic violence, their family, friends, colleagues, and others calling on their behalf. Tel. 0808 2000 247]. http://www.nationaldomesticviolencehelpline.org.uk/

Office for National Statistics. Domestic abuse in England and Wales: year ending March 2018. https://www.ons.gov.uk/peoplepopulationandcommunity/crimeandjustice/bulletins/domesticabuseinenglandandwales/yearendingmarch2018

Prison Reform Trust. 'There's a reason we're in trouble': domestic abuse as a driver to women's offending. 2017. https://www.prisonreformtrust.org.uk/publication/theres-a-reason-were-in-trouble/

Royal College of General Practitioners. Adult safeguarding toolkit. n.d. https://elearning.rcgp.org.uk/mod/book/view.php?id=12530

Walby S. The cost of domestic violence: update 2009. 2009. Lancaster University. https://eprints.lancs.ac.uk/id/eprint/88449/1/Cost_of_domestic_violence_update_4_.pdf

Women's Aid. Domestic abuse is a gendered crime. n.d. https://www.womensaid.org.uk/information-support/what-is-domestic-abuse/domestic-abuse-is-a-gendered-crime/

Chapter 11

Child and adolescent health in secure environments

Introduction

- All young people aged under 18 years whether in secure settings or elsewhere are defined as children. In prison service language they are referred to as 'juveniles'. 'Young offenders' are those aged 18–21 years. The current 'child first' agenda recommends that young people involved with the criminal justice system should be referred to as children or young people with offending behaviour rather than 'young offenders'.
- There are three main types of secure setting for children and adolescents in the UK:
  - Mental health (psychiatric intensive care units, low and medium secure units (LSUs and MSUs)).
  - 'Welfare' (secure children's homes (SCHs)).
  - Youth justice provision (young offender institutions (YOIs), secure training centres (STCs), and SCHs) also known as the children and young people's secure estate (CYPSE); at the time of publication advanced discussions are under way to create a new form of youth justice provision known as a 'secure school' from 2022.[1]
- This chapter of the handbook refers specifically to young people in youth justice settings although many of the general principles outlined apply across all settings.

Approach to working with children in secure settings

- The general approach to working with children in secure settings needs to take into consideration the fact that they are not 'small adults' and, as in all environments, require specific approaches to their health and general care.
- Those working with children should have special training to do so but if this is not the case, then they should demonstrate within their approach:
  - a recognition that young people are developing in a range of different areas (such as cognition, emotional, sexual, and moral development) and can therefore grow out of difficulties as well as into them
  - an understanding that all adults have a particular duty to ensure that children are safe and that their welfare is protected and that all safeguarding concerns are both reported *and* subsequently addressed
  - an understanding of the importance of family or significant others and the need to involve them in decisions about the child's care even when they are many miles away as is frequently the case within youth justice settings
  - an understanding that children's presentations both of physical and mental health conditions may differ considerably and be less clear-cut than in adults; a binary judgement relating to presence or absence of formal 'mental illness' may be inadequate
  - some knowledge of different statutory jurisdictions and legal frameworks relating to children; these are more comprehensive and complex than is the case for adults
  - an awareness of the differing roles of professionals working with children both in and outside secure institutions.

Young people in secure youth justice settings

- Young people in secure youth justice settings are generally placed there because of high-risk criminal behaviours. One of the best means whereby risk can be addressed is by assessment and meeting of general needs, including health needs, which are particularly high and frequently unmet in this population:
  - More than 25% have long-standing physical conditions including asthma, dental problems, STIs, BBVs, skin and musculoskeletal problems, epilepsy, and sickle cell anaemia.
  - The prevalence of all mental health disorders is at least three times that of under 18s in general, with conduct disorders, anxiety, and depression being particularly common; there are also high rates of psychosis, post-traumatic disorders, and self-harming behaviours.
  - Developmental disorders such as learning difficulties are evident in up to 50%; ADHD is more common (up to 10%); rates of acquired brain injury are high (>50%).
  - Substance misuse rates for smoking tobacco and use of illicit drugs and alcohol are high.
  - Exposure to traumatic experiences (serious maltreatment, being a victim of crime and bullying) are all more common than in other youth populations as are rates of local authority care (being a 'looked-after child').
- Complex presentations involving multiple health and other needs are common and frequently require cross-agency approaches rather than independent health decision-making.
- It is not uncommon for children with pronounced mental health, developmental, or other difficulties to enter a secure setting where they are vulnerable and cannot manage the day-to-day routines; in such circumstances the possibility of transfer to a more supervised setting should be actively considered.

Secure environments for children and young people within the youth justice system in England and Wales

(NB: different arrangements for youth custody exist in Scotland and Northern Ireland.)

- All types of youth justice custodial settings can accept young people on remand or following sentencing in court.
- All young people under 18 years in a custodial setting are automatically given the status of being 'looked-after children' because of their special circumstances.
- All custodial settings for young people under 18 years must provide appropriate educational, health, and welfare provision in line with education and safeguarding expectations elsewhere.
- The Youth Custody Service (YCS) was established in September 2017 as a distinct arm of HMPPS. YCS has operational responsibility for the CYPSE.

Young offender institutions

The majority of young people in youth justice custody are in YOIs (600–800 at any one time). There are five YOIs in England which each cater for between 40 and 300 young people aged 15–18 (and sometimes also for 18–21-year-olds). Of all secure settings, YOIs most resemble adult prisons in their fabric and general organization. In general, young people in YOIs are not considered unduly vulnerable although in practice this is sometimes not the case. One YOI (HMYOI Wetherby) has a special unit (the Keppel Unit) for young people who are considered particularly vulnerable and may have neurodevelopmental or other complex difficulties. Girls aged under 18 years are no longer detained in YOIs.

Secure training centres

There are three STCs in England. They are intended for younger people (from age 12) and those considered too vulnerable for YOIs. They have higher staffing ratios, lower overall capacity (60–100 places), and their buildings resemble an adult prison less than YOIs. Two STCs accept boys and girls; one is for boys only.

Secure children's homes

- There are eight SCHs in England and Wales. These cater for the youngest (from age 10 although only very rarely is a child under 12 years admitted) and the most vulnerable young people in youth justice custody (about 80–100 nationally) and have the highest staffing ratios. SCHs are much smaller than YOIs and STCs, with usually no more than 30 beds; some SCHs have both youth justice and 'welfare' places (for children detained on welfare rather than youth justice grounds under section 25 of the Children Act 1989).
- Decisions about in which type of establishment within CYPSE a young person is placed are made by the YCS on the basis of youth offending team recommendations are given in government placement guidance.[2]

Sections 53–56 of the recommendations provide the procedure for obtaining a placement review if the location is considered unsuitable.

References

1. Ministry of Justice. Secure schools vision. 2018. https://www.gov.uk/government/publications/secure-schools-vision
2. HM Prison and Probation Service. Placing young people in custody: guide for youth justice practitioners. 2017. https://www.gov.uk/guidance/placing-young-people-in-custody-guide-for-youth-justice-practitioners

Legislative frameworks relevant to children and young people in youth justice custody in England and Wales

(NB: different arrangements for youth custody exist in Scotland and Northern Ireland.)

Children Act 1989

- This is the most powerful and wide-ranging legislation for all those aged under 18 years. It covers parental responsibility and state intervention in family life, safeguarding, and detention in secure accommodation on welfare grounds.
- Aspects of particular importance for those working in custodial settings include:
  - safeguarding children process: ensuring young people are protected from others (either staff or peers), understanding duty to report concerns to relevant lead professional, and dealing with disclosure of harm
  - understanding who has parental responsibility when information needs to be shared or treatment decisions discussed (may be social worker or identified other if child subject to a full care order; section 31, Children Act 1989) or similar; will still be birth parent if child subject to 'voluntary' care order (section 20, Children Act 1989)
  - understanding the need to participate in a 'looked-after child' process with outside agencies for children entering custody subject to voluntary or 'full' care orders and the need to participate in similar process for others who become 'looked after' by virtue of being in custody.

Mental Health Act 1983

- This is particularly important as a means of transfer to hospital on the grounds of mental health need.
- It requires access to suitable mental health practitioners able to effect formal Mental Health Act[1] processes within the custodial setting and identify a relevant hospital bed.

Mental Capacity Act 2005

- This requires practitioners to be able to assess capacity in young people particularly in relation to decisions about their own treatment (short and long term) and about sharing information with others.[2]

In addition to this legislation, those working with young people should be aware of:

Education

- This is particularly important for this population: education/occupation is a major factor in subsequent reductions in offending for all young people. Routine and regular attendance are important for all and reasonable adjustments may be required to ensure access.

- Of particular relevance for those with disability, whether physical, mental health, or neurodevelopmental, is identification of special educational needs. This may already have been done within a current education, health, and care plan when a young person enters custody; if not, such needs should be identified within the custodial setting.

Youth justice

- Some understanding of the youth justice process post sentencing is required so that there is adequate participation in sentence planning and preparation for discharge.[3]

Common law

- Principle of necessity: this allows for emergency treatment decisions to be made for a young person in situations requiring rapid and immediate intervention to save life or prevent serious deterioration where their consent cannot be sought.[4]

References

1. Department of Health and Social Care. Reference guide to the Mental Health Act 1983. 2015. https://www.gov.uk/government/publications/mental-health-act-1983-reference-guide
2. Department of Health. Mental Capacity Act. London: HMSO; 2005. http://www.legislation.gov.uk/ukpga/2005/9
3. Gov.uk. Youth Justice Board. n.d. https://www.gov.uk/government/organisations/youth-justice-board-for-england-and-wales
4. General Medical Council. Decision making and consent. 2020. https://www.gmc-uk.org/ethical-guidance/ethical-guidance-for-doctors/decision-making-and-consent#paragraph-75

Other processes in secure custodial settings

Prison Service Orders (PSOs) and Prison Service Instructions (PSIs)

- These are comprehensive written procedures for all eventualities which occur within custodial settings.[1]
- They apply in YOIs and STCs but not SCHs; one such document—PSI 08/2012 'Care and management of young people'[2]—specifically covers the management of young people.
- They can be helpful but can hinder flexible practice in unusual crisis situations. In such circumstances, good established relationships with senior staff can be far more effective.

Assessment, Care in Custody and Teamwork (ACCT) process and documentation

- ACCT is the very important process for management of risk of self-harm/suicide in custody; requires sign up and written updates from all professionals working with identified young person as well as active participation in ongoing review process.[4]
- It is particularly important for vulnerable young people at the time of entry and in the days and weeks after entry into custody.

Framework for Integrated Care (also known as 'SECURE STAIRS')

- This is a new and comprehensive support and formulation process using trauma-informed and attachment-based principles.
- It ensures that all professionals working with a young person in a secure setting have a clear understanding of their needs and a single overall plan of care for them.[4]

References

1. HM Prison and Probation Service, Ministry of Justice. Prison service orders (PSOs). 2020. https://www.gov.uk/guidance/prison-service-orders-psos
2. HM Prison and Probation Service, Ministry of Justice. Caring for young people in custody: PSI 08/2012. April 2012 (updated January 2020). https://www.gov.uk/government/publications/caring-for-young-people-in-custody-psi-082012
3. Ministry of Justice. The Assessment, Care in Custody and Teamwork process in prison: findings from qualitative research. 2019. https://www.gov.uk/government/publications/the-assessment-care-in-custody-and-teamwork-process-in-prison-findings-from-qualitative-research
4. Taylor J, Shostak L, Rogers A, et al. Re-thinking mental health provision in the secure estate for children and young people: a framework for integrated care (SECURE STAIRS) Safer Communities. 2018;17(4):193–201.

Overview of health needs

Overview of health needs

A health-needs census undertaken in 2016 found that just under 1000 young people aged under 18 years old are detained in the secure estate in England and Wales at any one time.[1]

- The vast majority of these are boys/young men and only around 4% are girls/young women.
- Many are located a long way from home which is likely to affect adversely their ability to gain support from friends and family; information about health needs can also be difficult to obtain. Both factors can increase vulnerability.
- There are disproportionately more young people from black and minority ethnic (BAME) than from white backgrounds (51% BAME: 28% black, 13% mixed, and 11% Asian/other); 12% were born in a country other than the UK. One in ten secure establishments had a young person of BAME heritage who was the only such young person in that unit, resulting in potential cultural isolation.
- Certain disorders (e.g. sickle cell anaemia) are more common in those with a specific ethnic background and health staff are required to be aware of this. In addition, staff should also be aware of common culture-bound explanations for certain presentations (e.g. djinn possession to account for psychotic phenomena).

Health inequalities are evident among young people within the secure estate:

Physical health

They have often had lower level of access to general healthcare provision as younger children and may have missed out on routine vaccinations and health screens,[2] dentistry, eye tests, and access to services in relation to emotional/mental health needs, neurodevelopmental problems, and speech and language difficulties.[3]

The most widely cited study of 16–20-year-old young people in custody in England and Wales found that a quarter of males and a third of females had long-standing self-reported physical complaints[4] (Table 11.1). Other studies of females and males in YOIs have found high rates of physical morbidity.[5,6]

Injuries secondary to assaults including knife/sharp object attacks are becoming more common and there has been a rise in young people sustaining life-changing consequences such as stoma or paralysis. Some of these young people enter the secure estate and are likely to come to the attention of healthcare staff.

Mental health and neurodevelopmental difficulties

- The 2016 census found 24% of young people detained in the CYPSE had at least one mental health or neurodevelopmental diagnosis, 11% had two diagnoses, and 5% had three or more diagnoses; the prevalence of neurodevelopmental disorders and emotional dysregulation/emerging PD among those in the secure estate was found to be much higher than seen in the general adolescent population (Table 11.2).
- An assessment of mental health presentations identified a range of symptoms in young people in custody[5]; all are more common than in young people in community settings (Table 11.3).

Table 11.1 Prevalence of self-reported physical health complaints in 16–20-year-olds in custody in England and Wales

Type of physical health complaint	Male remand young offender (%)	Male sentenced young offender (%)	Female young offender (%)
Respiratory	10	11	18
Musculoskeletal	7	4	4
Nervous system	2	3	6
Skin	1	2	5
Any physical complaint	25	23	35

Table 11.2 Comparison of mental health disorders in male and female young people in secure care with known prevalence in general adolescent population

Prevalence of diagnosis	CYPSE (%)	General adolescent population (%)
Mental health/neurodevelopmental diagnosis	40.5	10
Autism spectrum disorder	4.9	1–2
ADHD	15.8	5
Intellectual disability	4.4	1–3
Emerging PD	6.4	0.9–3

Table 11.3 Health needs of male and female adolescents in custodial settings

Depressive symptoms	19%
Self-harm	10%
Anxiety	11%
Post-traumatic symptoms	11%
Psychotic symptoms	5%
Drug misuse	11%
Alcohol misuse	6%

- Rates of Traumatic Brain Injury (TBI) are also substantially greater than in the general population. A 2015 review[7] found that between 16.5% and 49% of incarcerated young people had experienced head injury with loss of consciousness. Such injuries can lead to a range of neurocognitive and developmental difficulties, including deficits in social communication, impulse control, regulation of aggressive responses to threat[8] leading to increased risk of criminality,[8] and increased risk of self-harm and suicide.[10]

A needs assessment study of young people in the secure estate in England in 2006 indicated that young people in secure settings have high levels of need across a range of domains: mental health (31%), educational (23%), and social (35%), many of which interact.[11]

References

1. Hales H, Warner L, Smith J, et al. Census of young people in secure settings on 14 September 2016: characteristics, needs and pathways of care. Ministry of Justice; 2016. https://www.engl and.nhs.uk/wp-content/uploads/2018/10/secure-settings-for-young-people-a-national-scop ing-exercise-paper-2-census-report.pdf

2. Kroll L, Rothwell J, Shah P, et al. Mental health needs of boys in secure care for serious or persistent offending: a prospective, longitudinal study. Lancet. 2002;359(9322):1975–1979.

3. Bryan K. Preliminary study of the prevalence of speech and language difficulties in young offenders Int J Lang Commun Disord. 2004;39(3):391–400.

4. Lader D, Singleton N, Meltzer H. Psychiatric Morbidity Among Young Offenders in England and Wales. Further Analysis from the ONS Survey. London: Home Office; 2000.

5. Youth Justice Board. Female Health Needs in Young Offender Institutions. London: Youth Justice Board; 2006. http://www.yjb.gov.uk/publications/Resources/Downloads/YJB_FH_12pp.pdf

6. Chitsabesan P, Lennox C, Theodosiou L, et al. The development of the comprehensive health assessment tool for young offenders within the secure estate. J Forensic Psychiatry Psychol. 2014;25(1):1–25.

7. Hughes N, Williams WH, Chitsabesan P, et al. The prevalence of traumatic brain injury among young offenders in custody: a systematic review. J Head Trauma Rehabil. 2015;30(2):94–105.

8. Catroppa C, Anderson V. Neurodevelopmental outcomes of pediatric traumatic brain injury. Future Neurol. 2009;4:811–821.

9. Ogilvie JM, Stewart AL, Chan RCK, et al. Neuropsychological measures of executive function and antisocial behavior: a meta-analysis. Criminology. 2011;49:1063–1107.

10. Chitsabesan P, Lennox C, Williams H, et al. Managing traumatic brain injury in young offenders: findings from the CHAT study and the development of a linkworker service. J Head Trauma Rehabil. 2015;30(2):106–115.

11. Chitsabesan P, Kroll L, Bailey S, et al. Mental health needs of young offenders in custody and in the community. Br J Psychiatry, 2006;188:534–549.

Identification of health needs and health promotion

Entering the CYPSE presents an opportunity for health assessment and interventions to address unmet need, with the potential of improving short- and long-term life chances. Young people in secure settings, as evidenced, have high rates of health need.

Identifying specific needs

The Comprehensive Health Assessment Tool (CHAT)[1] is a five-part comprehensive health assessment screen that is used by qualified healthcare staff with all young people entering the CYPSE to provide an assessment of immediate health needs followed by assessments of physical health, substance misuse, mental health, and neurodisability.

The CHAT results can be used as a starting point for evaluating a young person's needs. However:

- decisions regarding developing care plans and organizing further interventions should not be based on the CHAT alone
- such decisions should also be informed by more detailed interviews with the young person, their family, and other key professionals (e.g. wing/unit staff, drug and alcohol staff, education chaplaincy, and outside professionals such as youth offending services, children's social care, and child and adolescent mental health services (CAMHS))
- if a young person moves to a new secure setting, the CHAT assessment from the previous establishment should be reviewed. Healthcare staff need to remember that previous CHAT assessments may not be automatically visible on electronic records and may need to be specifically requested from the previous establishment
- a CHAT discharge plan outlining health assessments, interventions, and future needs must be completed and shared as part of any pre-release plan for the young person.

Creating a comprehensive consensus overview of need

- The new Framework for Integrated Care (SECURE STAIRS) approach,[2] recently adopted across the CYPSE, creates a multiagency formulation for each young person which aims to identify all relevant needs across a range of domains (e.g. education, physical and emotional health, reoffending) and improve the understanding of each young person.
- The process is designed to include the young person and is based on a trauma-informed approach developed by practitioners in youth justice and welfare settings.
- Once a consensus formulation of the young person has been agreed, a practical plan of care is developed and becomes subject to regular review.

Special circumstances requiring particular attention

- The healthcare needs of some young people in custody require particularly close attention, monitoring, and support. This applies to those being managed within a care and separation unit, via 'Rule 49', and those whose movements elsewhere are restricted (known as being 'on single unlock'). Both situations mean that the young person cannot leave their room when there are any other detainees out of their rooms and have the effect of removing the young person from peer association.

- The adverse consequences of time in isolation are well recognized and young people in such circumstances frequently have particularly complex needs. In addition to monitoring physical and mental health, consideration should also be given to facilitating access to the full range of entitlement to exercise, education, assessment, and planning according to the Framework of Integrated Care ('SECURE STAIRS').
- Local policies should be in place to guide provision of enhanced health services in such circumstances. Individual health practitioners in addition should be guided by their own clinical impression of such situations and *not* rely solely on protocol-based processes.

Health promotion

- The variable previous experience of health promotion and preventive measures of young people arriving in a secure setting means there is a valuable opportunity to rectify any measures which may not previously have been attended to and which may be identified within the CHAT and SECURE STAIRS process (e.g. general health checks, immunizations, dental check-ups, and eye tests).
- Poor health habits often start in adolescence and have a lifelong impact.[3] Custody offers an opportunity to provide reliable health information and improve health-related awareness and decision-making skills, with the potential to change the health trajectory of young people.
- Provision of information covering areas such as puberty, self-care/hygiene, diet, exercise, sleep, immunizations, smoking, alcohol and substance misuse, sexual health, dental health, eye health, stress management, parenting skills, and how to access health services (including after transition at the age of 18 to adult services) is particularly important and should form part of health promotion in all secure settings.

References

1. Offender Health Research Network. Comprehensive Health Assessment Tool (CHAT): Young People in Contact with the Youth Offending Service (YOS). Manchester: Offender Health Research Network; 2013.
2. Taylor J, Shostak L, Rogers A, et al. Re-thinking mental health provision in the secure estate for children and young people: a framework for integrated care (SECURE STAIRS) Safer Communities. 2018;17(4):193–201.

Physical health conditions

Acute medical presentations

See also Chapters 6 and 7.

Acute medical presentations as elsewhere among children and young people include:

- first presentations of diabetes or poor diabetic control leading to hypoglycaemia and ketoacidosis
- acute asthma
- first presentations or poor control of epilepsy
- sickle cell crises
- acute infections such as meningitis
- acute cardiovascular events
- acute trauma following assaults or serious self-harm.

With the exception of acute infections, many acute or emergency presentations represent exacerbations of chronic or potentially lifelong conditions. General principles of management in a custodial setting include the following:

- Awareness that management in young people can differ significantly from that in adults.
- A low threshold for involvement of outside specialist emergency provision. The special circumstances of young people in a secure setting can mean that health professionals can feel under pressure when a decision about the suitability of involvement of paramedics/ attendance at a local A&E department needs to be made; in such circumstances, a balance between their confidence in recognizing and optimally treating the condition and considering the benefits of treatment elsewhere is required and the best interests of the child should always be prioritized.
- A clear programme of training for all healthcare staff in recognizing and managing acute physical health presentations.

Long-term conditions

Many young people whatever their circumstances can struggle to come to terms with long-term physical (and mental health) conditions. This can result in denial of the need for long-term medication and appropriate preventive measures. Furthermore, the additional pressures of a move from a familiar home environment to a secure setting can lead to a range of emotional disturbance including neglect or active exacerbation of previously well-controlled conditions. Avoidance of such circumstances wherever possible is clearly a major priority for those providing healthcare provision. This can be achieved by:

- ensuring clear documentation of the condition within any healthcare and residential unit record
- ensuring that staff and the young person's involvement in and awareness of a clear management plan are established as soon as possible after the young person's arrival in custody

- ensuring that any overall plan for the young person includes consideration of the young person's emotional needs if there are difficulties with maintaining stability in line with a treatment plan; in such situations, as in community settings, involvement of mental health/ psychological support can be helpful within the context of an overall care plan.

Mental health conditions

As outlined in previously (see Chapter 8, p. 175), mental health conditions are more common in criminal justice populations than in the general community. In addition, untreated, they can contribute to increased levels of disturbance and increased vulnerability for young people within custodial institutions.

In a setting specifically catering for young people under 18 years, it is crucial that at least some staff within the healthcare provision have experience of working with children and young people and have had appropriate formal training; this should include input from a child and adolescent psychiatrist specifically to diagnose and implement treatment of mental health conditions in young people. In addition, the following should be in place:

• Clear protocols for assessment and treatment of mental disorders which are specifically child focused. Key disorders in this regard include:
  • ADHD
  • depression, anxiety, and bipolar disorder
  • disorders relating to specific or chronic trauma
  • psychosis
  • conduct disorder and emerging PD
  • autistic spectrum conditions
  • TBI
  • intellectual difficulties and disability
  • some of these key disorders are discussed in more detail in subsequent topics in this chapter.
• An emphasis within the healthcare team on engagement skills and persistence when there are concerns about a young person.
• Good liaison skills including:
  • ability to deal with polarization of opinion both within the secure environment but also with professionals who know the young person in their home setting
  • establishment of good relationships and communication between the mental health team and others in negotiating complex situations which cannot be resolved by formal protocols alone
  • knowledge of professional frameworks beyond the custodial setting and ability to ensure that clear arrangements are put in place for the young person when they are released.
• Access to specialist advice not available within the custodial institution itself including:
  • contact with the community teams and professionals previously involved with the young person
  • establishment of a working/advisory relationship with local specialist services such as the local regional community forensic CAMHS team.
• A willingness to remain involved in situations where a precise mental health disorder is difficult to identify/categorize but where there is evidence of major emotional and behavioural disturbance and a cross-disciplinary approach is required.

Emergency presentations

Emergency mental health presentations usually involve:
- concerns about serious self-harm or suicide
- acute psychosis: distress secondary to hearing voices and delusional thoughts
- reactions to specific changes in circumstances or events: entry into custody, bereavement, or response to bullying or assault.

Such presentations can be manifest as:
- high levels of overt distress associated with dramatic self-harm or suicidal gestures and other behaviours such as head-banging, destruction of property, and faecal smearing
- self-isolation, poor self-care, reduced intake of food and drink, and reduced communication with others
- sudden, unexpected behaviours not characteristic of the young person such as a serious unprovoked assault on another young person or member of staff.

In such circumstances there is frequently an underlying mental health or emotional cause. It is particularly important for there to be a concerted review of such cases by the mental health team to identify possible exacerbations of previous conditions or new presentations of major mental health concern. Even if there is not a formal mental health presentation at the root of the acute disturbance, it is likely that mental health input into future care-planning support for the young person will be required.

Responses from a healthcare team to emergency presentations:
- need to be prompt and involve mental health professionals working with other staff across the establishment
- require clarity regarding initial appraisal; this may identify a specific underlying mental health or neurodevelopmental condition or whether this is not immediately evident or is impossible to assess
- should include an immediate cross-disciplinary formulation of the situation
- should include development of an initial plan of care and support including:
  - clarity whether specific mental health interventions are immediately required
  - implementation of recognized support process such as ACCT in cases of self-harm or suicidal behaviours
  - ensuring that parents and carers or others with parental responsibility are informed of the concern and plan of care and that prompt contact with the young person by phone and, if possible, by an urgent face-to-face visit is organized
  - ensuring ongoing continuity of support from identified professionals for the young person to establish meaningful dialogue and trust
- may require emergency treatment under common law where the level of distress in response to psychosis is particularly acute and it is not possible to establish the young person's or significant other's consent to immediate treatment by medication.

Attempted suicide

- The processes are broadly similar to those employed with adults (see Chapter 15) but it is important to tailor interventions to children's needs.[1]
- Staff should also review the individual's integrated care (SECURE STAIRS) formulation and liaise with the family.

Transfer of a young person to an in-patient mental health setting

- Specific guidance for young people is provided within PSI 62.[2]
- Most mental health presentations can be managed within secure youth justice settings even when they involve significant levels of disturbance and concern.
- In rare cases, however, when either the initial presentation is such or when an agreed plan of care in custody proves insufficient to meet mental health need, a transfer to an in-patient mental health setting will be required. Such transfers to hospital occur under the Mental Health Act 1983 (sections 48/49 for young people on remand and sections 47/49 for those who have been sentenced).
- The decision to undertake a hospital transfer rests with mental health professionals within the healthcare team, and is usually guided by an experienced psychiatrist.
- Before making a final decision, a psychiatrist may wish to discuss the case with colleagues from the relevant community forensic CAMHS covering the young person's home area to get their support for a transfer and to ensure that they are aware of the young person's situation as they are likely to be involved in future follow-up of the case.
- This process is broadly similar to that employed with adults but includes two important differences in recognition of age—increased vulnerability and lack of maturity:
  - Parents or those with parental responsibility should be involved as much as possible in decisions about hospitalization of their children.
  - A shorter time frame (maximum 7 days) within which to effect the transfer from custody to hospital in recognition of increased vulnerability due to their youth and lack of maturity.
- Referrals can be made from the CYPSE to any of the units within the national MSU clinical network but would usually be made to the geographically closest one.
- Referrals should be made via the NHS England CAMHS Inpatient National Referral Forms[1] (if these forms are not immediately available, they can be accessed from any NHS England in-patient or community CAMHS provider).
- All referrals are discussed at weekly referrals of the national MSU network which has representation from all units.
- If a referral is considered appropriate, it will be allocated to a specific unit for assessment. This allocation will be made based on available treatment, geography, and current capacity to admit. If a young person

is considered for a national MSU bed, their transfer will be organized as soon as possible once the relevant Mental Health Act order is finalized.

- If the young person is not considered appropriate for an in-patient setting, the MSU assessor may advise the custodial setting further about recommendations for management. If the situation within does not improve or deteriorates further, the prison mental health team should not hesitate to re-refer to the MSU in-patient network.

References

1. Prisons and Probation Ombudsman for England and Wales. Independent investigations. Child deaths: learning from PPO investigations into the three recent deaths of children in custody. Learning Lessons Bulletin. March 2013. https://s3-eu-west-2.amazonaws.com/ppo-prod-stor age-1g9rkhjhkjmgw/uploads/2014/07/LLB_FII_03_Child_deaths.pdf
2. Twitchett C. Procedure for the transfer from custody of children and young people to and from hospital under the mental health act 1983 in England: PSI 62. Ministry of Justice; 2011. https://www.justice.gov.uk/downloads/offenders/psipso/psi-2011/psi-62-2011-transfer-children-under-mental-health-act.doc

Assaults

- A 2016/2017 survey[1] by HMIP found that 39% of children reported feeling unsafe at some point in their current YOI and 22% of children felt unsafe at some point since arriving at their STC.
- Approximately 2700 reported assaults occurred in 2016/2017 in the youth secure estate (which has a population of 900).[2]
- Assaults occur for a variety of reasons but, for young people, there is often a gang-related element to them. Gang disputes that arise outside the establishment can have consequences within it. Staff should also be aware that gang loyalties fluctuate and alliances can be formed within establishments that do not exist outside.
- Child sexual abuse also occurs within the youth secure estate and prevalence studies indicate there were around 200 alleged incidents between 2016 and 2017.[3]
- Young people sometimes try to manage their fear of being assaulted through hypervigilance, self-imposed cell confinement, deliberate projection of an image of self-confidence, going to the gym to 'bulk up', or forming alliances with other young people or staff whom they hope will be able to keep them safe. The onset of these types of behaviours should prompt sensitive exploration of whether fear of assault is the motivation behind them.
- A recent study[4] found that young people in custody had a poor understanding of what constituted sexually inappropriate behaviour and sexual 'banter'. They were much less likely to report sexual than physical abuse.
- When managing a young person about an assault, it is important that staff are aware of the further risks to which a young person may be exposed if the impression is inadvertently given to others that they are a 'snitch'.
- Where young people are involved in serious incidents, staff must ensure that local safeguarding and child protection procedures are followed as well as any other local investigation into the incident.

References

1. HM Inspectorate of Prisons. Children in Custody 2016–17. London: HM Inspectorate of Prisons; 2017.
2. Youth Justice Board. Youth justice annual statistics: 2016 to 2017. 2018. https://www.gov.uk/gov ernment/statistics/youth-justice-annual-statistics-2016-to-2017
3. Independent Inquiry into Child Sexual Abuse. INQ001769. 2018. https://www.iicsa.org.uk/key-documents/5554/view/INQ001769.pdf
4. Soares C, George R, Pope L, et al. Safe inside? Child sexual abuse in the youth secure estate. Independent Inquiry into Child Sexual Abuse; 2019. https://www.iicsa.org.uk/key-documents/9536/view/safe-inside%3F-child-sexual-abuse-youth-secure-estate-full-report.pdf

Autism and intellectual disability

Autism spectrum conditions (ASCs)

- ASCs represent a wide spectrum of impairment characterized by qualitative abnormalities in reciprocal social interactions and communication. It is often associated with markedly restricted, stereotyped patterns of behaviour and interests and unusual sensory sensitivities.
- The clinical expression of ASCs is not uniform but varies between individuals, their stage of development, changing environmental demands, and with the presence of comorbidities. However, people with ASCs typically experience difficulties or misunderstandings in their daily lives as a result of their condition.
- Imprisoned people with ASCs are at increased risk of bullying, confrontations, exploitation, anxiety, and social isolation as a result of ASC traits such as stereotyped behaviour, social naivety, and impaired empathy.[1]
- No studies conducted in English prison populations have been published although several researchers have suggested that there are likely to be many individuals with unrecognized ASCs in custody.[2,3] There have also been no published studies of the prevalence of ASCs among English adolescent offenders within secure settings or in the community.
- The difficulties experienced by people with autism can often lead to them attracting attention within custody. However, the underlying reasons for their behaviour are frequently not understood. This is particularly the case for those who are more verbally articulate.
- When faced with unexpectedly concerning or challenging behaviour, staff should consider whether the individual may have an ASC.
- Simply asking an individual whether it has ever been suggested that they might be on the autistic spectrum can sometimes flag up those who might benefit from further assessment.
- Pathways for obtaining autism assessments for individuals within youth (and adult) custodial settings are currently being developed.
- Some establishments have made (often simple) adjustments to their regimes, enabling them to become more sensitive to the needs of those on the autistic spectrum.[4]
- An emphasis on victim empathy is likely to be an unhelpful and inappropriate component of rehabilitation interventions undertaken with individuals with ASCs.

Intellectual disability

Intellectual disability is defined by three criteria:
- An IQ score of less than 70.
- Significant difficulties with everyday tasks.
- Onset prior to adulthood.

Generalized intellectual disability is significantly more common in young people in custody, mostly in the mild range of impairment.
- Many may not have had their intellectual disability recognized as it may have been overshadowed by their challenging behaviour or masked through the use of stock phrases.

- It has been suggested[5] that those with more severe intellectual disabilities are more likely to either have their 'challenging and/or offending behaviour ... excused by care providers' or to be diverted towards specialist services rather than entering the youth secure estate. As a result, the population within the youth justice system might be expected to demonstrate disproportionately high levels of mild or borderline intellectual functioning.
- Although the level of impairment may be mild, identification of intellectual disabilities is important as they may affect the ability of a young person to engage effectively with their court process and require adjustments to be made for a fair trial.
- A separate range of impairments are the specific intellectual difficulties which relate to reading, writing, or mathematics. Few prevalence studies exist in young people with offending behaviour. However, it appears that specific reading difficulties, such as dyslexia, are more common in young people who offend. Young people often feel ashamed by their reading difficulties and seek to conceal them.
- Studies of speech and language skills in young people with offending behaviour in the UK have found a high level of deficit in both receptive and expressive language skills, with rates of around 60%. This is likely to lead to difficulties in participating in education and offence-specific work as well as in day-to-day functioning. It may contribute to misunderstandings between peers and staff.

References

1. Alley C. Experiences of prison inmates with autism spectrum disorders and the knowledge and understanding of the spectrum amongst prison staff: a review. J Intellect Disabil Offending Behav. 2015;6(2):55–67.
2. McAdam, P. Knowledge and understanding of the autism spectrum amongst prison staff. Prison Serv J. 2012;26–30.
3. Myers F. On the Borderline? People with Intellectual Disabilities and/or Autistic Spectrum Disorders in Secure, Forensic and Other Specialist Settings. Edinburgh: Scottish Development Centre for Mental Health; 2004.
4. Lewis A, Foster M, Hughes C, et al. Improving the management of prisoners with autistic spectrum disorders. Prison Serv J. 2016;226:21–26.
5. Herrington V. Assessing the prevalence of intellectual disability among young male prisoners. J Intellect Disabil Res. 2009;53(5):397–410.

Attention deficit hyperactivity disorder

ADHD is the most common mental health disorder within the youth estate. It is a developmental disorder involving a combination of inattention, impulsivity, and restlessness. Not all of these core features are necessarily present to the same extent. ADHD is also associated with emotional instability, sleep problems, and organizational difficulties.

Symptoms will be evident (but are not necessarily recognized) before the age of 12 years. Clinically significant impairment persists beyond childhood in 65% of cases.[1] ADHD is associated with increased mortality,[2] criminality,[3] substance misuse,[4] and reduced quality of life.[5] It is also commonly comorbid with autism, other developmental disorders, conduct disorder, and anxiety.

Effective treatments exist for ADHD and custody offers an opportunity to evaluate symptoms and trial medication in a controlled and supervised environment.[6] Effective treatment results in significantly reduced[7] rates of challenging behaviour within secure establishments and reduced rates of offending in the community (by 32% in men and 41% in women).[8]

Presentation

Presentations that may suggest ADHD include:
- trouble waiting one's turn in queues or conversations
- reactive aggression
- blurting out inappropriate comments ('taking the joke too far')
- struggling to concentrate during sustained, repetitive, or unstimulating activities
- general disorganization such as losing possessions and poor time management
- exploitation by others as a consequence of impulsivity and poor consequential thinking.

NICE guideline NG87[6] covers the recognition, diagnosis, and management of ADHD in children, young people, and adults. Further practical advice, specifically tailored to working in adult and youth custodial environments, is also available.[9]

Many pharmacological treatments for ADHD are amphetamine derived and classed as controlled drugs. Prescription of sustained-release preparations is likely to reduce the number of daily doses required and be more convenient for all concerned. Such preparations are also less open to abuse than short-acting formulations.

Any decision to proceed to a trial of medication for ADHD can create challenges for staff working in the secure estate. These and other procedural difficulties can frequently obstruct a clearly justifiable trial of treatment and healthcare teams frequently need to be persistent in ensuring that the wider custodial setting establishes appropriate means for such needs to be met. Any treatment plan should ensure:
- means whereby regular and timely administration of prescribed medication is ensured—delayed administration of stimulant medication in the morning may cause sleep disruption later that night
- ongoing consistent enquiry about potential side effects of medication (some of which are short term in nature); establishment of a procedural

response to loss of appetite during the day and resultant increased appetite in the evenings in those subject to a trial of medication or those for whom medication has been identified as beneficial
- means of undertaking routine screening of cardiac and general health which may prove to a be a contraindication to starting medication
- means of ensuring regular monitoring of baseline indices (pulse, BP, weight, and height in young people).

Non-pharmacological interventions can have additional benefits for individuals with ADHD. These might include:
- provision of additional opportunities for physical exercise
- reasonable adjustments such as permitting additional breaks during tasks
- provision of less distracting environments for activities requiring higher levels of focus (e.g. education and rehabilitation activities).

References

1. Ogilvie JM, Stewart AL, Chan RCK, et al. Neuropsychological measures of executive function and antisocial behavior: a meta-analysis. Criminology. 2011;49:1063–1107.
2. Chitsabesan P, Lennox C, Williams H, et al. Managing traumatic brain injury in young offenders; findings from the CHAT study and the development of a linkworker service. J Head Trauma Rehabil. 2015;30(2):106–115.
3. Gudjonsson GH, Sigurdsson JF, Sigfusdottir ID, et al. A national epidemiological study investigating risk factors for police interrogation and false confession among juveniles and young persons. Soc Psychiatry Psychiatr Epidemiol. 2016;51(3):359–367.
4. van Emmerik-van Oortmerssen K, van de Glind G, van den Brink W, et al. Prevalence of attention-deficit hyperactivity disorder in substance use disorder patients: a metaanalysis and meta-regression analysis. Drug Alcohol Depend. 2012;122(1–2):11–19.
5. Peasgood T, Bhardwaj A, Biggs K, et al. The impact of ADHD on the health and well-being of ADHD children and their siblings. Eur Child Adolesc Psychiatry. 2016;25(11):1217–1231.
6. National Institute for Health and Care Excellence. Attention deficit hyperactivity disorder: diagnosis and management. NICE guideline [NG87]. March 2018 (updated September 2019). https://www.nice.org.uk/guidance/NG87
7. Young S, Gudjonsson GH, Wells J, et al. Attention deficit hyperactivity disorder and critical incidents in a Scottish prison population. Pers Indiv Dif. 2009;46(3):265–269.
8. Lichtenstein P, Halldner L, Zetterqvist J, et al. Medication for attention deficit-hyperactivity disorder and criminality. N Engl J Med. 2012;367(21):2006–2014.
9. Young S, Gudjonsson G, Chitsabesan P, et al. Identification and treatment of offenders with attention-deficit/hyperactivity disorder in the prison population: a practical approach based upon expert consensus. BMC Psychiatry. 2018;18:281.

Sexual health

Creating a healthy sexual identity is an important developmental task for adolescence. Coming into custody as a teenager can create obstacles to achieving this successfully. Sharing rooms may mean that opportunities for normal sexual behaviour such as masturbation are limited and there is a risk that discovery of such behaviour can lead to fear of punishment or being shamed and bullied.

Prior experiences

Many young people have not been exposed to positive relationship role models prior to coming into custody and may have acquired unhealthy attitudes and behaviours towards partners, sex, contraception, and parenting. Arrival in the secure estate offers an opportunity for these views to be challenged and for young people to helped to understand more about healthy relationships and sexual health. This creates the possibility for breaking the cycle of unhealthy intergenerational attitudes to relationships.

- Some young people may have previously experienced sexual abuse or exploitation (possibly gang related) and may be vulnerable to or fearful of this recurring in custody.
- Some young people may have had poor sexual education and this can make them vulnerable to exploitation or mean that they acquire ill-informed or unhealthy knowledge from their peers.
- The single-sex nature of secure establishments limits opportunities to start heterosexual relationships and this can be frustrating.
- Some young people may already be in relationships when they enter the secure estate but the enforced separation from their partner often leads to difficulties in maintaining their relationship and can become a source of distress. Other young people may be jealous of those who have partners and this can be a source of conflict.
- Some young people may have entered the secure estate before they had a chance to have a relationship or any sexual experience. This can lead to a sense of anxiety and shame.

LGBTQ+ considerations

- Some young people will be LGBTQ+ and may struggle to cope with this within a custodial environment and try and conceal their sexual identity from others for fear of being bullied. Larger establishments may provide LGBTQ+ support groups.
- Young people entering custody who identify as transgender will typically be placed into a mixed gender SCH or STC (section 46 of YCS placement guidance).[1]
- However, some transgender individuals may be placed in a YOI. In such cases, the young person should be referred automatically to the Complex Case Board in accordance with section 4.21 of the 'Policy Framework for the Care and Management of Individuals who are Transgender'.[2]
- Transgender young people transitioning from youth custody to the adult prison estate must be referred to the Complex Care Board in good time to enable transfer planning.

Promoting sexual health

An assessment of sexually transmitted diseases in 17–20-year-old men in an English YOI found that 52% had had a sexually transmitted disease within the last year and 16% had had two or more sexual partners in the previous 3 months.[3] Young people in custody have frequently also missed out on routine HPV vaccination and cervical screening.

Sexually transmitted diseases and BBVs are assessed routinely (via the CHAT) following entry into the secure estate. This offers a chance for treatment, partner notification, and safer sex education.

References

1. HM Prison and Probation Service. Placing young people in custody: guide for youth justice practitioners. 2017. https://www.gov.uk/guidance/placing-young-people-in-custody-guide-for-youth-justice-practitioners

2. HM Prison and Probation Service, Ministry of Justice. The care and management of individuals who are transgender. 2019. https://www.gov.uk/government/publications/the-care-and-management-of-individuals-who-are-transgender

3. David N, Tang A. Sexually transmitted infections in a young offenders institution in the UK. Int J STD AIDS. 2003 Aug;14(8):511-3. doi: 10.1258/095646203767869084. PMID: 12935377.

Safeguarding children and adolescents in secure environments

Introduction

Responsibilities for safeguarding children and young people up to the age of 18 years are enshrined in legislation which applies to all agencies providing services for children and young people and adults. All staff in prisons must take steps to prevent abuse from occurring, respond appropriately to any signs or allegations of abuse, and work effectively with others to implement protection plans. Fundamental to this is having in place policies consistent with the Local Safeguarding Children's Boards covering all aspects of safeguarding—safe recruitment, mental capacity, management of allegations, Prevent, information sharing, chaperone, whistleblowing, and escalation.

While the prison governor holds responsibility for safeguarding in the establishment, healthcare professionals (who must have a named safeguarding lead) have a duty to ensure that risks of harm are identified and to provide care and support to children and young people.

Legislation and guidance

- Safeguarding children is governed by the Children Act 1989, revised in 2004.
- 'Working Together to Safeguard Children' 2018 is statutory guidance.[1]

Identification of safeguarding issues

Children and young people in contact with the youth justice system are generally a socially excluded population with significant complex health needs. Immediate health needs, vulnerabilities, or risk of harm to self or others must be identified promptly on arrival by using the CHAT.[2]

Vulnerabilities in children and young people include:
- coming from a dysfunctional family with a history of offending
- past history of abuse:
  - physical abuse including TBI/female genital mutilation
  - emotional abuse—poor attachment/regulation/low self-esteem
  - sexual abuse—including child sexual exploitation/trafficking/prostitution
  - neglect—of health needs/education/self-neglect
- substance misuse
- learning difficulties/communication difficulties
- mental health problems—depression/anxiety/eating disorders
- self-harm and suicide attempts
- exploitation including radicalization/modern slavery
- bullying/victimization
- those who will struggle to cope in custody:
  - children and young people placed far from home
  - children and young people subject to restraint.

Management of vulnerabilities

The establishment must promote the welfare of children and young people, particularly those at most risk, and must protect them from all kinds of harm and neglect by:

- ensuring immediate safety of the child or young person
- clearly documenting vulnerabilities and risks
- care planning to include individual care and support
- opening ACCT if indicated
- discussing with healthcare safeguarding lead
- sharing information appropriately with safer custody team/officers
- informing the prison governor
- referral to or discussion with the Multi-Agency Safeguarding Hub (MASH)
- reporting any incidents as appropriate
- discussing at MDT meeting and in supervision.

Management of allegations of abuse in the establishment

- Ensure the immediate safety of the child or young person.
- Provide any urgent medical treatment.
- Remove the alleged perpetrator who may be a risk to others.
- Discuss with healthcare safeguarding lead and duty governor.
- If the child or young person has suffered or is likely to suffer significant harm, referral to be made to the MASH.
- Take part in strategy discussion, sharing information to inform next steps.
- Report incident and clearly document actions taken.

References

1. HM Government. Working together to safeguard children: a guide to inter-agency working to safeguard and promote the welfare of children. 2018. https://www.gov.uk/government/publications/working-together-to-safeguard-children--2
2. Offender Health Research Network. Comprehensive Health Assessment Tool (CHAT): Young People in Contact with the Youth Offending Service (YOS). Manchester: Offender Health Research Network; 2013.

Chapter 12

Foreign nationals in detention

Health needs of foreign nationals in detention

Introduction

Foreign nationals make up around 11% of the UK prison population. The most recent data available demonstrated that the majority are from other European countries (43% European Economic Area, 10% non-European Economic Area European countries), followed by Africa (18%) and Asia (14%). There are two prisons in England that detain only foreign nationals, but they are also held across the wider prison estate. Foreign national people in prison (FNPs) have shared health needs as per the general prison population but also have some specific needs that will need identifying and supporting. FNPs may well have come from countries where poor healthcare, poverty, violence, and war are prevalent. They may have endured arduous journeys before arriving in the UK. They may bear the health sequalae of these issues.

Health needs

a significant number of FNPs will be born or have lived in countries with a high incidence of TB and BBVs. BBVs—hepatitis B/C and HIV screening should be considered depending on the prevalence of the disease in the other country and additional risk factors, particularly sexual activity. Individuals should be helped to access screening for this (see HIV care in prisons, p. 150).

TB screening—symptoms of TB should be asked about and active TB be considered in anyone presenting with symptoms. Screening for latent TB infection (LTBI) should be carried out in those from a country with a high TB incidence or with a high clinical risk.

- Social risk factors such as homelessness, smoking, and drug and alcohol use are likely to be seen in FNPs as in the general prison population:
  - With this come the expected health sequelae (e.g. communicable diseases including BBVs, poor nutritional status, poorly managed chronic medical conditions, liver disease, respiratory disease, and cardiac disease).
- A significant number of FNPs will be born or have lived in countries with a high incidence of TB and BBVs.
- BBVs—hepatitis B/C and HIV screening should be considered depending on the prevalence of the disease in the other country and additional risk factors, particularly sexual activity. Individuals should be helped to access screening for this (see HIV care in prisons, p. 150).
- TB screening—symptoms of TB should be asked about and active TB be considered in anyone presenting with symptoms. Screening for latent TB should be carried out in those from a country with a high TB

For more details see:
- Asylum, p. 298.
- Assessing and reporting on torture and ill-treatment, p. 304.

incidence or with a high clinical risk[1] (see Management of tuberculosis in prisons, p. 146.
- MDR-TB is becoming a greater issue, particularly in Eastern Europe and Russia.
- Many FNPs will have been offered a different vaccine schedule in their home country—check what would have been offered on the WHO website (http://apps.who.int/immunization_monitoring/globalsummary/schedules).
- Mental health: language barriers, isolation, displacement, experience of violence, and immigration status uncertainty.

Sources of support
- A foreign national coordinator should be identified in the prison to champion the health and well-being of FNPs.
- Charitable organizations can provide support and guidance, such as the Association of Visitors to Immigration Detention (AVID).
- It is crucial that language line facilities are available and used. Staff may be unsure of how to use or unfamiliar with best practice when interacting through a translator—be open and support the team. There are free translating resources from organizations such as British Red Cross, Refugee Action, and Office for Health Improvement and Disparities (see Resources, p. 296).

Reference
1. National Institute for Health and Care Excellence. Tuberculosis. NICE guideline [NG33]. 2016 (updated September 2019). https://www.nice.org.uk/guidance/ng33/chapter/recommendations

Continuity of care

FNPs will be released either to the community or, more likely, deported back to their home country. Health interventions that will have been commenced in prison may need continuing on release.

See also Chapter 14.

Release

On release (whether being deported or released into the UK community) it is important to:
- provide a written summary of care
- provide the patient with a copy of medical records
- give general advice as to how the healthcare system works in the destination country (e.g. how to register with a GP in the UK)
- have a final consultation to discuss care provided and what follow-up is needed on return to home country/in the community
- provide at least a month of medication.

Resources

- Migrants Organise. Good practice guide to interpreting. 2010. http://www.migrantsorganise.org/?p=21539
- Office for Health Improvement and Disparities. Language interpreting and translation: migrant health guide. 2021. https://www.gov.uk/guidance/language-interpretation-migrant-health-guide
- Picture Communication Tool: http://www.picturecommunicationtool.com/
- World Health Organization. Immunization data: vaccine schedule. n.d. http://apps.who.int/immunization_monitoring/globalsummary/scheduleshttps://immunizationdata.who.int/listing.html?topic=vaccine-schedule&location=

Health and applications for asylum

Introduction

Asylum seekers are those who have left their home country and are claiming asylum under the 1951 UN Convention of the Status of Refugees or other forms of humanitarian protection, whereas refugees have had their protection status confirmed.

Conflict, persecution, and political instability continue to occur on a global scale, resulting in the significant displacement of people inside and across national borders. Many of those who traverse national borders to seek asylum at their destination arrive after treacherous, life-risking journeys. Those seeking asylum may have additional health needs resulting from their experiences during or prior to migration, poor access to healthcare in transit, lack of information and understanding of healthcare systems in the host country, and perceived or real barriers to healthcare.

UK asylum and appeal process

An asylum seeker is a person who has sought asylum in the UK and is awaiting a decision on that claim. Asylum seekers are required to demonstrate a well-founded fear of persecution and future risk on return due to their race, religion, nationality, political opinion, or membership of a particular social group, and an inability to seek protection from the authorities in their country of origin. Whether asylum should be granted depends on the risk to the applicant upon return, not on the demonstration of past persecution.

In the UK, asylum decisions are made by the UK Visas and Immigration (UKVI) department within the Home Office. An asylum seeker will have at least two official interviews. The first interview is called the Screening Interview. In this interview the applicant's personal details are recorded as well as an account of their journey to the UK. The second interview is the Substantive Interview. This interview provides the opportunity for the applicant to describe their past experiences and their future fear in the context of return to their country of origin.

Positive decisions will be made where UKVI finds the asylum seeker to have a well-founded fear of future persecution if they return. A person recognized as a refugee will usually be granted 5 years' leave to remain in the UK and can then apply for this to be extended and, ultimately, to seek citizenship. Time-limited leave to remain may also be granted on humanitarian or discretionary grounds. Following a refusal of an initial decision the applicant becomes a refused asylum seeker. Negative decisions may carry a right of appeal to an independent immigration tribunal, which can be exercised from within the UK.

Alleged victims of trafficking/modern slavery may be dealt with through the National Referral Mechanism (NRM). If they are initially found to have 'reasonable grounds' to be a victim of trafficking they are granted a short period of 'reflection and recovery' (45 days), while a 'conclusive grounds' decision is under consideration. If it is recognized that there are conclusive grounds that they were trafficked, they may be granted a time-limited period of leave. If there are ongoing support needs, they may be assessed for continued support via a Recovery Needs Assessment (RNA).

Victims of trafficking may also seek leave to remain through the asylum process outlined above.

The asylum process can be initiated from the prison or immigration detention setting. IRCs and some prisons may have legal surgeries to facilitate this. Where professionals working in these settings become aware of a patient's potential need to claim asylum, they can facilitate access to legal advice.

Foreign nationals in prison and immigration detention settings may have come from areas in which rates of ill-treatment/torture are relatively high (a recent US meta-analysis suggests up to 44% of asylum seekers may have been tortured). Furthermore, some foreign nationals (as well as UK nationals) may be victims of human trafficking/modern slavery. These forms of ill-treatment may involve coercion to engage in criminal activity and may in turn be the cause of their imprisonment. Victims of torture/trafficking may also be imprisoned or detained in relation to their use of false documents to enter and/or work in the UK.

In April 2022 the Nationality and Borders Act passed through Parliament which is expected to lead to significant changes in the asylum system in the UK.

Health problems associated with asylum seekers/refugees

Pre-migration difficulties

- Asylum seekers/refugees may have specific healthcare needs associated with what happened to them before they arrived in the UK.
- They may bear the physical and psychological consequences of human rights violations (see Assessing and reporting on torture and ill-treatment, p. 304).
- Histories of abuse and exploitation render asylum seekers more vulnerable to further such abuse and exploitation. Many may have come from areas where healthcare provision is already poor or has collapsed.
- Some may have come from refugee camps where nutrition and sanitation were poor.
- They may be at risk of malnourishment, anaemia, vitamin deficiencies, skin conditions and infestations, communicable diseases, and exacerbation of chronic medical conditions.

Peri-migration difficulties

- The journey to the UK can have effects on individuals through further violence and exploitation (often by human traffickers or smugglers), poverty, extremes of temperatures, length of the journey, overcrowded transport, and stress of leaving their country of origin.

Post-migration difficulties

Once in the UK, health needs of asylum seekers can develop or be significantly worsened because of barriers to healthcare and their socioeconomic situation, such as:

- lack of awareness of healthcare entitlement
- problems in registering and accessing primary and community healthcare services, particularly if their claim has been refused
- language barriers

- difficulties in disclosure of past traumatic experiences due to fear, shame, dissociative episodes, flashbacks, or poor memory (see Assessing and reporting on torture and ill-treatment, p. 304)
- loss of support from family and friends
- social isolation
- loss of status
- culture shock
- uncertainty
- racism and hostility
- housing difficulties
- poverty/destitution
- loss of choice and control.

Specific health concerns in asylum seekers/refugees

Mental health
- Emotional responses to trauma and grief.
- Depression.
- Anxiety and panic disorders.
- PTSD and complex PTSD (up to ten times the rate of PTSD than in the general population).
- Suicide/self-harm.
- Psychotic disorders.
- Substance misuse/abuse.
- Somatoform disorders and medically unexplained symptoms.
- Personality disorders.
- Learning difficulties.

Dental problems
- Dental problems are common due to poor dental care in the country of origin or may be due to trauma/torture.

Communicable disease
- Migrants may have greater risk of communicable disease due to the prevalence of a disease in their country of origin or during transit. For example:
  - TB, HIV, or hepatitis B/C
  - tropical diseases such as malaria and enteric and parasitic infections.
- Transmission and illness from exposure to communicable disease may be exacerbated by malnutrition, poor sanitation, overcrowding, and stress.
- Lack of access to full vaccination schedules may result in diseases (particularly diseases of childhood) not usually seen in host countries.
- General infectious diseases such as pneumonia.

Women's health
- Contraception and pregnancy: uptake of family planning services is low, and antenatal care frequently received late or not at all, resulting in poorer outcomes.
- Sequelae of sexual violence (see Assessing and reporting on torture and ill-treatment, p. 304).
- Screening: poor uptake rates for cervical and breast screening.

- Female genital mutilation: some women and girls may be arriving from areas with high female genital mutilation prevalence and can experience problems with childbirth, menstruation, urinary tract infections, fistulas, and psychological sequalae.

Chronic diseases

- Increase in incidence and severity of chronic diseases such as diabetes, COPD, ischaemic heart disease, and hypertension, which may not have been diagnosed or fully treated either in the country of origin, perhaps due to lack of healthcare services, or following arrival in the UK, due to difficulties accessing healthcare.
- Higher prevalence of diabetes and hypertension, particularly in older asylum seekers.

Chronic pain

Psychosocial stressors can compound physical injuries and illnesses resulting in chronic pain syndromes.

Medico-legal documentation of torture

In order to support the just determination of survivors' claims for asylum and thus maximize their prospects of recovery, doctors may be asked to document their physical and psychological findings and offer an opinion as to whether their findings are consistent with the claims. This may take the form of a professional report or an independent, Istanbul Protocol-compliant expert medico-legal report[1] (see Assessing and reporting on torture and ill-treatment, p. 304). No matter the reason for the assessment, a careful history is important in all assessments of alleged ill-treatment (see Assessing and reporting on torture and ill-treatment, p. 304).

Health and immigration removal centres

Immigration detention is the practice of detaining migrants and asylum seekers (see Immigration removal centres and immigration detention, p. 310).

Reference

1. Office of the High Commissioner for Human Rights. Istanbul Protocol: Manual on the Effective Investigation and Documentation of Torture and Other Cruel, Inhuman or Degrading Treatment or Punishment (2022 edition). New York: United Nations; 2022. https://www.ohchr.org/en/publications/policy-and-methodological-publications/istanbul-protocol-manual-effective-0

Further reading

Blackmore R, Boyle JA, Fazel M, et al. The prevalence of mental illness in refugees and asylum seekers: a systematic review and meta-analysis. PLoS Med. 2020;17(9):e1003337.

British Medical Association. BMA refugee and asylum seeker health resource. 2019. [This guidance is for doctors who may be uncertain about the specific health needs and entitlement to different types of care of patients who are refugees and asylum seekers.] https://www.bma.org.uk/media/1838/bma-refugee-and-asylum-seeker-health-resource-june-19.pdf

Burnett A, Ndovi T. The health of forced migrants. BMJ. 2018;363:k4200.

Doctors of the World. Primary care. In: Healthcare entitlement and charging in England—updated 2018. February 2018. https://www.doctorsoftheworld.org.uk/wp-content/uploads/2018/11/DoTW_Guide-to-Healthcare-entitlement-2018-2.pdf

Heslehurst N, Brown H, Pemu A, et al. Perinatal health outcomes and care among asylum seekers and refugees: a systematic review of systematic reviews. BMC Med. 2018;16:89.

Hunt J, Witkin R, Katona C. Identifying human trafficking in adults. BMJ. 2020;371:m4683.

Knights F, Munir S, Ahmed H, et al. Initial health assessments for newly arrived migrants, refugees, and asylum seekers. BMJ. 202:377:e068821.

United Nations High Commissioner for Refugees. Convention relating to the status of refugees (including text of 1967 protocol). https://www.unhcr.org/PROTECT/protection/3b66c2a a10.pdf

United Nations High Commissioner for Refugees. Global trends—forced displacement in 2018. United Nations; 2019. https://www.unhcr.org/en-au/ statistics/unhcrstats/5d08d7ee7/unhcr-global-trends-2018.html

World Health Organization. Female genital mutilation. January 2022. http://www.who.int/mediacen tre/factsheets/fs241/en/

Assessing and reporting on torture and ill-treatment

Introduction

Torture involves the deliberate infliction of pain or suffering (physical and/or psychological) by a perpetrator against an individual's will. This may be for a variety of purposes, which include obtaining information or exerting control. Although some legal definitions of torture emphasize the role of the state, from a clinical point of view it is widely accepted that torture includes a variety of cruel and inhuman or degrading treatment such as human trafficking/modern slavery, domestic abuse, and gender-based violence. All medical professionals working in a prison/detention setting have a primary responsibility to act in the best interests of their patients. They also have a professional duty to document and report any evidence of torture or other ill-treatment of detainees in their care.

Systematic documentation of the physical and psychological sequelae of torture by independent medical experts may also be critical in determining asylum claims and in criminal litigation. The Istanbul Protocol provides internationally recognized guidance on such documentation.[1]

Foreign nationals in prison and immigration detention settings may have come from areas in which rates of ill-treatment/torture are relatively high. Furthermore, some foreign nationals (as well as UK nationals) may be victims of human trafficking/modern slavery. These forms of ill-treatment may involve coercion to engage in criminal activity and may in turn be the cause of their imprisonment. Furthermore, victims of torture/trafficking may also be imprisoned or detained in relation to their use of false documents to enter and/or work in the UK.

If torture or ill-treatment is reported or suspected in detention (see below for indicative clinical features), the medical professional should:
- assess and document the alleged ill-treatment
- manage its physical and psychological sequelae
- initiate appropriate clinical investigation, management, and follow-up
- establish care needs and where they can best be met—in the prison healthcare setting or in the community (outpatient or inpatient treatment)
- consider legal protection needs.

Torture and its sequalae

Direct physical violence

Includes
- injuries seen from being beaten, punched, crushed, whipped, stabbed, burnt, scalded, cut, restrained, or suspended.

Sequalae include
- fractures, sprains, ligament damage, peripheral nerve injuries, dental and facial injuries, cigarette burns, scalds.

Sequelae of head injuries include
- headaches: stress, migraine, post-concussion syndrome
- haematoma (chronic subdural/intracerebral)

- epilepsy (incidence in general public 0.5%, incidence in torture victims 20%): grand mal seizures, or partial seizures
- anterograde or retrograde amnesia
- cognitive impairment.

Sexual violence
Includes
- violence to genitals
- molestation
- instrumentation
- rape.

Sequalae include
- STIs including BBVs
- pelvic inflammatory disease
- pregnancies, including ectopic pregnancies, enforced abortions
- lacerations, deformities to genital area
- pelvic pain
- vaginal bleeding
- fistulae
- testicular tenderness/pain
- dysuria
- anal issues—fissure, tags, haemorrhoids, rectal prolapse, bleeding, pain
- psychological issues including shame
- NB—male sexual abuse:
  - frequent in victims of torture
  - associated with intense shame so difficult to admit to.

Captivity/neglect
Includes
- small, overcrowded cells
- solitary confinement or other isolation
- unhygienic, damp, cold, or hot conditions
- irregular or contaminated food/water
- no privacy/forced nakedness
- sensory deprivation (sound, light, time)
- restriction of sleep, food, water, toilet, bathing, and lack of medical care.

Sequalae include
- chronic medical conditions/untreated existing conditions (e.g. hypertension, diabetes)
- untreated physical injuries
- malnourishment, anaemia, vitamin deficiencies
- infectious diseases (e.g. TB, chest infections, skin infections, gastrointestinal infections).

Environmental/work-related injuries
Includes
- working in harsh, unregulated conditions.

Sequalae include
- physical injuries; burns, lacerations, amputations, musculoskeletal and back pains
- effects of heat/cold/light exposure
- effects of chemical exposure.

Others
- Gunshots.
- Falaka: repeated beating on soles of feet. Can cause pain on walking even years later. Can be misdiagnosed as plantar fasciitis.
- Electric shock.
- Ears: perforated ear drums (slapping side of head).
- Eyes: directly targeted by blunt or sharp trauma, or chemicals. Kept in darkness or light exposure—photophobia, increased lacrimation, pain, retinal injury, keratitis, conjunctivitis.
- Chemical: salt, chili, gasoline—in eyes, wounds, body cavities.
- Asphyxiation: wet and dry methods, drowning, submersion, smothering, choking, chemical. Reported long-term issues include bronchitis/asthma.
- Hormonal: for example, forced contraception, hormones to speed up puberty for sexual exploitation purposes.
- Branding or tattooing: very degrading, permanent reminder.
- Medical/surgical: amputation of digits/limbs, harvesting of organs, forced 'aesthetic' procedures (e.g. breast enlargement).

Often NO observable physical sequalae
- Torturers may take care not to leave physical evidence.
- Even without such measures, *visible* evidence of past injuries may be absent if years have elapsed since the injury.
- Torture methods such as water boarding, electric shocks, and falaka can cause extreme pain and suffering without lasting visible lesions.
- Sexual assault often leaves no physical evidence.
- Severe bruising from blunt trauma may heal without residual evidence.

Specific psychological methods
There is an interaction between physical and psychological methods of torture. Physical attacks may leave no lasting marks but may have serious psychological impacts. Some forms of torture are specifically devised to increase the negative psychological impact and enhance psychological control over the individual.

Includes
- degrading/humiliating treatment (e.g. stripped naked, having to eat from the floor, no toilet facilities)
- constant threat of harm, death, or sexual violence (e.g. mock executions, threatened or actual rape)
- confinement in small spaces and/or isolation
- extremes of stimulation (noise, temperature, etc.)
- deprivation: sleep, light, food, healthcare
- forced confessions or repeated interrogations
- indefinite period of detention

- hearing abuse/torture of others
- threats made against loved ones/false information given about them
- being forced to harm/betray others.

Mental health sequalae of torture
Symptoms include
- extreme sadness, insomnia, nightmares, flashbacks, dissociation, emotional numbing, anger and irritability, fear, shame, guilt, and somatization.

Diagnoses include
- PTSD/complex PTSD
- depression
- anxiety and panic disorders
- psychosis
- suicidality and self-harm (increased in those with PTSD and major depression)
- substance abuse.

Guiding principles when taking a history

'Information is certainly important, but the person being interviewed is even more so, and listening is more important than asking questions.'
- Allow plenty of time and offer follow-up appointments if possible.
- Give a full explanation of your role, duty of confidentiality, and any process.
- Use a calm, empathetic manner and remain objective.
- Think of the space you are in, for example, as comfortable an environment as possible with no noisy interruptions.
- Beware of possible emotional reactions of victims recounting their story and risk of re-traumatization. If needed, take breaks or halt the interview.
- Make sure the interviewee is aware they can halt the interview at any point.
- Use open-ended questions, especially at the start of the clinical encounter.

Specific difficulties in recounting a history in torture and trafficking survivors

- *Factors during torture or trafficking* (e.g. blindfolding, drugging, loss of consciousness).
- *Disorientation* (being kept in the dark, moved frequently, solitary confinement, multiple episodes of ill-treatment over a prolonged time).
- *Memory impairment* due to organic causes (e.g. head injury, starvation, and suffocation).
- *Memory impairment* due to trauma-related mental ill health (e.g. depression, anxiety, and substance abuse, but, most notably, PTSD). People with PTSD have an impaired ability to recall clear and consistent chronologies and have trouble dealing with direct interviewing, especially in contexts which seem to them adversarial.

- *Shame*. PTSD (particularly when associated with sexual abuse) is associated with high levels of shame. Shame may also be linked to a sense that the victim 'gave in' to their torturer. The subsequent betrayal of others is particularly difficult to disclose.
- *Lack of trust* in the examiner.
- *Fear* of placing oneself or others at risk.
- *Coping mechanisms* such as denial and avoidance. Avoidance of reminders of trauma is a core feature of PTSD.

Remember that for all refugees, their journey and conditions in any destination country can compound the original traumas. For example, physical difficulties and abuse on journey; difficulties and delays in the asylum process, immigration detention, or prison; cultures of disbelief and racism; destitution; and separation from family, friends, and their own culture.

Reference

1. Office of the High Commissioner for Human Rights. Istanbul Protocol: Manual on the Effective Investigation and Documentation of Torture and Other Cruel, Inhuman or Degrading Treatment or Punishment (2022 edition). New York: United Nations; 2022. https://www.ohchr.org/en/publications/policy-and-methodological-publications/istanbul-protocol-manual-effective-0

Further reading

Busch JR, Hansen SH, Hougen HP. Geographical distribution of torture: an epidemiological study of torture reported by asylum applicants examined at the department of forensic medicine, University of Copenhagen. Torture. 2015;25(2):10.

Lunde I, Ortmann J. Prevalence and sequelae of sexual torture. Lancet. 1990;336(8710):289–291.

Orcutt M. Handbook of Refugee Health: For Healthcare Professionals and Humanitarians Providing Care to Forced Migrants. Boca Raton, FL: CRC Press; 2021.

Peel M, Lubell N, Beynon, J. Medical Investigation and Documentation of Torture: A Handbook for Health Professionals. Colchester: University of Essex; 2005.

Russell W, Hilton A, Peel M. Care and support of male survivors of conflict-related sexual violence: background paper. 2010. https://www.researchgate.net/publication/266376422_Care_and_Support_of_Male_Survivors_of_Conflict-Related_Sexual_Violence_Background_Paper_March_2010

Witkin R, Robjant K. Trauma informed code of conduct. Helen Bamber Association. 2018. https://www.helenbamber.org/resources/best-practiseguidelines/trauma-informed-code-conduct-ticc

World Health Organization. Refugee and migrant health. May 2022. https://www.who.int/news-room/fact-sheets/detail/refugee-and-migrant-health

Immigration removal centres and immigration detention

Introduction

The Home Office uses detention as a means of ensuring that those who seek to enter or stay in the UK illegally are prevented and deterred from doing so. It has, however, a legal duty to ensure that it deals humanely with all individuals who are detained, in particular those who might be considered vulnerable. Furthermore, doctors working in IRCs have duties defined in the General Medical Council's 'Good Medical Practice'[1] to protect vulnerable individuals. A duty of care to a patient is above that of any demands imposed by the institution, no matter how challenging this 'dual role' may be, and all care given should be equivalent to care given in any NHS setting. This overriding principle is easily forgotten but should be the main 'driver' for clinical decision-making in this context—just as it is in hospital, community, and prison settings.

Home Office detention policy, set out in Chapter 55 of the Home Office Enforcement Instructions and Guidance, states that certain categories of persons are normally considered suitable for detention only in *very exceptional circumstances*: minors; elderly; pregnant women; victims of trafficking; victims of torture; and those with a serious disability, medical condition, or mental illness.[2]

There are currently ten IRCs across the UK. At any time about 2000–3000 people are held in administrative detention in IRCs in the UK—about 30,000 a year.

- IRCs are 'closed' establishments which are locked and which detainees are not allowed to leave at will.
- There is no automatic judicial or independent oversight on the decision to detain or formal appeal process against such decisions.
- Detainees are not serving any criminal sentence.
- There is no time limit on detention and no pre-specified 'sentence'. Most detainees are held for less than 28 days, some are held for considerably longer.
- NB: the Nationality and Borders Act 2022 is likely to lead to a greater focus on detaining asylum seekers in immigration detention centres and in quasi-detention 'accommodation centres'. At the time of writing, this situation is unclear.

Since 2014, NHS England is responsible for commissioning healthcare for those detained in IRCs (which can hold people for prolonged periods) and short-term holding facilities whose main function is to hold newly arrived asylum seekers pending a decision on whether their claims will be processed in detention or in the community. All centres are obliged to have a GP attending.

Healthcare concerns

- People held in indefinite detention in IRCs are among the most vulnerable people in society.
- Many detainees have suffered torture or ill-treatment (see Assessing and reporting on torture and ill-treatment, p. 304).
- Significant and chronic health problems from pre-migration or post-migration difficulties (see Health and applications for asylum, p. 298).
- Age disputed minors are particularly vulnerable in an adult facility.
- Health, particularly mental ill-health, gets worse the longer a detainee is held.
- Detention for prolonged, indefinite, periods of time can cause mental health problems.
- Reduced sense of safety and freedom from harm.
- Reminder of past traumatic experiences.
- Aggravated fear of imminent return (reflected in the term 'immigration *removal* centre').
- Separation from support network.
- Disruption of treatment/care.
- Lack of access to appropriate healthcare in detention.
- Lack of an appropriate set of quality standards for healthcare in detention.

Adults at risk/safeguarding in IRCs

A new 'adults at risk' guidance came into effect in November 2021 which recognizes that vulnerable individuals may be at increased risk of harm from detention and states that vulnerable individuals ('adults at risk') should not normally be detained and can only be detained when immigration factors outweigh their indicators of risk.[3]

Indicators of risk include
- suffering from a mental health condition or impairment
- victims of torture
- victims of sexual or gender-based violence
- victims of human trafficking or modern slavery
- suffering from PTSD
- being pregnant
- suffering from a serious physical disability
- suffering from other serious physical health conditions
- being aged 70 or over
- being a transsexual or intersex person.

Several opportunities exist to identify such people before and during detention. These are summarized below.

Screening interview pre-detention
- Rule 34: outlines the obligation for a medical practitioner to conduct a physical and mental examination within 24 hours of admission (with consent).
- Rule 35: a mechanism which aims to ensure that particularly vulnerable detainees are brought to the attention of those with

direct responsibility for reviewing detention. Once a Rule 35 report is generated, the UKVI case owner must review the decision to detain. IRC GPs should raise a concern about detainees whose health would be injuriously affected by continued detention (see Assessing and reporting on torture and ill-treatment, p. 304).

Asylum interview

Despite these safeguards, problems include:
- inadequate training of detention centre and medical staff
- failure to investigate the possibility of vulnerability
- failure to properly assess and investigate sequalae of historical sexual violence
- failure to investigate and appropriately treat or refer significant medical problems
- Home Office caseworkers can override medical opinion given in Rule 35 reports on the basis of immigration factors
- poor documentation and treatment of harm on attempted removal—no patient-held record of diagnoses, investigation results, or treatment as well as insufficient medication, and no vaccinations/malaria prophylaxis given to take back to country of origin if removed from the UK.
- difficulty in accessing independent medical opinions
- difficulty in accessing appropriate interpreters
- poor communication with healthcare and difficulty in accessing healthcare on release leads to lack of continuity of care once in the community (again, no patient-held records)
- lack of consideration of mental capacity of detainees
- lack of appropriate training for IRC doctors, and barriers in raising concerns
- lack of appropriate time for assessment.

Mental health concerns in IRCs

The Royal College of Psychiatrists' position statement on people with mental disorders in IRCs[4] provides a useful summary of reasons why people with significant mental health problems should not be detained:
- People with a mental disorder constitute a 'particularly vulnerable' group.
- Detention is likely to precipitate a significant deterioration in mental health.
- IRCs are not appropriate therapeutic environments.
- There have been repeated examples of gross mismanagement of serious mental health problems in detention settings.
- Treatment of mental illness should take place in the *least restrictive environment*.

Capacity

Both pre-existing mental health disorders (which are likely to be aggravated by detention) and those arising in detention may result in detainees losing decision-making capacity with regard to healthcare and legal matters. This means that an already vulnerable population is less likely to receive appropriate healthcare for their mental health disorders and therefore may be impeded in accessing legal remedies leading to prolonged detention—which in turn leads to worse outcomes. Capacity assessments should be carried out where detainees need to make decisions and their capacity to do so is in doubt. If it is confirmed that they lack capacity, this should be taken fully into account.

Fitness to fly

Doctors in IRCs may be asked to comment on whether a detainee is fit to fly for the purposes of removal from the UK, from both a physical and a psychological standpoint. They should refer to specific guidance from the Civil Aviation Authority and the Regulation 3(2)b (The Immigration and Asylum (Provision of Accommodation to Failed Asylum-Seekers) Regulations 2005) where consideration is given to the possibility of being unable to leave the UK by reason of a physical impediment to travel or for some other medical reason.

The Civil Aviation Authority guidelines on fitness to fly[5] state that it is essential that psychiatric conditions are stable in order for people to fly. The guidelines highlight that the main areas for concern are people whose behaviour may be unpredictable, aggressive, disorganized, or disruptive.

References

1. General Medical Council. Good medical practice. 2013. https://www.gmc-uk.org/ethical-guida nce/ethical-guidance-for-doctors/good-medical-practice
2. Home Office. Management of adults at risk in immigration detention. 2022. https://www.gov.uk/government/publications/management-of-adults-at-risk-in-immigration-detention/management-of-adults-at-risk-in-immigration-detention-accessible-version
3. Home Office. Adults at risk in immigration detention. 2021. https://assets.publishing.service.gov.uk/government/uploads/system/uploads/attachment_data/file/1114803/Adults_at_risk_in_immigration_detention.pdf
4. Royal College of Psychiatrists. Detention of people with mental disorders in immigration removal centres (IRCs). 2021. https://www.rcpsych.ac.uk/docs/default-source/improving-care/better-mh-policy/position-statements/position-statement-ps02-21---detention-of-people-with-mental-disorders-in-immigration-removal-centres---2021.pdf
5. Civil Aviation Authority. Psychiatric conditions: information for health professionals on assessing fitness to fly. n.d. https://www.caa.co.uk/Passengers/Before-you-fly/Am-I-fit-to-fly/Guidance-for-health-professionals/Psychiatric-conditions/

Further reading

Shaw S. 'First do no harm': clinical roles in preventing and reducing damage to vulnerable immigration detainees. Medact submission to the review. Medact. 2017. https://www.medact.org/wp-content/uploads/2018/01/Medact-Submission-for-Shaw-FINAL-WEBSITE.pdf

Evidence base for mental health issues

Keller AS, Ford D, Sachs E, et al. The impact of detention on the health of asylum seekers. J Ambul Care Manage. 2003;26(4):383–385.
Pickles H, Hartree N. Fitness to fly in those being forcibly removed or deported from the UK. J Forensic Leg Med. 2017;47:55–58.
Royal College of Psychiatrists. Detention of people with mental disorders in immigration removal centres (IRCs). 2021. https://www.rcpsych.ac.uk/docs/default-source/improving-care/better-mh-policy/position-statements/position-statement-ps02-21---detention-of-people-with-mental-disorders-in-immigration-removal-centres---2021.pdf
Sultan A, O'Sullivan K. Psychological disturbances in asylum seekers held in long term detention: a participant–observer account. Med J Aust. 2001;175(11–12):593–596.
von Werthern M, Robjant K, Chui Z, et al. The impact of immigration detention on mental health: a systematic review. BMC Psychiatry. 2018;18(1):382.

Chapter 13

Ageing in prison

Ageing in prison: an introduction

In recent years there has been a dramatic rise in the number of older people in prison in the UK. The reasons for this include:

- harsher sentencing policies: people are now given longer sentences for crimes that in the past would have received a shorter sentence
- more stringent conditions for being released on temporary licence towards the end of a sentence
- willingness of the courts to imprison old people; 92% of those aged 80 or over in prison were sentenced at the age of 70 or older[1]
- a rise in the numbers of people convicted of 'historic' sexual offences; 45% of men aged over 50 and 87% of those over 80 are in prison for sexual offences[1]
- ageing populations: people who live in prison, like other populations, are living longer than in the past.

These factors mean that more people are growing old behind bars. In England and Wales, people over the age of 50 now account for 17% of the total prison population, and the over 60s are the fastest growing section of the prison population, their numbers having tripled in the past 15 years.[1] More people are also dying in prison; the rates of deaths from natural causes have increased by almost 60% in the last decade.[1]

Ageing in prison

The effects of ageing are magnified in the prison population because many people who are incarcerated have experienced a lifetime of health and socioeconomic disadvantage. It is widely accepted that long-term imprisonment causes premature ageing; the average 50-year-old in prison has an equivalent health status to a 60-year-old in the rest of the population.[2] Ginn[3] states that: 'the health of older prisoners is often poor, their social needs are inadequately addressed, and end of life care requires further attention' (p. 3). The average age at death from natural causes in prison is 56 years, compared with 81 years in the general population.[4]

Management of older people in prison

Older people often experience several diseases at the same time (multiple morbidity), and there are also some complex health states that tend to occur only in later life and that do not fall into discrete disease categories[5]; these include frailty, urinary incontinence, falls, delirium, and pressure ulcers.

Effective management of older people in prison is likely to require input from multiple providers from both inside and outside prison; some issues to consider are as follows:

- *Healthcare*: people in prison are NHS patients, and the 'principle of equivalence' as stated in the UN 'Nelson Mandela Rules' means that they should receive the same healthcare as people outside of prison.[6] Most prisons provide only primary care services, although a small proportion also have in-patient beds. People who reside within prisons usually have to be escorted to outside hospitals for appointments with specialist consultants or treatments such as chemotherapy.
- *Social care*: many older people in prison need help with ADLs. Since 2014, local councils have had a duty to assess people living in prison

with social care needs, and where appropriate agree a care and support plan. However, in practice, the provision of social care is still patchy, and often fellow people within the prison setting provide informal help to those who need it.

- *Palliative care*: those who are approaching the end of life in prison should have their palliative care needs assessed, and specialist palliative care staff from outside prison should be involved where needed.
- *Environment*: prison buildings typically feature long corridors, stairs, and small cells with bunk beds, which are not suitable environments for old, ill, frail, and dying people. Older people in prison report feeling highly vulnerable when housed with younger inmates and bullying and intimidation are common.[7] Some prisons have created 'older prisoner units' in an attempt to address some of these issues; more such initiatives are needed.
- *Equipment*: prison cells are often too small to accommodate equipment such as wheelchairs, pressure-relieving mattresses, hoists, etc. When such equipment is required, the patient may need to be transferred to a prison hospital wing or outside hospital or hospice.
- *Compassionate release*: early release on compassionate grounds is rarely granted, even at the very end of life.

References

1. Prison Reform Trust. Bromley briefings: prison factfile. Winter 2019. https://prisonreformtrust. org.uk/wp-content/uploads/2020/01/Bromley-Briefings-Prison-Factfile-Winter-2019.pdf
2. Hayes AJ, Burns A, Turnbull P, et al. The health and social needs of older male prisoners. Int J Geriatr Psychiatry. 2012;27(11):1152–1162.
3. Ginn S. Healthcare in prisons analysis: elderly prisoners. BMJ. 2012;345:e6263.
4. Independent Advisory Panel on Deaths in Custody. Avoidable natural deaths in prison custody: putting things right. September 2020. https://www.pslhub.org/learn/patient-safety-in-health-and-care/care-settings/prison-setting/independent-advisory-panel-on-deaths-in-custody-and-rcn-avoidable-natural-deaths-in-prison-custody-putting-things-right-september-2020-r3263/
5. World Health Organization. Ageing and health. 2020. https://www.who.int/news-room/fact-sheets/detail/ageing-and-health
6. United Nations General Assembly. United Nations Standard Minimum Rules for the Treatment of Prisoners (the Nelson Mandela Rules). Geneva: United Nations; 2015. https://undocs.org/A/RES/70/175
7. Turner M, Peacock M, Payne S, et al. Ageing and dying in the contemporary neoliberal prison system: exploring the 'double burden' for older prisoners. Soc Sci Med. 2018;212; 161–167.

Health and social care needs of older people in prison

Disease prevalence and complex comorbidities

- Approximately 85% of over 60s have one or more major illness; over 50% have three or more moderate or severe health conditions.
- *Non-communicable disease* prevalence in older people in prison is higher than younger people in prison and higher than community peers. Cardiovascular disease prevalence is 38% (hypertension 39%, ischaemic heart disease 21%, and stroke 6%), arthritis 34%, diabetes 14%, cancer 8%, COPD 8%, and asthma 7%.
- *Communicable disease* prevalence depends on high-risk lifestyle factors (e.g. IV drug use, multiple sexual partners, MSM, sex working, and length of time in prison).
- TB (0.12% active, 30% latent), hepatitis C (12.9%), and syphilis (1.1%) are more common in over 50s than under 50s.
- Mental illness prevalence in older people in prison is 38–61%; 50–59-year-olds have the highest prevalence and highest suicide risk; prevalence is higher than community peers.
- Depression (8–52%), PD (16–30%), anxiety (13–39%), and alcohol abuse (15.9%) are common.
- Schizophrenia and psychoses (3–12%), bipolar disorder (4.5%), and PTSD (6–9%).

Age-related or 'geriatric' syndromes

- *Age-related 'syndromes'*: falls, incontinence, sensory impairment, symptom burden, and dementia have multiple causes and a significant impact on older people.
- *Falls*: 30% of over 65s. Incidence rises with age.
- Risk factors:
  - Individual: multiple medications; cognitive impairment; poor vision; problems with gait, balance, muscle strength; foot problems; inactivity; physical demands of prison (e.g. climbing on to top bunk, queueing for meals or medication).
  - Prison environment: poor lighting, uneven floors, multiple steep steps, lack of lifts, seating, or adaptations.
- *Incontinence*: up to 40% in those over 60 years. Often underreported and undertreated. May lead to bullying, avoiding regime activities without easy access to toilets, social isolation, and depression.
- *Sensory impairment*: 65% have visual impairment, 28% have hearing loss; may cause difficulties with communication, following signs and verbal orders, social isolation, poor balance and falls, difficulty engaging in pre-trial preparation, and court.
- *Symptom burden*: may include chronic non-cancer pain, breathlessness, dizziness, constipation, emotional distress linked to cognitive impairment, adjustment, or 'institutionalization' ('biopsychosocial state' brought on by incarceration, characterized by anxiety, depression, hypervigilance, and a disabling combination of social withdrawal and/or aggression).

- *Dementia*: 8% in over 50s; higher prevalence than community (×2 60–69 years; ×4 over 70 years). Underdiagnosed due to repetitive regime, limited functional responsibilities (no cooking, managing money, laundry), and inexperienced wing staff.

Polypharmacy

- Multiple medicines are often co-prescribed to older people due to comorbidities, chronic pain, mental illness, and substance misuse. Prescribing more than four medicines (any type) concurrently increases the risk of falls, fear of falling, and cognitive impairment.
- Specific drugs/classes of drugs are particularly high risk for older patients including:
  - anticholinergics (urinary retention, constipation, impaired cognition and confusion, falls, and mortality)—be aware of other drug classes with anticholinergic properties and higher risk of toxicity/side effects if multiple anticholinergics co-prescribed
  - benzodiazepines (confusion, sedation, night falls, and hip fracture) and psychotropics.

Social care, suitable accommodation, and safeguarding

- Social care referrals should be made as soon as need is identified—in reception/secondary screening and when on the wing.
- Referrals can be initiated by healthcare, prison, or resident.
- Additional demands of the prison setting (e.g. walking distances between buildings, lack of seating, queuing to collect meals and medicine, and bunk beds) may uncover new needs.
- It is important that officers and healthcare staff working on wings are trained and remain vigilant for emerging physical or cognitive decline and frailty.
- It is essential to quickly identify and act on vulnerability, unmet need, and safeguarding concerns, including bullying which may relate to high-risk medicines, food, canteen supplies, and frailty.
- Appropriate notice and information should be provided to make necessary adaptations and acquire equipment to meet the needs of the older person prior to their:
  - discharge from hospital to prison
  - transfer to another establishment
  - release from prison to community.

Palliative and end of life care

See End of life care, p. 324.

Screening, immunization, and health checks

On arrival

- Identify and document (on SEAT template in English and Welsh prisons):
  - medical conditions needing urgent assessment and treatment
  - sensory, functional, and cognitive impairments
  - disabilities and social care needs, and mobility aids used (e.g. frame)

- issues not volunteered (e.g. incontinence, falls, and alcohol or drug dependence)
- immediate risk requiring safeguarding actions (e.g. risk of self-harm and suicide—open ACCT; frailty—locate in suitable accommodation with adaptations)
- prescribed, over-the-counter, and illicit drugs.

First week
- Use mental health screening, secondary screening, medicines reconciliation, and collateral information gathering to identify and document:
  - medical conditions not picked up on arrival, and new and emerging issues
  - past, current, and possible emerging mental health issues including adjustment difficulties
  - age-related problems (mobility issues, falls or difficulties with ADLs since arrival, incontinence, and sensory difficulties, e.g. reading signs, hearing instructions, cognitive impairment)
  - polypharmacy and problems with taking medication.
- Refer if required to in-house GP, mental health, substance misuse service, dentist, optician, audiology, podiatry, and diabetes.
- Ensure all outstanding hospital appointments and investigations have been identified and care continuity arrangements made.
- Make a referral to social care services if needed.
- Offer health promotion advice: keep active, exercise, choose healthy meal and canteen options, smoking cessation, sexual health, resources to support sleep hygiene, relaxation (yoga, mindfulness, reading, listening to music), and keep connected with friends/family (if possible).
- Offer vaccinations: hepatitis B (all), influenza (>65 years and <65 years at risk, annual), pneumococcal (>65 years, once; <65 years with a long-term health condition, every 5 years), COVID-19 (age, risk), shingles (>70 years, once).
- Offer screening tests: BBVs, vascular, bowel cancer, abdominal aortic aneurysm.

Medicines optimization

- Avoid dose omission of medicines in older patients who may quickly deteriorate.
- Assess in-possession risk in reception and at any necessary subsequent points (e.g. ACCT opened, cognitive decline, or poor concordance identified).
- Implement efficient medicines reconciliation to confirm community prescribing and obtain adequate collateral health information.
- Arrange early medicines review appointment to assess ongoing clinical need and priorities for treatment. Consider using decision aids such as STOPP/START tool to rationalize prescribing, and minimize iatrogenic morbidity (side effects and drug–drug interactions).
- Set up repeat medication ordering and monitoring to ensure safe continuity of medicines, as part of multimorbidity care pathway.

Access to specialist services

- Models of specialist care provision vary depending on the demographics of the individual prison population. Some services can be effectively delivered on site by visiting specialists, either in regularly scheduled clinics (e.g. psychiatry, optometry, podiatry, and physiotherapy), or for individual patient referrals (e.g. palliative care and memory clinic).
- Officers are needed to escort a patient to hospital. If an outpatient appointment has to be cancelled due to lack of escort staff, it is essential to reschedule the appointment at the earliest opportunity, to minimize the delay to accessing care.
- Some hospital specialties offer remote consultations to patients, via telephone or video calls. This avoids problems with escorts but requires a member of the healthcare team to be present. Patients with cognitive or sensory impairments may find remote consultations difficult.
- Good links with the local hospice team and palliative care consultant are important for prisons with older people serving long sentences.

Multimorbidity care delivery

- Ensure clear, timely communication and good partnership working between prison, health, and social care teams for older people with complex health and social care needs; consider setting out a memorandum of understanding to clarify roles and responsibilities.
- In the patient with multiple morbidities and frailty (e.g. angina, COPD, diabetes, poor hearing, memory loss, and reduced mobility), avoid multiple appointments with different practitioners for individual long-term conditions which can lead to polypharmacy, multiple investigations, duplication of monitoring, and episodes of unplanned care.
- Consider appointing a lead practitioner for older patients and consider using a multimorbidity care model in which health professionals (e.g. GP, nurse, pharmacist, and occupational therapist) and social care providers work together as a team to assess the older person, share information, and work with the patient to reach a shared decision on prioritizing their needs.
- Draw up a care plan which supports the patient to retain as much independence as possible. Map out agreed priorities for care. Include any self-management objectives, advance decisions to refuse treatment and DNACPR decisions. Share with all professionals and patient and revisit regularly to identify declining health and evolving needs.

Adaptations, buddy schemes, and voluntary sector input

- Needs of older people differ from the younger population in prison. Adaptations are required for:
  - regime activities (e.g. day care programmes, modified exercise)
  - accommodation and buildings (e.g. widening doorways, grab rails, seating, and signage).
- Some prisons have 'buddy schemes' in which selected residents assist (not intimate care) older, frail or disabled peers by, for example, collecting meals or pushing a wheelchair. Good training and ongoing supervision of peer carers (buddies) is essential, to avoid putting both patient and carer at risk.

- Partnerships with voluntary sector organizations enhance provision for older people through:
  - supervision and training of buddies
  - provision of modified exercise programmes and activities suitable for the over 50s (e.g. walking groups, gardening, bowls, modified gym sessions, board games, and community singing)
  - specific support groups (e.g. veterans family support, cognitive impairment, and support for families of residents with palliative care needs)
  - advice for resettlement (e.g. debt, housing advice, finance planning, and cooking skills).

Resettlement planning and release

- Planning and advice should be available from the point of entry into prison to avoid unsupported release (e.g. from court). Joined up working between probation, prison, health, social care, and voluntary sector providers should take place.
- In addition to meeting health, social care, and housing needs, tailored occupational therapy support will be needed to prepare for release (e.g. cooking, finance, and IT skills). This may be provided in partnership with voluntary organizations.
- Essential pre-release checklist:
  - Pre-registration with community GP practice.
  - Arrange appointments with community services (e.g. substance misuse, mental health, and GP).
  - Transfer of health and social care information to community teams.
  - Arrange up to 28 days of medications to take out with support (e.g. dosette box, arrangements for safe storage).

Further reading

Baillargeon J, Black SA, Leach CT, et al. The infectious disease profile of Texas prison inmates. Prev Med. 2004;38(5):607–612.

Crane J. Becoming institutionalized: incarceration and 'slow death'. Social Science Research Council; 2019. https://items.ssrc.org/insights/becoming-institutionalized-incarceration-and-slow-death/

Croft M, Mayhew R. Prevalence of chronic non-cancer pain in a UK prison environment. Br J Pain. 2015;9(2):96–108.

Di Lorito C, Völlm B, Dening T. Psychiatric disorders among older prisoners: a systematic review and comparison study against older people in the community. Aging Ment Health. 2018;22(1):1–10.

Fazel S, Hope T. Health of elderly male prisoners: worse than the general population, worse than younger prisoners. Age Ageing. 2001;30(5):403–407.

Hayes AJ, Burns A, Turnbull P, et al. The health and social care needs of older male prisoners. Int J Geriatr Psychiatry. 2012;27:1155–1162.

Forsyth K, Heathcote L, Senior J, et al. Dementia and mild cognitive impairment in prisoners aged over 50 years in England and Wales: a mixed-methods study. Southampton: NIHR Journals Library; 2020. https://www.ncbi.nlm.nih.gov/books/NBK558632/

Marcum ZA, Wirtz HS, Pettinger M, et al. Anticholinergic medication use and falls in postmenopausal women: findings from the women's health initiative cohort study. BMC Geriatr. 2016;16:76.

Munday D, Leaman J. The prevalence of non-communicable disease in older people in prison: a systematic review and meta-analysis. Age Ageing 2019;48(2):204–212.

National Institute for Health and Care Excellence. Multimorbidity: clinical assessment and management. NICE guideline [NG56]. 2016. https://www.nice.org.uk/guidance/ng56

National Institute for Health and Care Excellence. Physical health of people in prison. NICE guideline [NG57]. 2016. https://www.nice.org.uk/guidance/ng57

NHS England. Toolkit for general practice in supporting older people living with frailty. Appendix 5 STOPP, Screening Tool of Older Persons' potentially inappropriate Prescriptions; START, Screening Tool to Alert to Right Treatment. 2017. https://www.england.nhs.uk/wp-content/uploads/2017/03/toolkit-general-practice-frailty-1.pdf

Williams B, Ahalt C, Greifinger R. The older prisoner and complex chronic medical care. In: Enggist S, Møller L, Galea G, et al. (eds). Prisons and Health, pp. 165–170. Copenhagen: World Health Organization Regional Office for Europe; 2014. https://www.euro.who.int/__data/assets/pdf_file/0007/249208/Prisons-and-Health,-19-The-older-prisoner-and-complex-chronic-medical-care.pdf

World Health Organization. What are the main risk factors for falls amongst older people and what are the most effective interventions to prevent these falls? 2004. https://www.euro.who.int/__data/assets/pdf_file/0018/74700/E82552.pdf

End of life care

Introduction

The prison population is rapidly ageing and deaths in prison are rising annually with the majority being from natural causes. Therefore, most prison staff will at some stage need to provide end of life care. There are challenges in delivering high-quality healthcare especially around security arrangements, but the primary focus should always be on the patient's needs, respecting their wishes, and ensuring dignity at the end of life.

In 2011, the National End of Life Care Programme published a six-stage guide to improving end of life care in prisons titled 'The route to success'[1]:

End of life care pathway

1. Discussions as end of life care approaches

- Identification of people in prison approaching the end of life. Trigger points for initiating a discussion might include:
  - terminal diagnosis
  - deterioration in health with multiple hospital admissions
  - surprise question: 'Would I be surprised if this person were to die in the next 6–12 months?'.
- Register of patients requiring end of life care. Should be reviewed at least quarterly.
- Named GP, nurse, and case manager identified for each patient.

2. Assessment, care planning, and review

Advanced care planning is essential. Useful to have as a template in the medical records and must be easily accessible.

The care plan should include the following information:

- Name of patient and location.
- Medical conditions.
- Physical assessment—pain (including discussion of anticipatory medication), function, and social care needs.
- Psychological and spiritual needs.
- Wishes regarding future care.
- Resuscitation status—document the discussion clearly. If not for resuscitation, a DNACPR form must be completed and communicated to out-of-hours staff, ambulance service, the prison, and healthcare.
- Case manager, next of kin, and contact details—the family should be involved in care planning where appropriate.
- Consent to share medical information with the prison staff is important to enable appropriate care and is essential for release on compassionate grounds. This should be signed.
- Preferred place of care in the final days—prison, hospital, hospice, and who they want present.
- Application for early release on compassionate grounds should be made at the earliest opportunity if a prognosis of months.
- Refer to local hospice for advice and support.
- 'Just in case' medication should be ordered and kept in stock.

3. Coordination of care

The case manager (normally clinical services manager) should:

- ensure a family liaison officer is appointed early on
- arrange regular meetings with the healthcare team, the prison, and the patient; include the safer custody governor, wing officer, family liaison officer, chaplain, named GP, nurse, and hospice if involved
- inform out-of-hours team and the ambulance service
- ensure the prison facilitates escorts for all outside appointments and exercises judgement in appropriate use of restraints
- ensure security clearance for all external agencies
- work closely with pharmacy to ensure all medication, particularly anticipatory drugs, are kept in stock and accessible if during out-of-hours periods:
  - there should be a lockable safe in the patient's room where controlled drugs can be stored and accessed safely by the patient as required
  - there needs to be a plan in place for the safe delivery of pain relief when the patient becomes too frail or confused to self-administer
  - wing officers are not allowed to dispense medication
- ensure appropriate equipment is in place and a clear process for setting up a syringe driver if out of hours
- check early realease on compassionate grounds application has been completed.

4. Delivery of high-quality care

- Ensure the patient is involved at all stages.
- The patient's room will need to accommodate a wheelchair, hospital bed, hoist, and space for carers. Transfer to a more specialist setting (e.g. another prison with palliative care facilities) may need to be considered. The offender management unit may need apply for re-categorization early on which can take time to arrange.
- Develop an end of life care pathway as an operational policy to ensure consistency of care.
- Check systems in place for monitoring the quality of end of life care.
- Provide support to other people living in prison who may be affected by a terminally ill patient.
- Offer training in end of life care for all staff including prison officers.

5. Care in the last days of life

- The family liaison officer should enable regular visits. Strong support from family makes a significant difference to quality of life and all involved in the patient's care should be available to meet with the family for open discussions. Relatives also need to understand the procedure following a death in custody including certification and funeral arrangements.
- Drugs need regular stock checks to cover out-of-hours periods.

6. Care after death

It is useful to have a flowchart detailing what to do after death:

- Who to contact to verify death—normally the GP or out-of-hours service. The room is sealed, and the medical records locked as with a death in custody.

- Relatives need to be informed if not present along with prison staff and inmates.
- Outside services need to be informed and appointments cancelled by healthcare administrative staff.
- Details for bereavement support should be available to inmates, staff, and family.
- A debriefing session with healthcare and prison staff should be arranged to look at the care offered.

Reference

1. National End of Life Care Programme. The route to success in the end of life care—achieving quality in prisons and for prisoners. London: NHS; 2011.

Further reading

Bulman M. Why has the proportion of elderly prisoners risen so drastically? The Independent; 29 November 2017. https://www.independent.co.uk/news/uk/home-news/elderly-prisoners-jailed-over-50-age-numbers-increase-2002-figures-a8082921.html

Gold Standards Framework. https://www.goldstandardsframework.org.uk/

Prison Reform Trust. Prison: the facts. Bromley briefings. Summer 2018. http://www.prisonreformtrust.org.uk/wp-content/uploads/old_files/Documents/Bromley%20Briefings/old%20editions/Summer%202018%20factfile.pdf

Prisons and Probation Ombudsman. Learning from PPO investigations: end of life care. March 2013. https://www.ppo.gov.uk/app/uploads/2014/07/Learning_from_PPO_investigations_-_End_of_life_care_final_web.pdf

Dementia

Introduction

Prevention

Diagnosis

Dementia

Introduction

Dementia is an umbrella term for a range of progressive conditions that affect the brain. There are over 200 subtypes of dementia, but the five most common are Alzheimer's disease, vascular dementia, dementia with Lewy bodies, frontotemporal dementia, and mixed dementia.

People living in prison on average have a biological age of 10 years greater than that of the national population due to a variety of factors: lifestyle, substance misuse, poor mental health, low socio-economic grouping, learning difficulty, and so on. People living in prison who are over the age of 50 are the fastest growing age group in prison; it is therefore necessary to consider the specific healthcare needs of these people and for stakeholders to work together to meet these needs.

People with dementia will face a number of challenges by being in the prison environment—noise, disorientation, lack of family support, change in routine, and lack of accessibility.

Prevention

Preventative measures are in line with healthy heart advice: lowering BP, healthy eating, good diabetes control, weight management, smoking cessation, and alcohol and substance misuse support.

People in prison with single or multiple risk factors therefore need a focused healthy conversation regarding their health each time they have contact with the healthcare team using the principles of 'Making Every Contact Count' (MECC):

- It is recognized that keeping the mind active and challenged is important to maintain brain function.
- Collaboration with the prison, UK Health Security Agency, commissioners, and other stakeholders to support behaviour change programmes is required, such as diet/menu options, active regime, and gym access.
- Clear and relevant information needs to be displayed— use easy read/ infographics to support understanding.
- NHS Health Checks (England only) are an opportunity to discuss behavioural risk factors for dementia, disability, and frailty by tailoring the advice component of the NHS Health Check programme for different age groups.
- Effective care pathways should be established between the prison healthcare teams and specialist dementia diagnostic and memory services to facilitate diagnosis and ongoing support.
- Opportunity for virtual consults should be explored to avoid unnecessary change for the person with dementia and enable their prison key worker (if they consent) and healthcare team to input into the assessment.

Diagnosis

- Ask at the physical health check or other appropriate opportunities whether someone has a concern about their memory: if they answer yes, another appointment to discuss this further should be made.

- Record a history and corroborate this with wing staff or other prison staff where possible.
- Exclude reversible causes of cognitive decline, including delirium, depression, sensory impairment (such as sight or hearing loss), or cognitive impairment from medicines associated with increased anticholinergic burden.
- Tests to exclude reversible causes of cognitive decline include:
  - urine test
  - FBC test
  - calcium, vitamin D and bone profile
  - blood glucose level
  - renal function test
  - liver function test
  - TFTs for dementia screening
  - vitamin B_{12} level tests
  - folate level tests
  - BP.
- Complete a cognitive test using a validated brief structured cognitive instrument such as:
  - the ten-point cognitive screener (10-CS)
  - the six-item cognitive impairment test (6CIT)
  - the six-item screener
  - the Memory Impairment Screen (MIS)
  - the Mini-Cog
  - Test Your Memory (TYM).
- Refer the person to a specialist dementia diagnostic service/ neurological service where the diagnosis needs further assessment or the person has suspected rapidly progressive dementia.
- Minimize the use of medicines associated with increased anticholinergic burden such as solifenacin, tiotropium, and tolterodine.

Management in prison

- Work with the person with dementia to complete a 'This is me' leaflet early into the diagnosis.
- Run regular dementia friends training sessions for residents, officers, and other staff.
- Use the Royal College of Nursing five SPACE principles in order to promote dementia care in prison.
- Work with the prison to support the person with dementia to have a fixed cell and not to be moved from wing to wing.
- An application for clinical hold (detainee is not transferred or moved from the current prison due to health reasons) should be considered where their dementia is progressing and transfer could exacerbate their symptoms and disrupt their care.
- Refer for social services assessment and support as needed.
- Mental capacity assessments may be required to support court attendance/prison adjudication.
- Conversations regarding advanced care planning, including DNACPR, should be held while the person has the capacity to be involved in discussions.

- ReSPECT form should be completed as a recommended summary plan for emergency care and treatment and used as a best interests support tool.
- Consider applying for early release for the patient.
- Prepare to provide palliative and end of life care if early release is not an option—consider environment/nursing skill set.

References

Alzheimer's Society. https://www.alzheimers.org.uk

Dementia Action Alliance. Meeting the challenges of dementia in prisons. 2017. https://www.dementiaaction.org.uk/assets/0003/4619/Prisons_and_Dementia_-_DAA_briefing_paper.pdf

Dementia Friends. What is a Dementia Friends ambassador? 2022. https://www.dementiafriends.org.uk/WEBArticle?page=what-is-a-champion#.YGCmL9KSnlV

HM Prison and Probation Service. Model for Operational Delivery: Older Prisoners. April 2018. https://www.dementiaaction.org.uk/assets/0004/2423/MOD-for-older-prisoners__2_.pdf

Iacobucci G. Early release rules for prisoners at end of life may be 'discriminatory,' say doctors. BMJ. 2019;365:l4140.

Legislation.gov.uk. Equality Act 2010. 2010. https://www.legislation.gov.uk/ukpga/2010/15/contents

Legislation.gov.uk. Mental Capacity Act 2005. 2005. https://www.legislation.gov.uk/ukpga/2005/9/contents

Ministry of Justice. The needs and characteristics of older prisoners: results from the Surveying Prisoner Crime Reduction (SPCR) survey. 2014. https://assets.publishing.service.gov.uk/government/uploads/system/uploads/attachment_data/file/368177/needs-older-prisoners-spcr-survey.pdf

National Institute for Health and Care Excellence. Dementia. 2023. https://www.nice.org.uk/guidance/conditions-and-diseases/mental-health-behavioural-and-neurodevelopmental-conditions/dementia

Prison Reform Trust. Prison rules and adjudications. n.d. https://prisonreformtrust.org.uk/adviceguide/prison-rules-and-adjudications/

Public Health England. Physical health checks in prisons standards: a framework for quality improvement. 2017. https://www.healthcheck.nhs.uk/seecmsfile/?id=553

UK Health Security Agency. Adult weight management: short conversations with patients. 2021. https://www.gov.uk/government/publications/adult-weight-management-a-guide-to-brief-interventions

Osteoporosis: prevention of fragility fractures

Introduction

Osteoporosis is generally an asymptomatic condition that only presents with fragility fractures or abnormal imaging (dual-energy X-ray absorptiometry (DXA)).[1] It is a complex disease involving skeletal bone remodelling resulting in reduced bone density and abnormal bone architecture which causes an increased bone fragility and a susceptibility to fractures. Patients in the secure environment are less likely to present to healthcare professionals likely meaning reduced identification of fragility fractures and osteoporosis risk.

Fragility fractures

- Consider if fracture sustained from a low-impact injury (e.g. fall from standing height or less).
- Can be spontaneous in vertebrae.
- Commonly in wrist, hip, and spine.

Risk factors

- Female sex.
- Increasing age.
- Alcohol.
- Smoking.
- BMI of less than 18.5 kg/m^2.
- Chronic liver disease.
- COPD.
- Malabsorption (e.g. chronic pancreatitis, inflammatory bowel disease).
- Endocrine: menopause (including premature menopause), diabetes, hypogonadism, and hypothyroidism.
- Drugs (e.g. SSRIs, antiepileptics, proton pump inhibitors, oral corticosteroids).
- Rheumatological conditions.
- Previous fragility fracture (e.g. inflammatory arthritis).
- Parental history of fragility fracture.[2]

There is little research into osteoporosis in the prison environment. Reviewing the risk factors,[2] it can be seen that many people in prison are likely to be at greater risk of osteoporosis due to the high incidence of alcohol and tobacco use and in turn chronic liver disease/pancreatitis and COPD. Although there is limited research into substance misuse and osteoporosis, often substance misuse is associated with poor nutrition and low BMI. There is a high use of SSRIs in patients in the prison setting, which is an independent risk factor.

Clinical features

- Back pain.
- Kyphosis.
- Fragility fractures.

Assessment for osteoporosis

- DXA scan is the gold standard imaging method to show bone mineral density:
  - DXA scan for all those over 50 years with a fragility fracture.
  - DXA scan for those under 40 years with a major risk factor for osteoporosis.
  - Osteoporosis is diagnosed as a bone mineral density T-score less than −2.5.

Osteoporosis risk scores—used in all other patients
- QFracture.
- FRAX.
- Give a score for 10-year risk of developing osteoporosis:
  - High risk (10%): proceed to DXA scan.
  - Low risk: discuss lifestyle changes/risk factor modification.
  - Intermediate risk: clinician to consider overall risk factors.
- In hip/vertebral fracture and DXA is not feasible for your patient—can consider starting treatment without DXA.
- Secondary causes (see Risk factors, p. 332). Consider investigations:
  - FBC/bone profile/vitamin D level/TFTs/HbA1c/FSH/testosterone/ LFTs/coeliac screen/faecal calprotectin/BMI/chest X-ray/ spirometry.
- Non-osteoporotic fragility fractures must be ruled out, including:
  - myeloma
  - bone metastases
  - Paget's disease
  - osteomalacia.

Management

- Risk factor management including treating underlying causes, alcohol dependence, and smoking cessation.
- Lifestyle advice—regular exercise including balance and weight bearing, balanced diet, and vitamin D (see Nutrition and exercise, Chapter 4, p. 60).
- Falls prevention: can consider falls clinic, physiotherapy, and occupational therapy.
- Bone protection: first line is bisphosphonates to all those with a bone mineral density T-score less than −2.5.
- Calcium and vitamin D supplements as needed.
- Fracture treatment as needed.

References

1. BMJ Best Practice. Osteoporosis. July 2020. https://bestpractice.bmj.com/topics/en-gb/85
2. National Institute for Health and Care Excellence. Osteoporosis. Quality standard [QS149]. 2017. https://www.nice.org.uk/guidance/qs149

Compassionate release

Introduction

People sentenced to serve time in prison under the Criminal Justice Act (under section 39, 1991 and section 248, 2003) can be released on licence if the Secretary of State is satisfied that exceptional circumstances exist which justify early release on compassionate grounds. Consideration is based on the person's medical condition or as a result of tragic family circumstance. It is granted only in exceptional cases and the Secretary of State must consult the parole board, unless consultation is made impractical. Between 2012 and 2017, only 48 applications for compassionate release were successful while 845 deaths occurred from natural causes.[1] Each case is considered individually and must be approved personally by a Minister. Guidelines to compassionate release are outlined in PSO 6000[2] for determinate sentences and PSO 4700[3] for indeterminate sentences.

Initiating compassionate release application

- Considerations for compassionate release on medical grounds include all prognoses of less than 3 months including end of life care, cancer diagnosis, or where a condition renders the person incapacitated, such as a stroke.
- Discussions with the patient, and family, where appropriate, should take place and a record of the person's wishes should be undertaken as early as possible and preferably before the prognosis is less than 3 months.
- Consultant letters, hospital discharge letters, and prison healthcare MDT meetings discussing the patient's medical condition can serve as the initiation for compassionate release paperwork.
- A designated member of the healthcare team can communicate with the governor or appointed prison department such as the offender management unit to initiate the paperwork.
- The registered medical practitioner should complete section 4 and include any specialist reports from hospital.

Compassionate release on medical grounds

- When assessing a person for compassionate release, the medical practitioner should consider the following in their report:
  - How frail is the person? At what level are they performing ADLs? Are social services involved with care? What impact does the prison regime have on the person's ability to look after themselves?
  - At what rate is the deterioration of the person's health?
  - What level of vulnerability does the person have? What is the risk of serious harm to the person, above the expectations of being in the community?
  - Does the person have the strength and ability with their current health to be a threat of endangerment to the society if released? Do they have the ability to carry out the crime they have committed before?
- All of the following criteria must be met in order to receive compassionate release on medical grounds:

- The person is suffering from a terminal illness and death is likely to occur within a few months, or the person is bedridden or similarly incapacitated (e.g. severe stroke, paralysis, etc.).
- The risk of reoffending (particularly of a sexual or violent nature) is minimal.
- Further imprisonment would reduce the person's life expectancy.
- There are adequate arrangements for the person's care and treatment outside prison.
- Early release will bring some significant benefit to the person or his/her family.
- Financial costs for bed watches and caring responsibilities are not grounds for compassionate release.
- Self-induced harm such as hunger strike and refusal of treatment do not meet the criteria for compassionate release.
- A decision to reject compassionate release can be reconsidered with new evidence, such as a clearer prognosis.
- A report from the medical practitioner and consultant specialist, where appropriate, is required for an application.
- Application consists of six sections (on Form 210) to be completed and sent by the prison governor to the Early Recall and Release section of HMPPS:
  - Sections 1–3 completed by the governor.
  - Section 4 completed by the GP.
  - Section 5 completed by the prison probation officer.
  - Section 6 completed by the governor including the opinion of the medical director, prison health (at the Department of Health).

Compassionate release due to tragic family circumstance

- Medical practitioners should be aware of tragic family circumstances should they consult a person who meets this criteria for compassionate release. This can be escalated through the head of healthcare to the prison offender management unit.
- A medical report is not usually required for this application; however, supporting evidence may asked for.
- All of the following criteria must be met in order to receive compassionate release due to tragic family circumstance:
  - Circumstances of the person or the family has changed to the extent that continuing the sentence would result in exceptional severity of hardship, greater than the court could have foreseen.
  - The risk of reoffending is in the past.
  - The need for the person's permanent presence with his/her family can be demonstrated as real and urgent beyond doubt.
  - Early release will bring benefit to the person in prison or his/her family, which cannot be provided by another person or agency.
- Consideration may be given in exceptional circumstances such as a spouse dying or is seriously ill and there is no one to care for young children.
- A death of a relative would not usually be sufficient.
- Risk to welfare on children and the wider community will be considered.

- Available support from other family members, friends, or social services will be considered.
- Application consists of six sections to be completed (on Form 2161) and sent by the governor to the Early Recall and Release section.
  - Sections 1–3 completed by the discipline officer.
  - Section 4 completed by the prison probation officer.
  - Section 5 completed by the governor.
  - Section 6 completed by the person in prison.

Early Recall and Release section

- Case workers from the Early Recall and Release section liaise with the medical director, prison health at the Department of Health and decide to refuse or submit forms to Ministers for a decision.
- They consider the need for an additional licence including those recommended by courts.
- They notify the decision to the person.
- They release the person on licence if appropriate.

Further reading

Burtonwood J. Early release rules for prisoners at end of life need reform. BMH, 12 June 2019. https://blogs.bmj.com/bmj/2019/06/12/jim-burtonwood-early-release-rules-for-prisoners-at-end-of-life-need-reform/

Chapter 14

Creating person-centred, coordinated, and continuous care

Creating a person-centred biopsychosocial approach to care

Health and social care for individuals in contact with the criminal justice system is often complex due to both system and individual factors. Individuals need practitioners coming from multiple teams to have a coherent biopsychosocial understanding of their diverse interconnected problems. They need a single care and treatment plan based on available resources, and one that changes with needs over time. This is a formidable challenge in the face of a relatively poor evidence base, a paucity of practical frameworks for biopsychosocial formulations, and ongoing system turbulence.

This chapter is most relevant for the many individuals with complex problems who need coordination across teams and well-managed transfers to generate continuity but is also relevant for those with seemingly simple problems as taking into account social and system aspects can help ensure success in delivery of single disease-related interventions.

The problem from patient and practitioner perspectives

From the individual perspective, the following experiences for those with complex needs or specific ongoing healthcare requirements are likely to include[1]:

- bewilderment due to changes in location, system provider, and practitioner
- feelings of distrust due to past trauma and encounters with authority
- multiple practitioners being involved who appear not to be communicating
- being denied access to care due to seemingly arbitrary criteria
- changes to treatment without consultation
- a disruptive social context (homelessness, relationships) as a barrier to ongoing involvement both within prison and outside.

Practitioners' experience of care in the criminal justice system can include:

- relentless pressures of work to see more people in less time
- over-specified roles or job descriptions preventing engagement in whole person care
- a focus on following disease-based guidelines and/or organizational protocols which can feel at odds with providing whole person care
- being responsible for only one part of an individual's healthcare needs and not knowing about the rest of the care being provided
- being in a team with a very different culture from other teams
- a lack of easy access to both the written assessments and health and social care records in other teams and also to other practitioners
- reverting to putting up barriers to taking on new work due to workload stresses
- having limits to knowledge and skills suitable for working in prison
- liaising with multiple other organizations and practitioners which are hard to comprehend especially as they change repeatedly
- multiple incentives systems across services which are difficult to understand
- major separations between criminal justice system, third sector, and health in terms of governance and record keeping.

Reference

1. Quinn C, Denman K, Smithson P, et al. General practitioner contributions to achieving sustained healthcare for offenders: a qualitative study. BMC Fam Pract. 2018;19(1):22.

Building a shared understanding of an individual's biopsychosocial whole

- Many individuals seen in healthcare within the criminal justice system have complex social problems such as housing, unemployment, and particularly relationships, which impact health and the ability to engage in healthcare. These compound the challenge of supporting those with mental health problems, cognitive impairment, and increasingly frailty.
- For most individuals, this needs to be acknowledged with simple plans to ensure that specific treatment can be carried through. A shared understanding of how problems should be prioritized and how they interact can be extremely helpful to ensure the individual trusts that the system is working for them, can take responsibility for themselves more easily, and that practitioners can work together, particularly during key events or transitions.
- The aim is for individuals and their practitioners to have a coherent biopsychosocial understanding which can adapt in real time and form a plan of care.

Key steps for a person-centred biopsychosocial understanding and plan

The following three steps are described in the SHERPA model[1];
- Share ideas and agree together the most important problems.
- Understand how these link together.
- Develop and secure a plan

Practice tips for developing a biopsychosocial understanding

For each individual within the prison healthcare system, whether in primary care, mental health, substance misuse, or other areas, the following tips can guide practice for developing a shared understanding:
- Be aware of your role as a generalist bringing clinical problems together, such as a GP, or as a specialist providing specific diagnoses or recommendations for treatment:
  - Make a decision as to whether an individual has a relatively simple problem for which they are capable of ensuring ongoing engagement with care.
  - Whether one-to-one generalist care is needed now.
  - Whether one-to-one care is needed over time.
  - Whether a complex team is required to deal with the issues.
- Gather data from your own records and others' and the patient.
- Engage with the patient to listen to their narrative and ensure an understanding of their priorities, which may not be your own.
- Agree together what the key issues are to be prioritized, exchanging information and views so that both parties may change their ideas about what is most important.
- Discuss and agree together which issues are less relevant and can be shelved or postponed.
- Consider and agree how these issues link together, for example, is homelessness likely to lead to substance misuse? Is distress from flashbacks likely to lead to self-medication with substances? Is

homelessness likely to impact on ongoing hepatitis treatment after release?

- Liaise and gather information from other services who may already be or need to be involved both to check and adjust your understanding and to know who else is involved and what plans are already in place.
- Use either a diagram or list of causal links to summarize the key problems and links. Use language which is understandable.
- Secure the understanding within records for the individual to take away and to share with other services, ensuring it is easily accessible.
- Adjust as the situation changes.

In a busy practice context, practitioners will struggle to make time to do all these. Taking time, as part of a continuing professional development reflective practice case study, to attempt all steps may help embed them as a natural routine or checklist.

Ensuring an individual's biopsychosocial plan is put into action

A whole person plan needs to take account of the resources available, including the strengths of an individual. Within the complex world of prison healthcare, evidence, such as for mental health treatment, is often relatively weak. The plan needs to focus on the problems which are likely to be solvable.

The ideal situation is for each individual to take ownership for their specific plan and help ensure it is put into action. Many individuals lack capacity and a degree of support and organizational coordination is often required.

Practice tips

- Be clear as to whether you are responsible for a part of a plan to address a specific problem or diagnosis, or whether you also have a role for creating a coherent biopsychosocial plan and coordinating with others.
- Work through all the key problems in the biopsychosocial understanding and brainstorm the range of solutions required.
- Ensure that the emerging plan takes account of the evidence for effectiveness (where it exists) of proposed measures, make judgements together about whether interventions are likely to work, and share uncertainty.
- Be aware that individuals themselves may well have good ideas as to what may be effective for particular circumstances based on past experience, especially around social interventions where evidence from trials is even weaker or non-existent.
- Consider the motivation of the individual to engage in each option.
- For all components of a plan, consider how they will work together, who is responsible, and when each should start.
- Secure the plan in different locations including:
  - making sure the individual understands, and documenting on paper or electronic records accessible to you and others within the healthcare team
  - in communications to others who may need to be involved.

System enablers to ensure the development of secure biopsychosocial plans

Organizational systems and cultures have an enormous impact on practitioners' ability to operate in a person-centred way. For those managers and practitioner leaders with influence, the following are important to consider:

- Teams and leaders who communicate and trust each other.
- Records capable of showing shared understanding and plans clearly.
- Records capable of updating plans and exchanging with other organizations where sharing has been agreed by individuals.
- Opportunities to work with other teams to understand their role and cultural differences.
- Development of scales of engagement and clinical reasoning to bring together coherent biopsychosocial plans understandable to everyone.

Reference

1. Jack E, Maskrey N, Byng R. SHERPA: a new model for clinical decision making in patients with multimorbidity. Lancet. 2018;392(10156):1397–1399.

Coordinating care across teams

Coordination of care is important for those with complex care needs. Individuals in prison and in contact with the criminal justice system often have multiple teams within healthcare involved and also teams from organizations across the sector dealing with housing and substance misuse, the criminal justice system, as well as potentially social care.

While many patients with single problems or with good capacity and motivation to coordinate their own care can take control of the coordinating function, there are many others who, partly due to the constrained situation of prison and other criminal justice contact, as well as problems with cognitive capacity, emotional dysregulation, and social constraints such as homelessness, are unable to take on a coordinating role for their own care.

Many individuals have such significant health problems that, as in other settings, coordination is likely to be required. Examples include:

- individuals with frailty and dementia likely to require coordination between prison general practice services, mental health services, outpatient, and even inpatient care outside of prison within acute hospitals, and links with social care services which are developing in prisons
- individuals with long-term admissions and significant mental health problems and suicidal tendencies likely to be in and out of contact with prison in-reach mental health teams, have significant input from those in the prison service concerned with suicide risk, and may benefit from coordination with education as well as the range of third-sector opportunities
- individuals nearing release with difficult social situations requiring coordination between those involved in resettlement for housing, substance misuse services, GPs, and potentially ongoing mental health healthcare.

Coordination is an ongoing process often taken up by generalist workers, sometimes GPs in a more informal role, and at other times care coordinators with formalized processes under the care programme approach, or newer roles such as care navigators supporting the links between different services.

The practices of coordination require creative and systematic thinking, and action to set up the relationships required for a shared approach:

- Thinking about and making a decision as to whether an individual requires support with coordination or can manage alone.
- Supportive coaching to enable an individual to engage in different aspects of care.
- Active persistent engagement and liaison with other key practitioners.

Practitioner roles in setting up and continuing coordination

Practitioners supporting coordination need to be involved in the following activities:

- Creating a shared understanding of an individual's biopsychosocial whole through gaining perspectives from different health and social care practitioners with knowledge of or in contact with the patient.

- Coordination of views to create a single comprehensive plan with clarity about different roles.
- Having regular liaison meetings with other practitioners in teams with whom individuals are often shared.
- Liaison with other practitioners to revisit and reassess situations at regular intervals or after key events.
- Reviewing medication with different prescribers and pharmacists to ensure reviews are carried out in line with changing situations.

System facilitators

Good coordination by practitioners requires systems to work well together and the following are likely to be helpful[1]:

- Excellent relationships between team leaders and organizational leads, inspiring a sense of collaboration.
- Training to support staff to work together and supervision and mentoring to deal with the inevitable problems of dealing with multiple practitioners across multiple organizations.
- Excellent IT and electronic health records facilitating:
  - display of shared understanding and plan
  - listing responsibilities of the variety of health and social care workers involved
  - listing upcoming appointments with the variety of providers having one live list of current medication.
- Team meetings to support coming together of different cultures.
- Aligned incentives from commissioners.
- Routine reappraisal across teams at key events such as arrival in prison, prior to release, and sentencing.

Joined up medical and social care

Mr HP, a 62-year-old individual who has been in prison for 20 years and is unlikely to be released, had been a smoker for 40 years and developed a stroke and has early dementia. He has always been irritable with a low mood and now requires input from adult social care, a mental health team, a GP, and a pharmacist within the prison. Apart from the adult social worker, the other key professionals involved don't normally take on a proactive coordinating role. The social worker, who is new in post, takes it on himself to liaise with the GP and get a good understanding about the medical needs, ensures that the pharmacist provides medication in a suitable format, and is able to put in place two social interventions to support Mr HP to meet other individuals: attend the new dementia memory group within the prison and access one of the new wheelchairs for use on his wing.

Reference

Sheaff R, Brand SL, Lloyd H, et al. From programme theory to logic models for multispecialty community providers: a realist evidence synthesis. Health Services Delivery Research. 2018;6(24).

Creating onward continuity and transferring care

- Many individuals in contact with the criminal justice system have potentially problematic transfers: between police and courts, in and out of prison, between wings, and release when on remand to no ongoing care. These are all challenging situations.
- Continuity of care as a concept was developed within the mental health and general practice literature and included a range of issues:
  - Care over time with a single practitioner.
  - Care across teams.
  - Trust and relationships.
  - Considering the individual as a whole.
- For individuals in the criminal justice system with ongoing healthcare needs, continuity means getting to see another practitioner and that practitioner having the right information and understanding about the individual so care can be continued. Trusting relationships and providing a whole person approach will help all parties believe in and so ensure implementation.
- For individuals in the criminal justice system, practitioners may have limited opportunities to create continuity. Having access to previous records before or just after seeing someone and having a good understanding about where an individual will be going, which team care will be transferred to, and how to get the right information, are all vital for creating continuity of care.

Scenarios requiring continuity

The following scenarios are typical for individuals in contact with the criminal justice system:

- Coming into prison from care in the community.
- Leaving prison and returning to the community at the end of sentence.
- Leaving prison and all contact with the criminal justice system after release from the courts (e.g. if on remand and found not guilty).
- Transfer between wings and prisons.
- Transfer from contact with liaison and diversion teams.

The basics of continuity

In order to ensure continuity of care and ongoing quality of care, the following basics need to be in place:

- Transfer of records with a plan and preferably a shared understanding detailing who will be responsible for ongoing elements of care in the new setting.
- Continuity of a pathway of care—if an individual has started treatment then there is an assumption that this will be continued. While outpatient care might be relatively easy to continue if an individual is returning to where the care was offered, if an individual is leaving prison to a new setting or arriving in prison from a different setting then continuity is not ensured.
- Support after transfer of an understanding of the individual's goals across social, psychological, and physical domains.

Engager intervention: day of release

Individuals receiving the Engager intervention[1] are all offered a day of release package. In the pilot study, this was seen as an optional possibility, whereas in the full trial, because of the potential benefit, it was offered routinely to everyone and the majority took it up and received it. The Engager through the gate package involved working with individuals before release, making contact to build trust to understand their situation on release and to determine the likely problems on release. The scheme was particularly targeted at those with chaotic complex needs including unstable housing, ongoing substance use, and those with personality traits of paranoia and emotional instability likely to cause problems.

Release day work requires meticulous planning and working with the authorities to understand the date. Engager workers worked alone, after doing a risk assessment, and had the use of cars to drive individuals from appointment to appointment. Some simply wanted dropping home, others really valued support to attend their first substance misuse appointment, probation appointment, and housing appointments. The work could take 4–6 hours and on some occasions practitioners had to leave individuals on the street homeless, but even then the fact that they had taken the time was a huge generator of trust. The psychological and emotional work carried out by the practitioners on the day of release was continuous and sometimes involved sitting quietly together just to be calm while avoiding the pub or dealer, sometimes to carry out detailed planning, and was for some the start of deeper emotional work.

Tips for creating continuity

A range of key issues might be important when considering supporting continuity from different locations:

- Individuals who tend to be paranoid and distrustful of others require particular help when moving from one practitioner or team to another. Just ringing ahead and talking to a practitioner, and letting the individual know you have done that, or just writing a note can be helpful. Equally, coaching an individual regarding their tendency towards paranoia and thinking through different ways in which they might approach new situations can be helpful.
- Individuals with emotional lability are particularly difficult to support as they may appear calm in prison but be at risk of very significant increases in anxiety and anger at small precipitating events. Again, coaching an individual about this and the problems that are likely to occur on release, and the need to avoid substances as a way of coping, can be helpful, as can liaising with practitioners in teams they will be working with, particularly substance misuse, housing, and so on, and supporting the practitioners to understand the particular psychological profile of the individual.
- Individuals with a tendency to use substances on release need care and support to think about scenarios as well as prescribing support to reduce craving and the likelihood of using.

- Some individuals have a tendency to minimize problems and set themselves up to fail by not planning and making out that they will manage. In Engager, these individuals are called 'honeymooners'. Those using alcohol who were not drinking in prison but were likely to restart typified those who didn't engage fully with their situation or appreciate the need for self-reflection and to have support.
- Other individuals are pervasively low or depressed or have antisocial traits and will have a tendency not to engage with services and see them as negative or unnecessary. Again, being clear and open with individuals about their tendencies, as well as communicating about these issues as a part of transfer, can be helpful.

Release day package

Planning for specific medical problems on release is important. The last 10 years have seen a major improvement in substance misuse prescribing with routine provision of methadone prescription on release for those at risk of opiate misuse. Release day planning more generally for social issues such as housing is now more common and it should be feasible to link a range of packages together which might include:
- clear communication with GPs and other practitioners about not re-starting medication which has been deliberately stopped while in prison such as pregabalin, diazepam, or quetiapine
- opiate substitution
- contraception, particularly for women
- ongoing care, particularly for hepatitis treatment, as well as for other health conditions.

System facilitators

Providing high-quality ongoing care and continuity can be enhanced by a range of system facilitators. These include:
- joint commissioning of ongoing pathways, not just of physical health problems, but also mental healthcare
- easy transfer of records from one electronic system to another
- joint use of protocols and care plans so that an individual's shared understanding and plan can simply be transferred to another organization seamlessly without having to be repeated
- liaison and shared training programmes between teams, across the community–hospital interface in particular, in order to generate a shared culture and understanding
- an up-to-date list of teams, workers, team leaders, telephone numbers, bypass numbers, and so on, to facilitate liaison and discussion of cases.

Reference

1. Brand SL, Quinn C, Pearson M, et al. Realist formative process evaluation: prioritising and elaborating theory prior to full trial of a complex intervention for prison leavers with mental health problems. Evaluation. 2019;25(2):149–170.

Chapter 15

Prison health emergencies

Overdose

Drug overdose is often the result of an individual using multiple substances together. Sedating drugs can potentiate the effects of each other, so lower doses in combination can result in overdose.

Ensure appropriate mitigating actions are in place if clinically necessary to prescribe medications that could cause overdose if used inappropriately or in combination with other substances (see Abuse and diversion of medicines, p. 54).

The first few days in prison are a high-risk time for drug overdose:

- People may have been detained at the height of a chaotic time in their lives and may have taken multiple substances in the preceding days.
- They may be commenced on sedating medications such as chlordiazepoxide, methadone, and buprenorphine to manage dependence and withdrawal.
- They may internally conceal drug packages to smuggle them into prison. Package rupture can cause rapid life-threatening overdose.
- They are often not ready to be abstinent from drugs and are still in a 'drug-seeking' frame of mind which may lead to unsafe illicit drug use.
- They may be in a state of psychological distress and use drugs to cope.
- Monitoring should include frequent formal observations for signs of oversedation and acute withdrawal, as well as informal observation by healthcare and prison staff by placing people in an area where staff are present and can be easily contacted if a person feels unwell.
- Make patients aware of the risks of overdose from using illicit substances through open and frank discussions, and signposting to support information and organizations available in prison.

Intentional overdose

- Overdose is often accidental but may also be intentional.
- HCPs should be aware of the risks of suicide.
- HCPs should ensure they are familiar with the local ACCT processes for identifying and managing people in prison at risk of suicide.

Management of suspected overdose

Management of acute drug overdose should focus on treatment of the presenting clinical features—don't waste time trying to identify what substances have been taken (often the user won't even know).

Approach with caution: personal safety is paramount

- Ensure prison officers are present, and always carry a radio.
- Prison officers and healthcare staff have been known to succumb to the toxic fumes from PSs. If there is any smoke or smell of fumes, retreat and put on an FFP3 mask.

Primary assessment

- Use the ABCD approach as for any emergency.
- If the patient is unresponsive and lacks respiratory effort: request an ambulance, commence basic/immediate life support, and give naloxone (see below).

- A: airway adjuncts may be needed.
- B: stimulation may stimulate respiratory effort.
- C: consider IV access and IV fluids.
- D: check capillary glucose and temperature.

Naloxone
- Naloxone is an opioid antagonist used to treat opioid overdose.
- It is used if there is reduced conscious level or reduced respiratory effort.
- There is not a need to confirm opioids have been used before administration.
- Administer by intramuscular injection into the anterolateral thigh or deltoid.
- Dose: 400 micrograms every 2–3 minutes.
- Continue until patient has regained consciousness, is breathing normally, medical assistance is available, or contents of syringe are used up.
- If there is no response after 2 mg—reassess the diagnosis.
- Naloxone is shorter acting than most opioids, so repeated doses may be required.
- Patients who have received naloxone should be referred to hospital for monitoring and further assessment. They may require treatment with naloxone IV infusion.
- PS formulations have been known to contain fentanyl and fentanyl-like derivatives which can cause fatal overdose within a few minutes. Higher doses of naloxone and more rapid escalation of dosing may be required.

Secondary assessment
- Look for drug paraphernalia, needle track marks, and smells of alcohol or fumes.
- Is there evidence of self-harm or trauma?
- Pupils: may be pin-point (opioids), enlarged (stimulant use), or transiently unequal.
- Eye movements: may be dysconjugate (benzodiazepines) or nystagmus (dissociatives).
- Abnormal posturing may be present; however, lateralizing neurological deficit suggests an alternative diagnosis.
- Pre-hospital toxicological testing (blood or urine) is not recommended as it may delay transfer to hospital and will rarely change management.

Seizures
- Seizures caused by drug overdose should be managed as per NICE guidelines.[1]
- Note the time and protect the patient from injury if possible; do not restrain them.
- If prolonged or recurrent seizures, treat with benzodiazepines (buccal midazolam preferred).
- Once seizure has terminated, place the patient in the recovery position, and monitor and manage ABCs; do not leave them alone until fully recovered or handed over care to paramedics.

Indications for hospital transfer

These include:
- reduced conscious level
- reduced breathing
- hypotension
- tachycardia, bradycardia, or irregular pulse
- treated with naloxone
- hypo- or hyperthermia
- seizure
- healthcare staff not present on site to monitor (e.g. at some sites overnight).

Reference

1. National Institute for Health and Care Excellence.

Self-harm by ligature

Introduction

Deliberate self-harm (DSH) is any act of self-injury carried out by an individual, irrespective of their motivation.[1] Patients who self-harm are not always intent on taking their own lives; however, there is a proven link between self-harm and suicide with over half of those who die by suicide having a history of DSH. Self-harm could also a cry for help, so it should never be trivialized or ignored.

The most common method of suicide in the UK is hanging, strangulation, and suffocation (grouped as one method). In 2018 it accounted for 59.4% of male suicides and 45% of female suicides.[2]

Mechanism of injury

In a hanging or ligature injury, a device is placed around the neck preventing blood and oxygen from reaching the brain. It is possible that a person in prison will find means to hang themselves from a point; other, more common methods involve tying a ligature around their neck with the other end secured to a fixed object and twisting the body until strangulation occurs.

If the patient has experienced a drop equal to or greater than their own height, it is most likely that the cervical spine fractures and the spinal cord is transected, generally resulting in instant death. This type of injury, where the body is suspended off the floor, is called a complete hanging.

Should the patient be suspended, and part of the body touches the floor, this is classed as an incomplete hanging. Arterial and venous obstruction may be evident, resulting in decreased cerebral perfusion and hypoxic injury—unconsciousness will quickly follow. Muscular tone will decrease which will increase obstruction of the airway and arterial blood flow. Bradycardia and hypotension can be caused by vagal stimulation on the carotid sinus. Cardiac arrest may follow.

Initial scene assessment

Following an episode of serious self-harm, it is important to be mindful about what language is used. It is never appropriate to discuss the reasons why the patient has harmed themselves during treatment. This can be supported when the patient has received treatment and stabilized. The HCP should:

- ensure an emergency ambulance is en route—be prepared to change the response level as the patient is assessed in line with the Ambulance Response Programme
- be mindful of your personal safety—never enter a cell alone
- ensure the cell door is locked back in the open position
- try to gain as much information as possible without delaying treatment
- consider the environmental factors and what space is needed to work in
- maintain dignity and safety at all times.

Primary survey

Remove ligature using prison-issued safety knife if required; if patient is suspended, lower to the ground taking care not to cause further injury.

Any patient who has suffered ligature injury should be assessed and life-threatening conditions dealt with rapidly. The <C>ABCDE approach as suggested by NICE[3] should be used, with each of the following aspects being assessed and treated:

• C: catastrophic haemorrhage.
• A: airway maintenance and cervical spine consideration.
• B: breathing, ventilation.
• C: circulation, further haemorrhage control.
• D: disability, assessment of neurological state.
• E: exposure, undress patient for full examination and assessment.

Patient management

• Airway—look, listen, feel. Talk to patient for response—do they sound hoarse, any cough, stridor, or muffled voice?
• In an unconscious patient, the airway should be maintained—initially with appropriate manual manoeuvres, then an oropharyngeal airway (if tolerated) or a nasopharyngeal airway.
• Consider cervical spine immobilization if the patient has been suspended. Ligature injuries are primarily hypoxic events with no spinal cord/vertebrae involvement unless there has been a long drop into a ligature. Manual in-line stabilization is recommended for unconscious patients from hangings. It is the clinician's decision to use a hard collar or not, this is to be considered following assessment of any increase in intracranial pressure and cerebral oedema.
• Assess airway for foreign objects, secretions, and laryngeal injury. Any foreign objects to be removed with Magill's forceps, secretions should be removed with postural drainage (bearing in mind possible cervical spine injury) and/or suction.
• Assess breathing; if no breathing, commence resuscitation as per Resuscitation Council (UK) guidelines,[4] and within scope of practice. If patient is breathing, assess for respiratory distress and mental status changes indicating hypoxic injury.
• Once airway is patent and patient is breathing, give high-flow oxygen (15 L/min) with 100% non-rebreathable reservoir mask.
• Assess for other pulmonary complications by auscultation—respiratory distress syndrome, pulmonary oedema.
• Check for skin petechiae (including Amussat's sign, Simon's sign, and Martin's sign) which may indicate the severity of strangulation injury. Assess if any injury or potential injury requires further observations or hospital treatment.
• Other complications—hyperthermia, seizures. Unless there has been a significant amount of blood loss, fluids are restricted to prevent exacerbation of cerebral oedema.
• Complete a full secondary survey of the patient.

Aftercare

• The welfare of staff involved in the incident must be considered as soon as possible. This will involve hot debriefs in line with prison protocols.
• If there is a Trauma Risk Management (TRiM) practitioner on site, staff are to be referred immediately.

- PSI 64/2011 requires that any person in prison identified as at risk of suicide or self-harm must be managed using ACCT.
- Work with prison staff who will implement the ACCT case management system.
- ACCT is a person-centred, multidisciplinary approach to support, care, and risk identification.
- Consider liaising with prison mental health services.

References

1. National Institute for Health and Care Excellence. 2011.
2. Office for National Statistics. 2019.
3. National Institute for Health and Care Excellence. 2019.
4. Resuscitation Council (UK). Resuscitation guidelines. 2021. https://www.resus.org.uk/library/2021-resuscitation-guidelines

Poisoning

Overview

Consult TOXBASE or the UK National Poisons Information Service for management advice.

Patients who have features of poisoning, or who have taken poisons with delayed action should generally be admitted to hospital. Delayed-action poisons include aspirin, iron, paracetamol, tricyclic antidepressants, and modified-release drug preparations.

In the prison environment, because of the potential for diversion and trading of prescribed medication, or of illicitly brought in substances, it is important to consider that the patient may not know, or may choose not to disclose, what has been taken. Accidents or intentional ingestion may involve domestic and industrial products, or 'hooch' (an illicit alcohol made in prisons), the contents of which may not be known. Therefore, a low threshold for hospital admission is needed as the course and effects of the poisoning may not be predictable. The patient may need constant monitoring in a clinical setting—something which is usually not possible in the prison environment (especially overnight).

A note of all relevant information, including initial assessment and any treatment given, should accompany the patient to hospital.

It is not uncommon for poisoned patients to refuse hospital admission, or to self-discharge before treatment or monitoring is complete. In these circumstances, it is essential to fully assess and record the patient's capacity to make the decision. A decision in the patient's best interests may need to be made, involving the wider prison and healthcare teams in a multidisciplinary forum.

Further resources

TOXBASE, the primary clinical toxicology database of the National Poisons Information Service, is available on the internet to registered users at https://www.toxbase.org (a backup site is available at https://www.toxbasebackup.org if the main site cannot be accessed). It provides information about routine diagnosis, treatment, and management of patients exposed to drugs, household products, and industrial and agricultural chemicals.

Specialist information and advice on the treatment of poisoning is available day and night from the UK National Poisons Information Service on the following number: Tel. 0344 892 0111.

Advice on laboratory analytical services can be obtained from TOXBASE or from the National Poisons Information Service. Help with identifying capsules or tablets may be available from a regional medicines information centre or from the National Poisons Information Service (out of hours).

General management of the poisoned patient

In most patients, treatment is directed at managing symptoms as they arise. Only a few poisons (such as opioids, paracetamol, and iron) have specific antidotes and few patients require active removal of the poison.

Nevertheless, knowledge of the type and timing of poisoning can help in anticipating the course of events. All relevant information should be sought from the poisoned individual, bearing in mind that it may not be complete or entirely reliable.

Sometimes symptoms arise from other illnesses and patients should be assessed carefully. For example, hypoglycaemia may present with altered behaviour, reduced consciousness, sweating, and tremor, which could mimic intoxication.

On initial assessment, a full set of observations, including Glasgow Coma Scale score and blood glucose, should be taken. A NEWS2 score can be useful for the prison doctor and may be requested by the ambulance control.

Undertake an ECG and carry out a focused examination, as appropriate. Where possible, take a history, to include:
- what has been ingested/inhaled, including doses and quantity of tablets
- what time this occurred, including if there was a staggered ingestion
- any symptoms experienced
- existing medical problems
- other medications usually taken (consider interactions).

If the patient is unresponsive and not breathing normally, commence CPR, initiate a 'Code Blue', and call 999.

Airway and respiration

Respiration is often impaired in unconscious patients. An obstructed airway requires immediate attention. In the absence of trauma, use simple measures such as chin lift or jaw thrust. An oropharyngeal or nasopharyngeal airway may be useful in patients with reduced consciousness, provided ventilation is adequate. Most poisons that impair consciousness also depress respiration, so assisted ventilation using a bag-valve-mask device may be needed.

Inhalation of toxic gases, such as chlorine and ammonia, can cause upper respiratory tract irritation, usually presenting as dyspnoea. Give high-flow oxygen and arrange hospital admission.

Blood pressure

Hypotension is common in severe poisoning with CNS depressants. A systolic BP of less than 70 mmHg may lead to irreversible brain damage or renal tubular necrosis. Hypotension should be corrected initially by raising the patient's legs and administering IV fluids, where facilities for this exist.

Hypertension may be associated with sympathomimetic drugs such as amphetamines and cocaine.

Cardiac effects

Cardiac conduction defects and arrhythmias can occur in acute poisoning, notably with tricyclic antidepressants, some antipsychotics, and some antihistamines. ECG changes may also occur as a result of electrolyte abnormalities or myocardial ischaemia following poisoning.

An approach to the ECG in toxicology—check the following

- Rate and rhythm—P wave and QRS morphology may also be affected, depending on the substance ingested.
- PR interval—is there any degree of heart block?
- QRS duration in lead II.
- New right axis deviation of the QRS—may indicate sodium channel blockade.
- QT interval—a prolonged QT interval predisposes to the development of torsades de pointes. This is more likely to occur where there is coexisting bradycardia.
- Signs of myocardial ischaemia.
- Signs of increased cardiac ectopy or automaticity.

Body temperature

- Hypothermia may develop if the patient has been unconscious for some hours, or had a 'long lie'. Hypothermia should be managed by prevention of further heat loss and re-warming, as clinically indicated.
- Hyperthermia can develop in patients taking CNS stimulants, serotonergic drugs, or antimuscarinic drugs.
- Hyperthermia is initially managed by removing all unnecessary clothing and using a fan. Sponging with tepid water will promote evaporation.
- Both hypothermia and hyperthermia require urgent hospitalization for assessment and supportive treatment.

Serotonin syndrome

This may be seen in SSRI/serotonin–norepinephrine reuptake inhibitor overdose, or after dose increases or a new agent being started. Effects include neuromuscular hyperactivity (such as tremor, hyperreflexia, clonus, myoclonus, rigidity), autonomic dysfunction (hyperthermia, tachycardia, BP changes, diaphoresis, shivering, diarrhoea), and altered mental state (agitation, confusion, mania).

Treatment consists of withdrawal of the serotonergic medication and supportive care; admit.

Neurological effects

Patients may have reduced responsiveness, as measured using the Glasgow Coma Scale. There may be changes in mental state, including drowsiness or agitation. Assess their pupils; these may be pinpoint (e.g. in opiate poisoning) or dilated (e.g. in stimulant or benzodiazepine poisoning).

Convulsions during poisoning

Single short-lived convulsions (lasting <5 minutes) do not require treatment. If convulsions are protracted or recur frequently, benzodiazepines should be given according to local policy (usually midazolam via the buccal route, or diazepam via the rectal route).

Measures to reduce absorption

Given orally, activated charcoal can bind many poisons in the gastrointestinal system, thereby reducing their absorption. The sooner it is given, the more effective it is, but it may still be effective up to 1 hour after ingestion of the poison. It is particularly useful for the prevention of absorption of poisons that are toxic in small amounts, such as antidepressants.

If vomiting occurs after dosing, it should be treated (e.g. with an antiemetic drug) since it may reduce the efficacy of charcoal treatment.

Activated charcoal should *not* be used for poisoning with petroleum distillates, corrosive substances, alcohols, malathion, cyanides, and metal salts, including iron and lithium salts.

Follow-up

Consider a multidisciplinary approach to following up the poisoned patient after initial treatment or discharge from hospital. Depending on the circumstances, it may be appropriate to consider any or all of the following:
• Refer the patient to the substance misuse team.
• In episodes of intentional poisoning, ensure the patient has an ACCT opened so that they are supported and followed up by the prison and the mental health team.
• Inform the medicines management team and request a medicines reconciliation check and/or cell search, in conjunction with the prison.
• Review the patient's prescribed medication.
• Review the patient's in-possession risk assessment.
• Submit a prison security intelligence report.
• Submit a clinical incident report.
• Submit a prison safeguarding referral.

Refusal of hospital admission

It is not uncommon for poisoned patients to refuse hospital admission, or to self-discharge before treatment or monitoring is complete. The frequency, nature, and duration of monitoring advised will be dependent on the substances involved. Consider seeking advice from the emergency department team and discussing how this could be undertaken with the on-site healthcare and prison teams (e.g. duty governor/Oscar 1). For example, it may be appropriate to use a constant supervision cell for continuous observation.

In these circumstances, it is essential to fully assess the patient's capacity to make the decision in question, using the Mental Capacity Act. This should include a discussion of the risks of not accepting treatment and of remaining in the prison setting where continuous clinical monitoring is not possible.

If a person is assessed as not having the capacity to make the decision in question, a best-interests meeting involving any other appropriate parties may be helpful. This may include the prison's Safer Custody team, the mental health, primary care, and substance misuse teams.

Further reading

Holstege CP, Eldridge DL, Rowden AK. ECG manifestations: the poisoned patient. Emerg Med Clin North Am. 2006:24(1):159–177.

Joint Formulary Committee. British National Formulary. 2020. https://bnf.nice.org.uk/treatment-summary/poisoning-emergency-treatment.html

National Poisons Information Service. TOXBASE. https://www.toxbase.org

Nickson C. ECG in toxicology. Life in the Fastlane; 2021. https://litfl.com/ecg-in-toxicology/

Self-harm

Introduction

Being sentenced to go to prison is a transition from normal life to a system behind walls and closed doors. This can affect people in different ways and many struggle to adjust which can impact their mental health and behaviour. There are pathways to offer support to those affected and this can stop people from harming themselves. As a healthcare provider, it is common occurrence to treat victims of DSH within the prison environment.

Initial approach

Be mindful of personal safety—never enter a room or cell without prison staff presence and assurance that it is safe to do so. The prison staff will search the patient and ensure no weapons are present. The room/cell door should never be closed and should be locked back in an open position.

Assessment

Consider the immediate environment

- Is it appropriate to offer treatment where the person is residing—consider cell mates, onlookers, and regime (e.g. association).
- Offer a treatment room where appropriate to do so, attempting to maintain confidentiality and dignity at all times. Can the patient be treated on site or is hospital necessary?

Any life- or limb-threatening injuries should be dealt with in a timely and appropriate manner using the <C>ABCDE algorithm as suggested by NICE.[1]

- Catastrophic haemorrhaging: venous or arterial bleed should be treated with the application of a haemostatic tourniquet.
- Airway: check for foreign objects, secretions, and so on (including cervical spine if indicated by mechanism of injury).
- Breathing: assess breathing, any chest injuries?
- Circulation: deal with non-life catastrophic bleeds, hypovolaemic shock may occur with extensive bleeding.
- Disability: other associated injuries.
- Environmental: guard against hypothermia with major blood loss.

Take a brief history of the incident paying attention to the patient's mental state. Attempt to gather as much information about the patient as possible, this will help support someone else in knowing the best way to engage with the patient. If the patient is a prolific self-harmer, try not to embark on a conversation about why they self-harm. This is a conversation they will have had many times—instead, talk about other topics to distract them.

Concentrate on the following

- Events and circumstances leading to self-harm incident.
- Intention of DSH (i.e. preparation, tools used).
- Outcome of DSH—what treatment is required?
- Current social stresses, any debts? Personal or family issues?
- Alcohol/drug misuse.
- Be mindful of language used while treating an injury—many people in prison with PD may be triggered or excited by any reaction to the injury.
- Do not engage in conversation about the severity of the injury.

Aftercare

- Give clear guidance on wound management and possible risks, such as infection. Where appropriate, offer clean dressings for the patient to reapply.
- Work with prison staff who will implement the ACCT case management system.
- PSI 64/2011 requires that any person identified as at risk of suicide or self-harm must be managed using ACCT.
- ACCT is a person-centred, multidisciplinary approach to support, care, and risk identification.
- Consider liaising with prison mental health services.

Suicide risk

The NICE guideline 'Preventing suicide in community and custodial settings'[2] gives clear guidance on suicide prevention within prisons, which includes recommendations for assessment and treatment of patients within the first 48 hours after having self-harmed.

Suicide within UK prisons is substantially higher than among society in general. During a 3-year period (2009–2011), self-inflicted deaths within English prisons were recorded at 69 per 100,000 inmates. At inquest, over 80% of these received a suicide or open verdict.

Middle-aged men from a lower socioeconomic background are at most risk from suicide, whereas young people are more at risk of DSH. The prison population is at increased risk from suicide and DSH—this can happen at any time during their remand or sentence, but evidence suggests the risk is increased in such occasions as:

- early days and weeks in prison, either on remand or sentence
- post sentencing
- post transfer from other prisons (away from friends and family)
- post recall to prison.

Factors suggesting suicidal intent

- Careful planning and intent.
- Finalizing acts such as suicide notes and final statements.
- DSH carried out in secret or at night when unlikely to be found.
- Not asking for help following DSH.
- A sustained wish to die.
- Recent change in relationships.
- Bereavement.
- Physical illness.
- Drugs/alcohol.

The clinician should carry out a studied suicide risk assessment which will link in with the patient's ACCT. Suicide risk tools should be used for increasing care pathways, but not to determine who should or should not be referred for treatment. Tools include the Columbia Suicide Severity Rating (Fig. 15.1).

References

1. National Institute for Health and Care Excellence. 2019.
2. National Institute for Health and Care Excellence. Preventing suicide in community and custodial settings. NICE guideline [NG105]. September 2018. https://www.nice.org.uk/guidance/ng105

COLUMBIA-SUICIDE SEVERITY RATING SCALE
(C-SSRS)
Posner, Brent, Luca, Gould, Stanley, Brown, Fisher, Zelazny, Burke, Oquendo, & Mann
© 2008 The Research Foundation for Mental Hygiene, Inc.

RISK ASSESSMENT VERSION
(* elements added with permission for Lifeline centers)

Instructions: Check all risk and protective factors that apply. To be completed following the patient interview, review of medical record(s) and/or consultation with family members and/or other professionals.

Suicidal and Self-Injury Behavior (Past Week)		Clinical Status (Recent)	
☐	Actual suicide attempt ☐ Lifetime	☐	Hopelessness
☐	Interrupted attempt ☐ Lifetime	☐	Helplessness*
☐	Aborted attempt ☐ Lifetime	☐	Feeling Trapped*
☐	Other preparatory acts to kill self ☐ Lifetime	☐	Major depressive episode
☐	Self-injury behavior w/o suicide intent ☐ Lifetime	☐	Mixed affective episode
Suicide Ideation (Most Severe in Past Week)		☐	Command hallucinations to hurt self
☐	Wish to be dead	☐	Highly impulsive behavior
☐	Suicidal thoughts	☐	Substance abuse or dependence
☐	Suicidal thoughts with method (but without specific plan or intent to act)	☐	Agitation or severe anxiety
☐	Suicidal intent (without specific plan)	☐	Perceived burden on family or others
☐	Suicidal intent with specific plan	☐	Chronic physical pain or other acute medical problem (AIDS, COPD, cancer, etc.)
Activating Events (Recent)		☐	Homicidal ideation
☐	Recent loss or other significant negative event	☐	Aggressive behavior towards others
	Describe:	☐	Method for suicide available (gun, pills, etc.)
		☐	Refuses or feels unable to agree to safety plan
☐	Pending incarceration or homelessness	☐	Sexual abuse (lifetime)
☐	Current or pending isolation or feeling alone	☐	Family history of suicide (lifetime)
Treatment History		**Protective Factors (Recent)**	
☐	Previous psychiatric diagnoses and treatments	☐	Identifies reasons for living
☐	Hopeless or dissatisfied with treatment	☐	Responsibility to family or others; living with family
☐	Noncompliant with treatment	☐	Supportive social network or family
☐	Not receiving treatment	☐	Fear of death or dying due to pain and suffering
Other Risk Factors		☐	Belief that suicide is immoral, high spirituality
☐		☐	Engaged in work or school
		☐	Engaged with Phone Worker*
		Other Protective Factors	
		☐	
Describe any suicidal, self-injury or aggressive behavior (include dates):			

Lifeline Version 1/2014

Fig. 15.1 (Contd.)

SUICIDAL IDEATION				
Ask questions 1 and 2. If both are negative, proceed to "Suicidal Behavior" section. If the answer to question 2 is "yes", ask questions 3, 4 and 5. If the answer to question 1 and/or 2 is "yes", complete "Intensity of Ideation" section below.	**Lifetime: Time He/She Felt Most Suicidal**		**Past 1 month**	
1. Wish to be Dead Subject endorses thoughts about a wish to be dead or not alive anymore, or wish to fall asleep and not wake up. *Have you wished you were dead or wished you could go to sleep and not wake up?* If yes, describe:	Yes ☐	No ☐	Yes ☐	No ☐
2. Non-Specific Active Suicidal Thoughts General non-specific thoughts of wanting to end one's life/ commit suicide (e.g., *"I've thought about killing myself"*) without thoughts of ways to kill oneself/associated methods, intent, or plan during the assessment period. *Have you actually had any thoughts of killing yourself?* If yes, describe:	Yes ☐	No ☐	Yes ☐	No ☐
3. Active Suicidal Ideation with Any Methods (Not Plan) without Intent to Act Subject endorses thoughts of suicide and has thought of at least one method during the assessment period. This is different than a specific plan with time, place or method details worked out (e.g., thought of method to kill self but not a specific plan). Includes person who would say, *"I thought about taking an overdose but I never made a specific plan as to when, where or how I would actually do it...and I would never go through with it."* *Have you been thinking about how you might do this?* If yes, describe:	Yes ☐	No ☐	Yes ☐	No ☐
4. Active Suicidal Ideation with Some Intent to Act, without Specific Plan Active suicidal thoughts of killing oneself and subject reports having some intent to act on such thoughts, as opposed to *"I have the thoughts but I definitely will not do anything about them."* *Have you had these thoughts and had some intention of acting on them?* If yes, describe:	Yes ☐	No ☐	Yes ☐	No ☐
5. Active Suicidal Ideation with Specific Plan and Intent Thoughts of killing oneself with details of plan fully or partially worked out and subject had some intent to carry it out. *Have you started to work out or worked out the details of how to kill yourself? Do you intend to carry out this plan?* If yes, describe:	Yes ☐	No ☐	Yes ☐	No ☐
INTENSITY OF IDEATION				
The following features should be rated with respect to the most severe type of ideation (i.e., 1-5 from above, with 1 being the least severe and 5 being the most severe). Ask about time he/she was feeling the most suicidal. Lifetime - *Most Severe Ideation:* ___ Type # (1-5) ___ Description of Ideation Recent - *Most Severe Ideation:* ___ Type # (1-5) ___ Description of Ideation	**Most Severe**		**Most Severe**	

Fig. 15.1 (Contd.)

Frequency *How many times have you had these thoughts?* (1) Less than once a week (2) Once a week (3) 2.5 times in week (4) Daily or almost daily (5) Many times each day	——	——
Duration *When you have the thoughts how long do they last?* (1) Fleeting - few seconds or minutes (2) Less than 1 hour/some of the time (3) 1-4 hours/a lot of time (4) 4-8 hours/most of day (5) More than 8 hours/persistent or continuous	——	——
Controllability *Could/can you stop thinking about killing yourself or* *wanting to die if you want to?* (1) Easily able to control thoughts (2) Can control thoughts with little difficulty (3) Can control thoughts with some difficulty (4) Can control thoughts with a lot of difficulty (5) Unable to control thoughts (0) Does not attempt to control thoughts	——	——
Deterrents *Are there things - anyone or anything (e.g., family, religion,* *pain of death) - that stopped you from wanting to die or* *acting on thoughts of committing suicide?* (1) Deterrents definitely stopped you from attempting suicide (2) Deterrents probably stopped you (3) Uncertain that deterrents stopped you (4) Deterrents most likely did not stop you (5) Deterrents definitely did not stop you (0) Does not apply	——	——

Reasons of Ideation
What sort of reasons did you have for thinking about
wanting to die or killing yourself? Was it to end the pain or
stop the way you were feeling (in other words you couldn't
go on living with this pain or how you were feeling) or was it
to get attention, revenge or a reaction from others? Or both?
(1) Completely to get attention, revenge or a
      reaction from others
(2) Mostly to get attention, revenge or a reaction
      from others
(3) Equally to get attention, revenge or a reaction
      from others and to end/stop the pain
(4) Mostly to end or stop the pain (you couldn't go
      on living with the pain or how you were feeling)
(5) Completely to end or stop the pain (you
      couldn't go on living with the pain or how you
      were feeling)
(0) Does not apply
	——	——

C-SSRS—Lifetime Recent - Clinical (Version 1/14/09)

Fig. 15.1 (*Contd.*)

SUICIDAL BEHAVIOR *(Check all that apply, so long as these are separate events; must ask about all types)*	Lifetime		Past 3 month	
Actual Attempt: A potentially self-injurious act committed with at least some wish to die, *as a result of act.* Behavior was in part thought of as method to kill oneself. Intent does not have to be 100%. If there is *any* intent/desire to die associated with the act, then it can be considered an actual suicide attempt. ***There does not have to be any injury or harm,*** just the potential for injury or harm. If person pulls trigger while gun is in mouth but gun is broken so no injury results, this is considered an attempt. Inferring Intent: Even if an individual denies intent/wish to die, it may be inferred clinically from the behavior or circumstances. For example, a highly lethal act that is clearly not an accident so no other intent but suicide can be inferred (e.g., gunshot to head, jumping from window of a high floor/story). Also, if someone denies intent to die, but they thought that what they did could be lethal, intent may be inferred. *Have you made a suicide attempt? Have you done anything to harm yourself? Have you done anything dangerous where you could have died? What did you do? Did you ____ as a way to end your life? Did you want to die (even a little) when you ____? Were you trying to end your life when you ____? Or Did you think it was possible you could have died from ____? Or did you do it purely for other reasons / without ANY intention of killing yourself (like to relieve stress, feel better, get sympathy, or get something else to happen)?* (Self-Injurious Behavior without suicidal intent) If yes, describe:	Yes ☐ Total # of Attempts _____	No ☐	Yes ☐ Total # of Attempts _____	No ☐
Has subject engaged in Non-Suicidal Self-Injurious Behavior?	Yes ☐	No ☐	Yes ☐	No ☐
Interrupted Attempt: When the person is interrupted (by an outside circumstance) from starting the potentially self-injurious act (*if not for that, actual attempt would have occurred).* Overdose: Person has pills in hand but is stopped from ingesting. Once they ingest any pills, this becomes an attempt rather than an interrupted attempt. Shooting: Person has gun pointed toward self, gun is taken away by someone else, or is somehow prevented from pulling trigger. Once they pull the trigger, even if the gun fails to fire, it is an attempt. Jumping: Person is poised to jump, is grabbed and taken down from ledge. Hanging: Person has noose around neck but has not yet started to hang - is stopped from doing so. *Has there been a time when you started to do something to end you life but someone or something stopped you before you actually did anything?* If yes, describe:	Yes ☐ Total # of interrupted _____	No ☐	Yes ☐ Total # of interrupted _____	No ☐
Aborted or Self-Interrupted Attempt: When person begins to take steps toward making a suicide attempt, but stops themselves before they actually have engaged in any self-destructive behavior. Examples are similar to interrupted attempts, except that the individual stop him/herself, instead of being stopped by something else. *Has there been a time when you started to do something to try to end your life but you stopped yourself before you actually did anything?* If yes, describe:	Yes ☐ Total # of aborted of self-interrupted _____	No ☐	Yes ☐ Total # of aborted of self-interrupted _____	No ☐

Fig. 15.1 *(Contd.)*

Preparatory Acts or Behavior: Acts or preparation towards imminently making a suicide attempt. This can include anything beyond a verbalization or thought, such as assembling a specific method (e.g., buying pills, purchasing a gun) or preparing for one's death by suicide (e.g., giving things away, writing a suicide note). *Have you taken any steps towards making a suicide attempt or preparing to kill yourself (such as collecting pills, getting a gun, giving valuables away or writing a suicide note)?* If yes, describe:		Yes ☐ No ☐ Total # of preparatory acts		Yes ☐ No ☐ Total # of preparatory acts

	Most Recent Attempt Date:	Most Lethal Attempt Date:	Initial/First Attempt Date:
Actual Lethality/Medical Damage: 0. No physical damage or very minor physical damage (e.g., surface scratches). 1. Minor physical damage (e.g., lethargic speech; first-degree burns; mild bleeding; sprains). 2. Moderate physical damage; medical attention needed (e.g., conscious but sleepy, somewhat responsive; second-degree burns; bleeding of major vessel). 3. Moderately severe physical damage; *medical* hospitalization and likely intensive care required (e.g., comatose with reflexes intact; third-degree burns less than 20% of body; extensive blood loss but can recover; major fractures). 4. Severe physical damage; *medical* hospitalization with intensive care required (e.g., comatose without reflexes; third-degree burns over 20% of body; extensive blood loss with unstable vital signs; major damage to a vital area). 5. Death	*Enter Code*	*Enter Code* _____	*Enter Code*
Potential lethality: Only Answer if Actual Lethality = 0 Likely lethality of actual attempt if no medical damage (the following examples, while having no actual medical damage, had potential for very serious lethality; put gun in mouth and pulled the trigger but gun fails to fire so no medical damage; laying on train tracks with oncoming train but pulled away before run over). 0 = Behavior not likely to result in injury 1 = Behavior likely to result in injury but not likely to cause death 2 = Behavior likely to result in death despite available medical care	*Enter Code* _____	*Enter Code* _____	*Enter Code* _____

C-SSRS—Lifetime Recent - Clinical (Version 1/14/09)

Fig. 15.1 Columbia Suicide Severity Rating. Reproduced from the Columbia Lighthouse Project with permission.

Victims of assault

Introduction

Assaults in public prisons have been increasing steadily between 2014 and 2019.[1] These include a significant number of violent and sexual assaults occurring while in custody.

If an incident occurs within the prison, healthcare staff should always be called to attend. Clinical teams have a number of responsibilities to consider in these situations:

First aid and medical response

As soon as it is safe to do so, the responsible clinician should attend and assess any injured parties. The order of priority should be clinically triaged, all individuals involved should see a HCP irrespective of their alleged role in the incident.

Arrange to see the patient in a suitable healthcare room for a full examination and assessment. Offer appropriate emergency and first-aid care, including a thorough top-to-toe assessment of the individual.

Document/record

Record verbatim what is reported or disclosed by the patient including the following:
- *What* has happened?
- *When* did it happen?
- *Where* did it happen?
- *Who* was involved?

Record any injuries

Record site and nature of any injuries on the clinical system, using body maps or detailed description.

Treat minor injuries on site

Small wounds can often be dressed, glued, or sutured on site by suitably trained staff. Provide first-aid treatments, ice packs, and simple analgesia as required.

Consider the BBV status and risk of transmission for individuals involved in bite injuries and other incidents where there have been potential percutaneous exposure involving blood (see Hepatitis B, p. 158, Hepatitis C, p. 162, and HIV care in prisons, p. 150).

If there are any concerns or if the clinician is unable to exclude serious underlying injuries or fractures, arrange admission to hospital just as in any other primary care setting.

Work with prison staff to facilitate escort to A&E/hospital via ambulance or prison transport depending on the level of concern.

Head injury

NICE recommends immediate referral to a hospital emergency department if there are any risk factors which may indicate an intracranial complication or cervical spine injury such as:
- a Glasgow Coma Scale score less than 15
- evidence of shock

- a history of bleeding or coagulation disorders, or current anticoagulant medication
- current alcohol or drug intoxication
- any loss of consciousness after the injury
- any post-traumatic seizure
- any previous brain surgery
- amnesia (antegrade or retrograde) lasting more than 5 minutes
- persistent headache since the injury
- vomiting
- any focal neurological deficit
- a suspected open or depressed skull fracture
- a suspected basal skull fracture (haemotympanum, cerebrospinal fluid leakage from ear or nose, Battle's sign, bilateral black eyes)
- signs of a penetrating injury or visible trauma to the scalp or skull
- suspected cervical spine injury.

For patients remaining in justice settings who have sustained a head injury, consider the need for 24-hour supervision. Options may include ensuring a shared cell or increased observations.

Burns, chemical burns, and scalds

Immediate first aid for a burn depends on the cause of injury, but should include immediate cooling with cool or tepid water for at least 30 minutes.

In an assault, chemicals and hot water are sometimes targeted at the head and neck. If this has occurred, assess the person's airway, breathing, and circulation, begin cooling, and arrange immediate hospital admission.

In the event of a chemical burn, remove affected clothing, irrigate copiously, and identify the causal chemical if possible to inform the ambulance team.

NICE recommends immediate admission for any patient with:
- complex burn injuries and full-thickness burns
- deep dermal burns affecting more than 5% of total body surface (palm of the hand size)
- all chemical and electrical burns
- burns affecting the face, hands, feet, genitalia, or perineum, or any flexural surface.
- circumferential deep dermal burns.

When cooling burns, be aware of the risk of hypothermia and keep the patient warm.

Admission to hospital

These can be highly contentious situations where multiagency teams have conflicting priorities. Although rare, duty clinicians may occasionally feel under pressure to avoid admission, rush assessments, or collude with assumptions about an individual's well-being.

The HCP should take time to ensure they have assessed the patient fully before giving clinical advice. Remember the principle of equivalence: 'People in prison should be provided with treatment which is at least consistent in range and quality with that which is available to the wider community'.[2]

If the HCP is not able to fully assess the patient due to safety concerns raised by prison staff, the HCP should always follow the prison staff's instructions but document the incomplete assessment, with a plan to review the patient as soon as it is safe to do so. The HCP should advise prison staff on any signs of deterioration that they should be watchful for.

Conflicting priorities

Work with prison colleagues to agree maximum time frames for transfer to hospital or frequency of required clinical observations and document the decision in the patient's notes.

Be clear about the medical recommendation and the rationale. If the prison staff are unable to facilitate the recommendation, agree with operational staff to escalate this to the duty governor, who holds ultimate responsibility to follow medical advice in all but exceptional circumstances.

Document the recommendation and who this has been discussed with.

Report

An Incident Report should be completed for any assault or injury to a person in prison. This will usually be completed by the first attending officer. However, if the incident is disclosed to the HCP, as the first person informed, they should complete an Incident Report.

Involving the police

The custodial staff have the primary responsibility for the safety and security of the people living in prison, and will have protocols to facilitate a process of adjudications and consequences on any resident involved in a violent or threatening incident on the wing. They will also facilitate the involvement of police if the victim wishes to press charges.

However, victims of assault may choose to report the incident to the police immediately, later, or not at all. Some may not feel sufficiently safe while in custody and will consider pressing charges after they have been released. Healthcare staff should always offer support to a patient to report assaults in confidence to the police.

Sexual assault

In the event of a serious or sexual assault, forensic evidence may need to be collected by trained staff. Advise the patient not to wash or change their clothes until specialist advice has been sought.

The SARC team will advise on the need for forensic samples and will usually arrange to see the patient to facilitate examination and sample collection.

It is important to be familiar with local SARC protocols. Up-to-date details of 'Rape and Sexual Assault referral centres' searchable by location/postcode are available at https://www.nhs.uk/.

Aftercare

SARCs will also support and assess the need for the following:
- Emergency contraception.[3]
- Test and treat for STIs including consideration of prophylactic cover.[4]

- If indicated, post-exposure prophylaxis after sexual exposure to HIV should be started withing 72 hours of the assault.[5]
- BBV screening and early vaccination for hepatitis A and B.[5]

Emotional support

Anyone experiencing violence or assault should be offered emotional support.

People living in prison have access to listening support 24 hours a day:
- Peer-trained listeners.
- Chaplaincy.
- Samaritans phone line.

This can also be provided by prison mental health teams and locally commissioned specialist counselling services.

Safety of the person in prison

Following an assault in custody, the person in prison may have concerns about their ongoing safety in the establishment. Violence between people living in the prison is often related to the illicit economy[6] and these conflicts can be ongoing and prolonged.

Work with prison staff in your 'safer custody' team to ensure the patient has been adequately supported to discuss their concerns, disclose issues placing them at risk, and is provided with appropriate strategies to keep them safe for the remainder of their sentence. This may include:
- single cell status
- self-isolation
- 'vulnerable prisoner units'
- transfer of assailants or victim
- treatment for substance misuse difficulties.

References

1. Gov.uk. Prisons data: safety and order. n.d. https://data.justice.gov.uk/prisons/safety-and-order
2. RCGP Secure Environments Group. Position statement on 'Equivalence of care in secure environments in the UK'. 2018. https://www.rcgp.org.uk/representing-you/policy-areas/care-in-secure-environments
3. Faculty of Sexual and Reproductive Health. Clinical guidelines on emergency contraception. 2017. https://www.fsrh.org/documents/ceu-clinical-guidance-emergency-contraception-march-2017/
4. British Association of Sexual Health and HIV. Guidelines. https://www.bashh.org/guidelines
5. British Association of Sexual Health and HIV. UK guidelines for the use of HIV post-exposure prophylaxis 2021. 20121. https://www.bashhguidelines.org/media/1308/pep-2021.pdf
6. HM Prison and Probation service. Guidance: violence reduction in prison. 2019. https://www.gov.uk/guidance/violence-reduction-in-prison

Sharps injury in secure environments

Introduction

The term 'sharps injury' applies to any incident where a needle, blade (such as a scalpel), or other sharp instrument or object causes injury by penetrating the skin. In clinical practice this relates predominantly to needlestick injuries (NSIs). In the secure environment, while there is no documented greater incidence, there are a number of additional considerations in the management of sharps injuries. These include the higher prevalence of BBVs and also the greater possibility for adverse behaviours and poor understanding of the resident, associated with mental health illness and learning difficulties.

Needlestick injuries

Routine data on NSIs occurring specifically in secure settings is not available; however, the UK Health Security Agency does monitor significant occupational exposure (SOE) through non-mandatory reporting. Through this it received reports of 8765 SOEs in England, Wales, and Northern Ireland between January 1997 and June 2018.[1] The majority of these exposures were due to non-compliance with standard infection control precautions for the handling and safe disposal of clinical waste.

The main risk from these injuries occurs when the sharp has been used, and contaminated by bodily fluids, and therefore may cause exposure to infection. Certain features of a percutaneous injury carry a particularly high risk such as a deep injury, poorly controlled HIV infection in the source patient, visible blood on the device which caused the injury, and injury with a needle which had been placed in a source patient's artery or vein.

Possible outcomes

- Physical injury.
- Local infection.
- Transmission of BBVs.

While the major pathogens of concern are HBV, HCV, and HIV, there are many others that may be transmitted. These include but are not limited to human T-lymphotropic retrovirus (HTLV)-I and HTLV-II, hepatitis D virus (HDV, or delta agent) which is activated in the presence of HBV, cytomegalovirus, Epstein–Barr virus, toxoplasmosis, and malarial parasites.

Of note: the average estimated seroconversion risks from published studies and reports are:

- 0.3% for percutaneous exposure to HIV-infected blood
- 0.1% for mucocutaneous exposure to HIV-infected blood
- 0.5–1.8% for percutaneous exposure to HCV-infected blood with detectable RNA
- 30% for percutaneous exposure of a non-immune individual to an HBeAg positive source.

The risk of acquiring hepatitis B from a carrier after NSI is 2–40%, and the risk of hepatitis C infection from NSI is 3–10%, and for HIV is 0.2–0.5%. The total number of HCV seroconversions from SOEs in the UK is 23 (as of 2020), and there have been no further confirmed HCV seroconversions reported in the UK since 2015, and in the case of HIV, the last reported seroconversion from SOEs was in 1999. However, the effects of the injury and the anxiety about its potential consequences, including the adverse side effects of post-exposure prophylaxis, can have a significant personal impact on an injured employee.

Who is at risk?

In the context of secure environments, healthcare workers are particularly vulnerable. This includes those who directly handle sharps (undertaking phlebotomy, vaccination, and minor surgical procedures) but also those workers who may inadvertently be put at risk when sharps are not stored or disposed of correctly. It is also possible that patients in prison could also suffer a NSI (e.g. in their cells or while working or in the healthcare department).

Management

It is important to explain to the recipient of the NSI about what has happened, the potential risks involved, and what action should be taken next, and inform the healthcare manager. The incident should be documented in healthcare records (if appropriate), as well as on an incident reporting software (such as Datix). This will ensure a review and investigation of the incident, and possibly facilitate any changes (policy, practices, or equipment) which could prevent future incidents. It may be advisable that the person who has had the sharps injury is brought back or contacted within 1–2 days to address any questions or anxiety about the outcome and onwards management and to provide psychological support.

Immediate action

- First aid:
  - Encourage the wound to gently bleed, but do not squeeze, ideally holding it under running water.
  - Wash the wound using running water and plenty of soap.
  - Don't scrub the wound while washing it.
  - Dry the wound and cover it with a waterproof plaster or dressing.
- Assess the extent of the wound, if any, or the probability of exposure of open skin lesions or mucous membranes to blood.
- Determine immunization status for tetanus and HBV. Tetanus vaccine, with or without tetanus immunoglobulin, should be given if indicated. Consider the need for antibiotics and hepatitis B vaccine.
- Document the circumstances of the injury (the date and time of injury or exposure, where the needle was found, circumstances of the injury, type of needle, whether there was a syringe attached, whether visible blood was present in or on the needle or syringe, whether the injury caused bleeding, and whether the previous user of the needle is known).
- Notify the healthcare manager and then contact the occupational health department (if available) or attend the A&E department (if incident occurs out of hours).
- Testing needles and syringes for viruses is not indicated. Results are likely to be negative, but a negative result does not rule out the possibility of infection.
- Take blood from the injured person for virology (HIV, hepatitis B, and hepatitis C) as a baseline/storage.

- If possible, identify the source of the contaminant:
  - Obtain consent to access the medical records of the patient or staff member.
  - It can be very helpful to test source patients, with their informed consent, for HIV, HBV, and HCV, regardless of risk factors, unless very recent results are available.
  - Testing should only be done after appropriate discussion and counselling. Robust systems should be in place for ensuring that the source patient is are made aware of the results and that any positive results are managed appropriately.
  - If source patient tests negative for BBVs and is not thought to be high risk then reassure them; no additional follow-up is required.
- If unknown source of contaminant:
  - Re-check HIV status 3 months later and hepatitis serology 3 and 6 months later.
  - LFTs should be performed and repeated at 3 and 6 months.

Hepatitis B

- If donor is HBV surface antigen positive then advice should be sought from a hepatology consultant who will conduct a risk assessment to decide if hepatitis B immunoglobulin is required in addition to vaccine (accelerated course). Concurrent administration does not impact the development of immunity. If hepatitis B immunoglobulin is indicated, it should be given as soon as possible, ideally at the same time or within 24 hours of the first dose of vaccine, but not after 7 days have elapsed since exposure.
- Follow up recipient at 6-month screen serum for HBV surface antigen and surface antibody.

Hepatitis C

Effective oral treatments are now available for hepatitis C, with minimal side effects and high success rates. Any needlestick donors or recipients found to be living with hepatitis C should be encouraged to receive treatment.

If donor is HCV RNA positive, test recipient as follows:

- 6 weeks: serum sample for HCV antibodies.
- 2 weeks: serum sample for HCV antibodies and RNA.
- 6 months: serum for HCV antibodies.

HIV

In the case of definite exposures to blood or other high-risk body fluids known or considered to be at high risk of HIV infection, contact a local genitourinary medicine consultant. High risk is determined by assessment of the person who has had a NSI (immunity) or identification (or probability) of the source of the contaminant. If identified or probability that the source is a known HIV patient, has HIV but is on medication, or is in a demographic that may have HIV or has high probability of acquiring the illness (e.g. IV drug user).

Post-exposure prophylaxis should be commenced as soon as possible if clinically indicated, preferably within 1 hour of the incident. It may still be worth considering up to 72 hours after the exposure, but the relative benefit of prophylaxis diminishes with time. Clinical indication for post-exposure prophylaxis is based on information such as HIV viral load, resistance profile, and treatment history. Post-exposure prophylaxis is no longer recommended if the source is on antiviral treatment with a confirmed and sustained (>6 months) undetectable plasma HIV viral load.

The British Association of Sexual Health and HIV recommend the use of Truvada (tenofovir/emtricitabine) and raltegravir as the regimen of choice for post-exposure prophylaxis.[1]

Prevention is better than cure!

The healthcare employer in secure environments must provide a safe working environment: they should prevent exposure and if not possible, control the risk of exposure. This is in accordance with legislation. There should be a local protocol which guides the HCP in what to do and who to contact if there is an NSI.

The clinical team must ensure

- standard precautions for infection control are in place; this includes washing hands with soap and water before and after procedures, and using protective barriers such as gloves, gowns, aprons, masks, and goggles where there is direct contact with blood and other body fluids
- safe use and disposal of sharps:
  - use of new, single-use disposable injection equipment for all injections is highly recommended; sterilizable injection should only be considered if single-use equipment is not available and if the sterility can be documented with time, steam, and temperature indicators
  - sharps should not be passed directly from hand to hand and handling should be kept to a minimum
  - used needles must not be bent or broken before disposal and must not be recapped
  - used sharps must be discarded immediately by the person generating the waste sharps into a sharps container conforming to current standards
  - increased use of suitable equipment, for example, safer needle technology, may also help to reduce instances of NSIs.
- clear procedures for response to sharps injury, including speedy access to appropriate prophylaxis treatments
- improved education and training and higher levels of awareness of the risks and preventive measures are also likely to contribute to reducing the numbers of NSIs in the UK.
- reduce the incidence of these injuries by following *safe working practices*.[2]
- Hepatitis B vaccination.

Hepatitis B vaccination for HCPs has been recommended since the 1980s. From UK Health Security Agency data, 98.4% of those who had SOEs were known to have been vaccinated with at least one dose of hepatitis B vaccine. New employees should complete a pre-employment health assessment and any at-risk HCP (by medical history or job specification) should be offered and actively encouraged to have the hepatitis B vaccination. Hepatitis B vaccination should also be offered to people in prison who are in high-risk groups, with consideration of the accelerated course to ensure compliance. While there have been no confirmed HBV seroconversions as a result of SOEs among HCPs and ancillary staff reported in the UK, this is largely due to the hepatitis B vaccination programme. It is therefore imperative that the high rates of vaccination continue and health promotion remains active.

The law

- Health and Safety at Work etc. Act 1974: employers need to assess the risk to their staff and others.
- Control of Substances Hazardous to Health Regulations (COSHH) 2002: employers to assess risks from exposure to hazardous substances and protect workers from those risks.
- Management of Health and Safety Regulations 1999.
- Reporting of Injuries, Diseases and Dangerous Occurrences Regulations 1995 (RIDDOR).
- Health and Safety (Sharp Instruments in Healthcare) Regulations 2013.

References

1. British Association of Sexual Health and HIV. UK guidelines for the use of HIV post-exposure prophylaxis 2021. 20121. https://www.bashhguidelines.org/media/1308/pep-2021.pdf
2. Health and Safety Executive. Avoiding sharps injuries. n.d. https://www.hse.gov.uk/biosafety/blood-borne-viruses/avoiding-sharps-injuries.htm

Further reading

Department of Health. HIV post-exposure prophylaxis: guidance from the UK Chief Medical Officers' Expert Advisory Group on AIDS. 2008. https://assets.publishing.service.gov.uk/government/uploads/system/uploads/attachment_data/file/203139/HIV_post-exposure_prophylaxis.pdf
National Institute for Health and Care Excellence. Healthcare-associated infections: prevention and control in primary and community care. NICE Clinical guideline [CG139]. 2012 (updated February 2017). https://www.nice.org.uk/guidance/cg139
Northamptonshire Healthcare NHS Foundation Trust. Sharps management, needlestick injuries and exposure to blood borne viruses: procedure ICPr005. https://www.nhft.nhs.uk/download.cfm?doc=docm93jijm4n1418
Public Health England. Eye of the needle: United Kingdom surveillance of significant occupational exposures to bloodborne viruses in healthcare workers. December 2014. https://www.gov.uk/government/publications/bloodborne-viruses-eye-of-the-needle
UK Health Security Agency. Hepatitis B: the green book, chapter 18. February 2022. https://www.gov.uk/government/publications/hepatitis-b-the-green-book-chapter-18

Cell fires

Introduction

Deliberate fires remain a significant risk within prisons and present an increased hazard within closed environments, such as prison cells. People in prison may start fires with a view to gaining a move, as a protest, or in order to cause self-harm. Deliberate cell fires have the potential to place people and staff within prisons in significant danger.

Any cell fire incidents must be controlled by the incident commander (who will be a member of operational security staff) prior to medical staff approaching the area. Prison staff will put on Cell Snatch Rescue Equipment—specially designed smoke hoods giving an oxygen supply for up to 15 minutes—before attempting fire-fighting and rescue of cell occupants.

Situation

The timely assessment of burns sustained during a cell fire is crucial. Determining the nature, cause, and location of the fire will help the clinician establish the mechanism of injury, but this must not delay treatment. History taking should include the following:

- Was there an explosion (e.g. aerosols)?
- What was the fire fuel (i.e. causing toxic gases)?
- Was the fire inside the cell (i.e. an enclosed space)?
- What was the time of the fire and of patient extraction?
- How long was the patient exposed to conditions?
- Was there any loss of consciousness?

Initial assessment

Physical assessment of a patient should follow the <C>ABCDE algorithm as suggested by NICE[1]:

- Catastrophic haemorrhaging.
- Airway: check for burns (including cervical spine if they have been thrown or jumped onto netting to escape fire).
- Breathing: inhalation of hot gases or full circumferential burns to torso which may restrict chest movement.
- Circulation: hypovolaemic shock may occur with extensive burns.
- Disability: other associated injuries.
- Environmental: guard against hypothermia when cooling burns.

Attention should be paid to the patient's airway and breathing as they have been inside an enclosed environment where the heat and smoke will have been intensified. Signs of inhalation injury include:

- burns to face
- increased respiratory rate
- respiratory distress
- increased effort of breathing
- change in mental state
- carbonaceous sputum
- singeing of nasal hairs
- soot around mouth and nose
- stridor
- hoarseness.

Burns assessment

Assessing the depth and surface area of burns is important. Burns are classified as follows:

- Superficial: minor burns affecting the epidermis, high degree of pain.
- Partial thickness: affects dermis, blood capillaries, nerve endings, sweat glands, looks wet. Painful, can blister.
- Full thickness: epidermis and dermis complete destruction, tissue and nerves, often less painful due to nerve damage.

Tools to assess total body surface area include:

- Wallace's rule of nines—for medium to large burns in adults (Fig. 15.2):
  - arm (each)—9%
  - head and neck—9%
  - leg (each)—18%
  - genitalia and perineum—1%
  - anterior trunk—18%
  - posterior trunk—18%.
- the Lund and Browder chart—more accurate measure of burns (Fig. 15.3)
- the person's palmar surface (including fingers extended)—can be used as a guide for small or scattered burns, or for assessing the amount of unburnt skin in very extensive burns. This is equivalent to ~1% of the person's total body surface area.

NB: do not include simple erythema when estimating total body surface area.

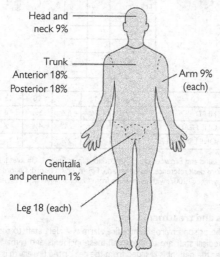

Fig. 15.2 Wallace's rule of nines in adults. Reproduced from Crouch et al. (Eds), Oxford Handbook of Emergency Nursing, Figure 12.1, Oxford: Oxford University Press. Copyright © 2010, by permission of Oxford University Press.

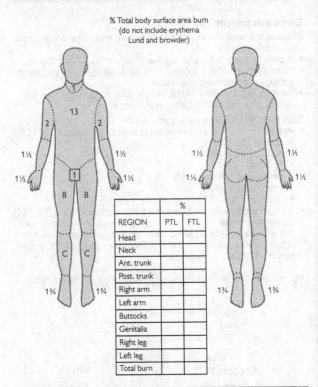

% Total body surface area burn
(do not include erythema
Lund and browder)

	%	
REGION	PTL	FTL
Head		
Neck		
Ant. trunk		
Post. trunk		
Right arm		
Left arm		
Buttocks		
Genitalia		
Right leg		
Left leg		
Total burn		

AREA	Age 0	1	5	10	15	Adult
A-1½ OF HEAD	9½	8½	6½	5½	4½	3½
B-1½ OF ONE HEAD	2¾	3¼	4	4½	4½	4¾
C-1½ OF ONE LOWER LEG	2½	2½	2¾	3	3¼	3½

Fig. 15.3 Lund and Browder chart. Reproduced from Smith J, Greaves I, Porter KM (eds). Oxford desk reference: major trauma, Figure 22.7, Oxford: Oxford University Press. Copyright © 2007, with permission from Oxford University Press.

Actions and treatment

Within the prison environment a fire alarm will alert staff to the incident. Prison medical staff are to attend all these incidents and remain on scene until either the patient is rescued from the cell or the fire alarm is cancelled.

• Ensure rescuer safety—prison officers will use specialized cell fire extraction kit and fire-fighting equipment.

- Ascertain ambulance attendance has been requested.
- Once patient is removed from cell environment, if clothes are smouldering or burning, ensure flames are extinguished with fire blankets or by rolling patient on floor.
- Protect airway and provide high-flow oxygen.
- Remove clothing and assess burns.
- Cool burns with tepid water or burns applications for 20–30 minutes with tepid water.
- Do not use ice or very cold water, as this may cause vasoconstriction, exacerbate the wound, and cause hypothermia.
- If water is not available, use wet towels or compresses.
- Cover burns with cling film or specialized dressings.
- Consider hydration and fluids as scope of practice allows.
- Analgesia to be given appropriately as scope of practice allows.
- Guard against hypothermia with appropriate blankets and covers.
- Reassess burns regularly.
- All patients with exposure to smoke should be conveyed to hospital for observations due to possible inhalation injury.

Reference

1. National Institute for Health and Care Excellence. 2019.

Managing resuscitation scenarios in prisons

Introduction

Currently in the UK, there are ~60,000 out-of-hospital cardiac arrests (OHCAs) each year. Of these, UK ambulance services initiate resuscitation on ~28,000 people—less than half of all OHCA. Resuscitation may not take place because of advanced directives being in place, evidence of irreversible death, or simply because suitably trained persons were not available within a reasonable timeframe.[1]

There are around 300 deaths in custody per year.[2] It is not known how often CPR is attempted, or how successful it is. However, it is crucial that all staff are suitably trained in CPR in order to ensure that anyone experiencing OHCA within prison settings has the best chance of receiving care.

Background

Cardiac arrest situations are stressful and challenging, and so having a systematic and well-practised approach to their management is important. Resuscitation Council (UK) guidelines[3] are produced and updated periodically, ensuring a system is available for all grades of staff to follow in line with their scope of practice and training.

Training

It is vitally important that healthcare staff employed within the prison system have good theoretical, underpinning knowledge of basic CPR. Skills used in cardiac arrest scenarios need expert teaching and instruction. It is highly recommended this should be done in the form of a Resuscitation Council (UK) approved course, such as *Basic Life Support*, *Immediate Life Support*, or *Advanced Life Support* depending on clinical grade (see http://www.resus.org.uk). These courses should be completed prior to commencing work within the prison.

Prison healthcare staff should make themselves familiar with the communication system for calling an emergency within the establishment they are working in, as this could differ from prison to prison.

A cardiac arrest within a prison is an OHCA, therefore a direct link to the ambulance service is required to obtain the fastest response for expert help in the resuscitation of a patient.

Skills required

Cardiac arrest skills, such as chest compressions and defibrillation, are the technical skills required to attempt resuscitation of a patient. The Resuscitation Council (UK) advocates the inclusion of non-technical communication skills also. This will enable effective communication, command of a resuscitation scenario, and working as an effective team. These skills are covered in resuscitation courses but should be practised regularly and reinforced as ongoing continuing professional development.

Cardiac arrest recognition

Cardiac arrest is a clinical diagnosis. All HCPs should be capable of recognizing cardiac arrest. Checks as described by the Resuscitation Council

(UK) should be carried out to confirm cardiac arrest upon arrival on scene. These are:
- ensure personal safety
- check patient for response (no response—call for help)
- open airway and check for normal breathing
- check for carotid pulse
- if no signs of life commence CPR appropriate to clinical grade.

General management of cardiac arrest in prisons

The principles of managing a cardiac arrest within the prison environment are as for any OHCA. There are constraints upon the management of the scenario which prison healthcare staff must be aware of:
- Communication to officers and ambulance service must be early and succinct.
- Ensure to specifically say 'cardiac arrest' which will ensure the correct ambulance response (C1).
- Attempt to gain good access to the patient—360° if possible.
- Communication must be continuous and robust.

Survival of OHCA is affected by following the 'Chain of Survival' (Fig. 15.4).[4] This commences with early recognition and call for help, early and effective CPR, early defibrillation, and good post-resuscitation care.

Management features of cardiac arrest in prisons

The successful management of a cardiac arrest within a prison depends on several factors including the following:
- A strong team approach: an experienced team leader must be quickly identified as soon as an OHCA is recognized, who will delegate tasks, while controlling, coordinating, and organizing the team.
- Skills of first responders: may be non-clinical or inexperienced, therefore team management and communication must be assertive and clear.
- Location: it is advised to gain 360° access to the patient to aid in the team approach to resuscitation—in many areas of the prison environment (e.g. cells, landings) it is not possible to gain 360° access

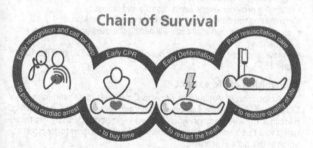

Chain of Survival

Fig. 15.4 Chain of Survival. Reprinted from Adult Basic Life Support (2017) with permission. Full version available from www.resus.org.uk. See plate section.

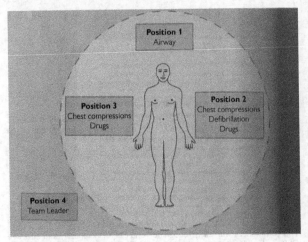

Fig. 15.5 Team member positions to ensure 360° access to the patient. Reproduced from Advanced Life Support (2017) with permission. Full version available from www.resus.org.uk

due to limited space and furniture being fixed to the floor. Do not attempt to move the patient unless they are in an unsafe environment as this will delay administration of CPR (Fig. 15.5).

• The lead clinician must be aware of special limitations to scene access and egress and plan accordingly. Ensure advanced plans are in place to manage such scenarios, and that operational security staff are aware of what will be required in the event of an OHCA.

CPR must focus on
• high-quality chest compressions
• changing provider every 2 minutes to avoid fatigue
• minimizing the time off the chest for necessary checks.
• a calm and collected approach will benefit the management of the scenario
• follow advanced, immediate, or basic life support algorithm (Figs. 15.6 and 15.7).

Recognition of life extinct

The Association of Ambulance Services Chief Executives[5] and Joint Royal Colleges of Ambulance Liaison Committee[6] have provided clear clinical guidelines on when not or when to stop resuscitation. Prison healthcare staff should be aware of this and able to take the decision to stop resuscitation in this difficult scenario.

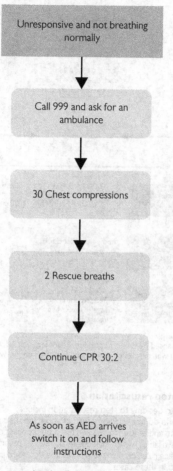

Fig. 15.6 Basic life support algorithm. Reprinted from Adult Basic Life Support (2017) with permission. Full version available from www.resus.org.uk

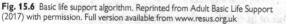

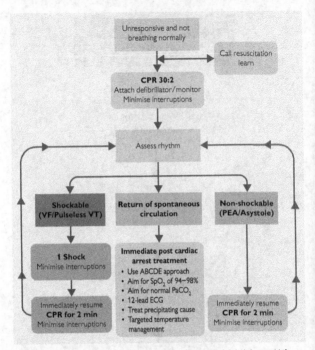

Fig. 15.7 Advanced life support algorithm. Reprinted from Adult Advanced Life Support (2017) with permission. Full version available from www.resus.org.uk

When to stop resuscitation

Key triggers to deciding to stop resuscitation include:
- patients who do not achieve return of spontaneous circulation despite appropriate and efficient advanced life support being carried out (if provider available), which includes evaluation of reversible causes
- Home Office rules on management of the deceased patient must be adhered to in these cases.

Out of hospital post-resuscitation care

A patient who has been successfully resuscitated following a cardiac arrest is now the focus of post-resuscitation care which concentrates on optimum perfusion of the heart and brain. Monitoring is to include:
- pulse oximetry: 94–98%
- capnography: end-tidal carbon dioxide of 4.6–6 kPa (if available)
- BP: minimum systolic 100 mm/hg

- 12-lead ECG where appropriate and if available
- blood glucose
- temperature.

The patient should not be moved until return of spontaneous circulation has been observed and monitored for 10 minutes.

Staff welfare

Staff should be debriefed immediately with appropriate support offered; avoid staff leaving premises immediately and being alone.

References

1. University of Warwick. 2020.
2. Gov.uk. 2020.
3. Resuscitation Council (UK). Resuscitation guidelines. 2021. https://www.resus.org.uk/library/2021-resuscitation-guidelines
4. Resuscitation Council (UK). What is the chain or survival. 2019. https://www.resus.org.uk/home/faqs/faqs-basic-life-support-cpr
5. Association of Ambulance Chief Executives. Resuscitation to recovery. 2017. http://aace.org.uk/wp-content/uploads/2017/03/FINAL_Resuscitation-to-Recovery_A-National-Framework-to-improve-Care-of-People-with-Out-of-Hospital-Cardiac-Arrest-in-England_March-2017.pdf
6. Joint Royal Colleges Ambulance Liaison Committee (JRCALC). UK Ambulance Services Clinical Practice Guidelines. Bridgwater: Class Publishing; 2019.

Index

For the benefit of digital users, indexed terms that span two pages (e.g., 52–53) may, on occasion, appear on only one of those pages.

Tables and figures are indicated by t and f following the page number